Register Now for Onl[ine Access] to Your Book!

W9-BBA-770

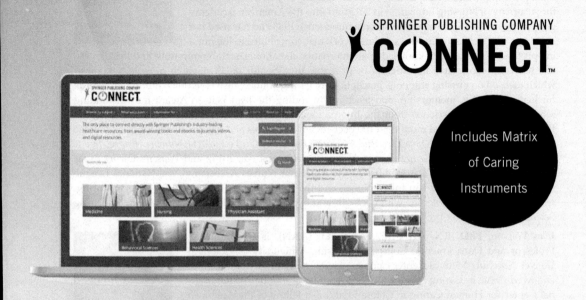

SPRINGER PUBLISHING COMPANY
CONNECT™

Includes Matrix
of Caring
Instruments

Your print purchase of *Assessing and Measuring Caring in Nursing and Health Sciences, 3e,* **includes online access to the contents of your book**—increasing accessibility, portability, and searchability!

Access today at:

http://connect.springerpub.com/content/book/978-0-8261-9542-5
**or scan the QR code at the right with your smartphone
and enter the access code below.**

68T56JHV

*Scan here for
quick access.*

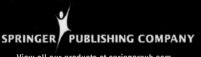

SPRINGER PUBLISHING COMPANY

View all our products at springerpub.com

Kathleen L. Sitzman, PhD, RN, CNE, ANEF, FAAN, is Professor, Undergraduate Nursing Science, East Carolina University, Greenville, North Carolina. Previous to her current position, she held dual appointments at Weber State University in Ogden, Utah: director, Bachelor of Integrated Studies Program, and faculty in the School of Nursing. She was inducted into the Academy of Nursing Education in 2015 and into the American Academy of Nursing in 2016. Dr. Sitzman has been a nurse since 1983 and has used her extensive experience to produce scholarly work that contributes to the nurs-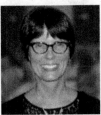

ing profession and body of knowledge on international, national, state, community, and local levels. She has been coprincipal investigator or principal investigator on 14 research projects, several of which focused on nursing students' perceptions of caring online. She has received numerous awards for her scholarship, mentorship, and teaching, including the Jean Watson Award for outstanding scholarship in caring science from the International Association for Human Caring (2007–2008). Dr. Sitzman has published more than 100 peer-reviewed articles and has coauthored four textbooks: *Understanding the Work of Nurse Theorists: A Creative Beginning* (2nd ed.; 2011); *Nursing History: Trends and Eras* (2nd ed.; 2014); *Caring Science, Mindful Practice* (1st ed.; 2014); and *Watson's Caring in the Digital World*, (2017). She is a member of the American Nurses Association, the National League for Nursing, Sigma Theta Tau International, and the International Association for Human Caring. Dr. Sitzman has been generous with her skills and expertise by serving on a wide variety of Caring Science–related service projects.

Jean Watson, PhD, RN, AHN-BC, FAAN, LL (AAN), is Distinguished Professor and Dean Emerita, College of Nursing, University of Colorado Denver Anschutz Medical Center campus, where she held the nation's first endowed Chair in Caring Science for 16 years. She is founder of the original Center for Human Caring in Colorado and is a fellow of the American Academy of Nursing; past president of the National League for Nursing; and founding member of the International Association of Human Caring and International Caritas Consortium. She is founder and director of the nonprofit foundation, Watson Caring Science Institute (www.watsoncaringscience.org).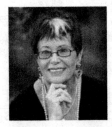

Dr. Watson has earned undergraduate and graduate degrees in nursing and psychiatric-mental health nursing and holds her PhD in educational psychology and counseling. She is a widely published author and recipient of many national/international awards and honors, including the Fetzer Institute Norman Cousins award, in recognition of her commitment to developing, maintaining, and exemplifying relationship-centered care practices; an international Kellogg Fellowship in Australia; a Fulbright Research award in Sweden; the Hillebrand Center for Compassion Care in Medicine award, Notre Dame University; the Academy of Integrative Health and Medicine award for pioneering work in Caring Science; and the Japanese International Society of Caring and Peace Chair. She holds 15 honorary doctoral degrees, including 12 international honorary doctorates (Sweden, United Kingdom, Spain [2], British Columbia and Quebec, Canada, Japan, Turkey, Peru [2], Colombia, and South America).

Clinical nurses and academic programs throughout the world use her published works on the philosophy and theory of human caring and the art and science of caring in nursing. Dr. Watson's caring philosophy is used to guide transformative models of caring and healing practices for hospitals, nurses, and patients alike, in diverse settings worldwide

At the University of Colorado, Dr. Watson held the title of Distinguished Professor of Nursing, the highest honor accorded its faculty for scholarly work. In 1999 she assumed the Murchison-Scoville Chair in Caring Science, the nation's first endowed chair in Caring Science, based at the University of Colorado Denver Anschutz Medical Center.

As author/coauthor of over 30 books on caring, her latest books range from empirical measurements and international research on caring, to new postmodern philosophies of caring and healing, philosophy and science of caring and caring science as sacred science, and global advance in caring literacy. Her latest work is *Unitary Caring Science: Philosophy and Praxis of Nursing.* Her books have been AJN Books of the Year awards and seek to bridge paradigms as well as point toward transformative models for the 21st century. In October 2013, Dr. Watson was inducted as a Living Legend by the American Academy of Nursing, its highest honor.

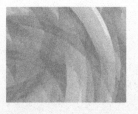

Assessing and Measuring Caring in Nursing and Health Sciences

Watson's Caring Science Guide

Third Edition

Kathleen L. Sitzman, PhD, RN, CNE, ANEF, FAAN

Jean Watson, PhD, RN, AHN-BC, FAAN, LL (AAN)

EDITORS

SPRINGER PUBLISHING COMPANY

Watson Caring
Science Institute

Springer Publishing Company, LLC
11 West 42nd Street
New York, NY 10036
www.springerpub.com

Acquisitions Editor: Margaret Zuccarini
Compositor: S4Carlisle

ISBN: 978-0-8261-9541-8
ebook ISBN: 978-0-8261-9542-5
Supplementary Material: Master Matrix of All Measurement Instruments: 978-0-8261-9539-5
DOI: 10.1891/9780826195425

A supplementary Master Matrix of All Measurement Instruments is available from Springerpub.com/sitzman3e

19 20 21 22 / 5 4 3 2 1

The author and the publisher of this Work have made every effort to use sources believed to be reliable to provide information that is accurate and compatible with the standards generally accepted at the time of publication. The author and publisher shall not be liable for any special, consequential, or exemplary damages resulting, in whole or in part, from the readers' use of, or reliance on, the information contained in this book. The publisher has no responsibility for the persistence or accuracy of URLs for external or third-party Internet websites referred to in this publication and does not guarantee that any content on such websites is, or will remain, accurate or appropriate.

Library of Congress Cataloging-in-Publication Data

Names: Sitzman, Kathleen, editor. | Watson, Jean, 1940- editor.
Title: Assessing and measuring caring in nursing and health sciences:
  Watson's caring science guide / Kathleen Sitzman, Jean Watson, editors.
Description: Third edition. | New York : Springer Publishing, [2019] |
  Preceded by Assessing and measuring caring in nursing and health sciences
  / Jean Watson. 2nd ed. 2009. | Includes bibliographical references and
  index.
Identifiers: LCCN 2018060324| ISBN 9780826195418 | ISBN 9780826195395
  (supplementary material) | ISBN 9780826195425 (ebook)
Subjects: | MESH: Nursing Audit | Nursing Care–standards | Nurse-Patient
  Relations | Quality Indicators, Health Care
Classification: LCC RT42 | NLM WY 100.5 | DDC 610.73--dc23 LC record available at
  https://lccn.loc.gov/2018060324

Contact us to receive discount rates on bulk purchases.
We can also customize our books to meet your needs.
For more information please contact: sales@springerpub.com

Publisher's Note: **New and used products purchased from third-party sellers are not guaranteed for quality, authenticity, or access to any included digital components.**

Printed in the United States of America.

I dedicate my work on this book to Jean Watson. Watson's work has provided the structure, lexicon, and deep philosophical foundation that has informed my scholarly pursuits since 1981. She is the inspiration for every one of the 14 research studies I have cocreated and published over the last 17 years. Her vision, genius, generosity of spirit, and guiding insight continue to fuel my passion for examining caring through rigorous research, and then disseminating results widely to others. Illuminating the intricacies and profound impact of caring in multiple settings and disciplines is critical in facilitating the creation of a world where caring is routinely cultivated and enacted in service to all humankind.
—Kathleen L. Sitzman

I am grateful to Kathleen L. Sitzman for her sustained devotion to caring science scholarship, practice, education, and research, and for her willingness to take on the editorial leadership for this third edition. My appreciation goes to all the original authors and new authors continuing to develop and expand approaches to assessing and measuring caring. My special gratitude goes to Springer Publishing Company for support and assistance with this third edition; with deep regard for the personal interest and support of Margaret Zuccarini, Publisher Emerita. Without this combined team effort and sustained interest, this edition would not have been possible.
In loving kindness and thanks,
—Jean Watson

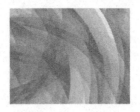

Contents

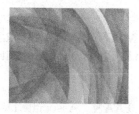

Contributors

David G. Arthur, PhD, RN, CMHN, MACMHN   Professor and Dean, School of Nursing and Midwifery, The Aga Khan University, Karachi, Pakistan; Adjunct Professor, Peking Union Medical College, Beijing, China

Lisa A. Bagnall, PhD, RN, CNL   Clinical Assistant Professor, Biobehavioral Nursing Science, University of Florida-College of Nursing, Gainesville, Florida

Carolie Coates, PhD   Research and Measurement Consultant

Sylvie Cossette, PhD, RN   Professor, Faculty of Nursing, University of Montreal, Researcher, Research Center, Montreal Heart Institute, Montreal, Quebec, Canada

Sherill N. Cronin, PhD, RN-BC   Professor and Chair of Graduate Nursing, Lansing School of Nursing and Health Sciences, Bellarmine University, Louisville, Kentucky

Joanne R. Duffy, PhD, RN, FAAN   Visiting Professor, Indiana University, Indianapolis, Indiana; Executive Vice President and Senior Consultant, QualiCare, Winchester, Virginia

Guillaume Fontaine, MSN, PhD Candidate, RN   Faculty of Nursing, University of Montreal, Research Center, Montreal Heart Institute, Montreal, Quebec, Canada

Anne-Marie Goff, PhD, RN   University of North Carolina Wilmington, School of Nursing, College of Health and Human Services, Wilmington, North Carolina

Pamela Hinds, PhD, RN, FAAN   Director, Nursing Research and Quality Outcomes, Children's National Medical Center, Washington, District of Columbia

Amandah Hoogbruin, PhD, MScN, BScN, RN   Retired, Bachelor of Science in Nursing Faculty, Kwantlen Polytechnic University, Surrey, British Columbia, Canada

Sharon D. Horner, PhD, RN, FAAN   Associate Dean for Research, The University of Texas at Austin, School of Nursing, Austin, Texas

Linda Hughes, PhD, RN‡

Patricia Larson, DNSc, RN, FAAN

Christine L. Latham, DNSc, RN   Professor Emerita and Director of the Center for Nursing Workforce Excellence, School of Nursing, California State University, Fullerton, California

Barbara H. Lee, MSN, MEd, RN-BC, CWOCN   Associate Professor of Nursing (Emeritus), Lansing School of Nursing and Health Sciences, Bellarmine University, Louisville, Kentucky

Anna M. McDaniel, PhD, RN, FAAN   Dean and the Linda Harman Aiken Professor, University of Florida, College of Nursing, Gainesville, Florida

John W. Nelson, PhD, MS, RN   President and Data Scientist, Healthcare Environment, St. Paul, Minnesota

Ngozi O. Nkongho, PhD, RN   Former Chair, Department of Nursing, Lehman College, The City University of New York, Bronx, New York

Jan Nyberg, PhD, RN (retired)

Jacinthe Pepin, PhD, RN   Professor, Faculty of Nursing, University of Montreal, Director, Center for Innovation in Nursing Education, University of Montreal, Montreal, Quebec, Canada

Janet F. Quinn, PhD, RN, FAAN   Director, HaelanWorks, Lyons, Colorado; Faculty Associate, Watson Caring Science Institute, Boulder, Colorado; Adjunct Faculty, University of Colorado College of Nursing, Boulder, Colorado; University of Arizona College of Nursing, Tucson, Arizona

Marilyn A. Ray, PhD, RN, CTN-A, FSFAA, FAAN, FESPCH (Hon.), FNAP
Professor Emeritus, Florida Atlantic University, The Christine E. Lynn College of Nursing, Boca Raton, Florida

---

‡Deceased

Gwen Sherwood, PhD, RN, FAAN, ANEF   Professor Emerita, University of North Carolina at Chapel Hill, School of Nursing, Chapel Hill, North Carolina

Kathleen L. Sitzman, PhD, RN, CNE, ANEF, FAAN   Professor of Nursing, East Carolina University College of Nursing, Greenville, North Carolina

Denise Testa, PhD, CRNA   Clinical Associate Professor, Connell School of Nursing, Boston College, Chestnut Hill, Massachusetts

Marian C. Turkel, PhD, RN, NEA-BC, FAAN   Watson Caring Science Post Doctoral Scholar, Associate Professor, Florida Atlantic University, Christine E. Lynn College of Nursing, Fort Lauderdale, Florida

Jean Watson, PhD, RN, AHN-BC, FAAN, LL (AAN)   Founder/Director, Watson Caring Science Institute, Distinguished Professor Emerita and Dean Emerita, University of Colorado Denver, College of Nursing, Anschutz Medical Center—Retired

Roger Watson, PhD, RN, FAAN   Professor of Nursing, Faculty of Health Sciences, University of Hull, Hull, East Yorkshire, United Kingdom

Zane Robinson Wolf, PhD, RN, CNE, FAAN   Dean Emerita and Professor, Adjunct Faculty, School of Nursing and Health Sciences, La Salle University, Philadelphia, Pennsylvania

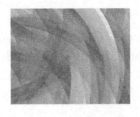

Foreword

The third edition of *Assessing and Measuring Caring in Nursing and Health Sciences* expands on content from the first two editions and adds two new measures for assessing caring behaviors of online instructors and relationship-based care environments. Measures within the text provide perspective from multiple viewpoints, including those of students, staff, and patients, regarding their own caring behaviors as well as those of others.

As we confront an increasingly value-based healthcare reimbursement environment, never has it been more critically important to be able to provide empirical evidence of the value of environments based on theory-based behaviors. Without theory-guided actions, our behaviors are less deliberate and far less repeatable. While no single way of evaluating human caring experiences can provide an adequate or comprehensive understanding of an environment, whether it be an online classroom or an acute care hospital, quantitative measures are necessary to build empirical evidence. When quantitative measures are integrated with other ways of knowing, such as qualitative and artistic expressions, we begin building a comprehensive understanding of the human caring experience and nursing science.

The third edition comes during the 40th anniversary year of Dr. Jean Watson's groundbreaking book, *Nursing: The Philosophy and Science of Caring*, and is a testament to Dr. Watson's distinguished career as a nurse theorist and advocate for human-to-human caring as an ontology and epistemology. In addition to human caring measures and assessment tools, this edition contains chapters in which human caring theory is discussed in the context of today's healthcare environments and provides a philosophical foundation for asking critical questions to assess clinical practice. The measures are applicable to nursing as well as other healthcare disciplines.

As the research advisor to the board and a board member of the Watson Caring Science Institute, I am often consulted regarding instruments students and researchers may use to capture human caring from multiple perspectives. I have often guided individuals who are seeking measures to the earlier editions of this book, which have provided content regarding the psychometric foundation of the caring measures as well as the measures themselves. This edition builds on the earlier versions with added detail as well as new measures that reflect the current environment in which we teach and practice. As the earlier editions have been, I am certain that the third edition will become an invaluable resource for those interested in the assessment of human caring perspectives of self and others.

Barbara B. Brewer, PhD, MALS, MBA, RN, FAAN
Associate Professor
The University of Arizona College of Nursing

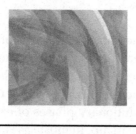

Preface

This third edition of *Assessing and Measuring Caring in Nursing and Health Sciences* is designed to continue to provide nursing leaders, students, clinicians, and scholars with the latest compilation of up-to-date instruments, along with new ones not included in the second edition. Further, in this edition, Dr. Kathleen Sitzman has joined me as first editor. She has taken the responsibility of tracking down new instruments, as well as researching authors' updates of earlier versions of their instruments. This edition also includes an update from Dr. Carolie Coates, a measurement expert scholar, who provides a continuing critique and challenge for future directions of construct validity issues, as well as an update of her Caring Efficacy Scale.

This edition encompasses a comprehensive compilation of all the extant instruments for assessing/measuring caring currently found in the nursing literature. The continuing framework is Caring Science—providing concrete tools and guidelines for assessing, researching, and selecting specific indicators of caring. Different instruments are based on one's phenomena of interest, form of inquiry, objects of analysis, particular population, setting, and so on. This updated edition has relevance for caring among students, faculty, patients, and nurses, thus allowing use in educational and clinical care research. Other instruments include caring in administration relational-system level; still others a population of family and computerized options. All of these instruments provide an opportunity for students and measurement scholars to contribute new depth by extending reliability, validity, and integrity of use of any of these tools.

It is necessary to have access to a full range of valid and reliable instruments to capture some of the dynamics, challenges, vicissitudes, and opportunities to make tangible what otherwise remains elusive and nonmeasurable. Diverse concepts such as quality of care, patient/client nurse perceptions of caring, caring behaviors, and abilities are included. They are all part of this comprehensive compilation. The theoretical or atheoretical origin of each instrument is explored to provide context for whether each instrument is inductive, deductive, or empirically or theoretically derived.

As in previous editions, the framework matrix of each instrument is provided, which includes information as to origin, development, and use; key citations; as well as copies of the instruments wherever possible. This matrix of information is located at the end of the book. This allows the reader to see the chronological development and the evolutionary phases of each instrument as well as the evolution of the author's scholarship. In most cases, the authors of each measurement tool request that users contact them to seek permission to use. The request is made with the hope that researchers will inform the author of results to assist in further validity–reliability studies. *The Master Matrix of All Measurement Instruments is also available at Springerpub.com/sitzman3e.*

As Magnet® hospitals are increasingly grounded in professional practice models that embrace caring as a core focus, there is increasing demand for outcomes associated with patient experiences of caring. It is our hope that these caring assessment tools will help systems and clinicians to capture core quality indicators of caring, guiding some of the nursing research and transcending conventional standard patient satisfaction surveys that are devoid of any information of human caring.

At the disciplinary level, the development and evolution of these instruments contribute to a backstory of nursing theory and knowledge development, merging theoretical and empirical—working between and beyond existing paradigms. This evolution is paving the way to new forms of evidence, guided by nursing's relational ontology of caring. This collection stands as a testimony to nursing caring scholars, nationally and internationally, experimenting with expanding epistemological–methodological directions for forms of caring inquiry.

At another level, this work may be considered controversial, in that it is not the answer to the question of how to "measure caring." Nevertheless, empirical indicators of caring help us move closer to spotlighting nursing's caring work, which warrants attention, research, and study as a major contributor of patient care. The phenomenon of human caring can be assessed through different measurement lens; thus, different caring measurements are required. As caring is such an elusive concept, it is helpful to have valid options to select for research.

The earlier edition of this book was translated into Japanese; other individual instruments have been translated, extending this paradigm of caring assessment and research into a global reach. It is our hope that knowledge and research on caring will continue to expand and grow. Having an updated collection of valid and reliable instruments for assessing and measuring caring is one step forward in transforming patient caring and outcome research.

Jean Watson

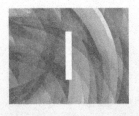

Overview

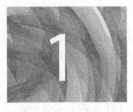

Introduction: Measuring Caring

Jean Watson

During this era when new formal models of healthcare are emerging, human caring remains a critical indicator of patient experience and related outcomes. Assessing and measuring human caring is a complex and dynamic phenomenon. While theories of caring and theoretical critiques surrounding the concept of caring abound, it is more or less agreed that human-to-human caring involves an expression of openness, a consciousness, an intentionality, a receptiveness, and authenticity within a personal, intersubjective context. Due to the urgency of a worldview shift for sustaining humanity and planet Earth, the concept of Unitary Caring is increasingly posited as one of the seminal theoretical, expanded paradigm concepts for the discipline of nursing. (For more exploration of these points, see Benner & Wrubel, 1989; Bowden, 1997; Brilowski & Wendler, 2005; Brody, 1988; Brown, Kitson, & McKnight, 1992; Cowling, Smith, & Watson, 2008; Fry, 1989; Kuhse, 1993; Newman, Smith, Pharris, Dexheimer, & Jones, 2008; Nyman & Sivonen, 2005; Rosa, Horton-Deutsch, & Watson, 2018; Smith, 1999; Stockdale & Warelow, 2000; Swanson, 1999; Van der Wal, 2006; Watson, 1988, 1990, 1999, 2005a, 2005b, 2018; Watson & Smith, 2002.)

When the institutional norm is to obtain external, observable criteria, one may continue to ask: "What do you mean by assessing and 'measuring caring'"? How can we justify having empirical, objective measures about such an elusive, nonmeasurable, existential (even spiritual), human relational phenomenon as human caring in nursing and healthcare practice? With this line of thinking there is concern of attempts to reduce human caring to a commodity. These are the questions that one hears within corporate healthcare circles. The ethical concern is that in trying to measure caring, one is drawn into a process of reducing a complex subjective, intersubjective, relational, often private, and invisible human phenomenon to a level of objectivity that exhausts, trivializes, and dilutes its authenticity and deeper meaning.

© Springer Publishing Company DOI:10.1891/9780826195425.0001

Because of its highly subjective, intersubjective nature, trying to reduce the very nature of caring to external outer-world empirical measures, such as a set of behaviors, tasks, or physical–physiological indicators, is often considered contradictory. (However, these connections are increasingly being made in broader arenas of biomedical science and noetic sciences.)

The very paradigm in which caring is located, with its ambiguity and ubiquitous nature, emphasized in the caring theory literature, has tended to make caring almost unmeasurable, both ethically and practically, unless by some qualitative standards that seek to capture its elusive, phenomenological, subjective dimensions.

This dilemma is part of the debate about measuring such a soft phenomenon of the human realm. For example, in summary, human caring is often considered an ethical worldview, an ontology, an intentionality, a consciousness, a way of being, in contrast to an "outward-doing" of something that can manifest itself in the physical, external, objective corporate realm (Watson, 1999, 2005a, 2005b, 2008, 2018).

So, at one end of the continuum, some view human caring as a basic way of being; a motive; a moral-imperative, philosophical starting point; an existential, spiritual intent that cannot be defined in terms of external objective criteria; rather it is "each nurse's own honest authenticity, a way of Being and Becoming, an informed moral consciousness" (Watson, 2008, 2012, 2018).

On the other hand, there is a continuous call for nursing to advance its knowledge of caring by advancing "the empirical measurement of caring in a way that withstands the scrutiny of the scientific community" (Brewer & Watson, 2015; Duffy, 2009; Valentine, 1991, p. 100). There remains an interest and need in nursing caring research to mediate between paradigms and worldview. We can now do this by examining the frequency of caring behaviors, and uncovering the clinical conditions that affect the delivery of caring. Such empirical caring knowledge not only makes the study of caring visible in the U.S. cost-driven corporate system of sick care, but also generates new indicators of whole-person health outcomes, leveraging data with administrators and policy makers (Brewer & Watson, 2015; Duffy, 2009; Lee, Larson, & Holzemer, 2006, p. 8; Watson & Brewer, 2015).

Healthcare systems and society are increasingly dependent on having new standards of human caring to assure ethical, relational integrity as core to human health and healing. Capturing human caring is diverse and complicated, especially when the dominant biotechnical culture tends to focus on external indicators of treatment and cure. Human caring often remains in the background as those private, invisible, unidentified, and unnamed relational occasions.

Indeed, in the last few decades, there is an interest in capturing the patient's subjective experience of caring with original mediating measures versus objective criteria alone. The Watson Caritas Patient Score (WCPS; www.watsoncaring science.org) is one example of a theory-based subjective measure that mediates between objective and subjective indicators, allowing for translating, quantifying, and assessing the objective/subjective intersection of human caring. The WCPS is designed to offer objective insight into a patient's subjective experience of caring/caritas and staff behaviors. There remains the challenge to continue to develop and translate subjective patient/human caring experiences into objective criteria. Such approaches capture system-wide indicators of caring and patient data, moving beyond conventional institutional objective external indicators alone. "Without indicators of caring and patient experiences, it is not reliable nor possible for systems to have data relating caring process of nursing to authentic meaningful outcomes" (Brewer & Watson, 2015).

Duffy's Quality-Caring Model (2002, 2009) is another example that demonstrates the value of caring in nursing within the evidence-based practice milieu of modern/postmodern healthcare. It favors a process, or way of being, that challenges modernist conventions and highlights the power of relationships. By reaffirming the nature of nursing's work as relationship centered, her work has meditated between worldviews and paradigm dissonance. Relational caring dimensions can be incorporated as empirical indicators for validation.

Such efforts, which are highlighted in this measurement book, seek to validate the so-called invisible, often unnamed and unknown relational caring work of nursing and healthcare providers. By empirically validating and researching human caring in nursing and healthcare, the health–healing relational, subjective/intersubjective dynamics of nursing and healthcare are revealed; this caring is made visible and tangible toward the goal of improving patient care and transforming healthcare systems. Showcasing human caring as a core value, with economic and scientific implications, is an important step forward in honoring the ethical, philosophical, and relational dimensions of the patient experience.

As we review empirical measures of caring, it is important to note the necessity of exploring coherence between theory, philosophy, and empirics as foundational to developing disciplinary knowledge (Chinn, 2016). To view these instruments strictly as empirical evidence alone would be incomplete without exploring the underlying philosophical–theoretical constructs, the nature of worldview or paradigm in which these measures are located. Indeed by viewing these instruments as empirical evidence alone does not suffice as adequate when deeper philosophical–theoretical issues are imbedded behind the development of each measure (Chinn, 2016, p. 291).

By moving from caring theory at a metalevel to empirical measures, one can highlight linkages between theory, measurement, and selected outcomes. Since most of the measurement tools in this compendium were developed from theories and/or derived from conceptual systems, it is anticipated that new measures will continue to evolve that will offer closer ontological–methodological congruency and/or make the places where the reconciliations were made overt. The more recent instruments developed by Nelson, Watson, and Inova Healthcare (2006), Persky et al. (2008), and the Ray, Turkel, and Marino (2002), Watson (2008), and Sitzman (2018) tools are recent examples.

Each conceptual–theoretical system of caring used to inform the developments of the different tools could be traced back to implied philosophical assumptions, as well as related middle   range theory, practice, or research tradition. The research traditions are the "designs, methods, data forms, and analytic processes that best help the scientist develop and test the middle range theories emerging from the broader grand theory or conceptual model" (Smith & Reeder, 1998, p. 34). Here we can acknowledge that a context for research and use of measurement for the phenomenon of caring holds the foundational ontological, philosophical, and epistemological assumptions implied or made explicit; while those assumptions inform design and methods and data forms for a study, the "ontological paradigms within the discipline may be consistent with more than one epistemic paradigm" (Smith & Reeder, 1998, p. 34), allowing for both older and newly developed instruments, data forms, and combinations of qualitative and quantitative data that best capture the complexities of the nature and quality of human caring.

Measuring caring within this context takes on a different meaning and may allow researchers to be more explicit so that the manifest key indicators of empirical caring still contain and honor the non-manifest field that is emergent and unseen behind the observable empirics. We remind ourselves that the empirical objective evidence of caring measurements is not the phenomenon itself, but only an indicator. The empirical indicators cannot be understood by themselves but must be located back into the conceptual system or model from which they were derived. In other words, the part that becomes objectively present in the manifest field must be placed within the context of the whole non-manifest field from which it emerged. The findings can then be interpreted/reinterpreted within an authentic theoretical–conceptual context and not stand alone as isolated evidence, void of context and meaning. It is through such efforts to connect research traditions, designs, methods, measurements, and findings that new interpretations, new knowledge, and new theories can be generated. Therefore, new insights can be obtained, and the shortcomings as well as strengths of existing tools can be identified, paving the way for a new generation of measurements and design as well as theory evolution.

Access to sensitive, nursing–healthcare indicators of care/caring, which many of the caring instruments in this third edition represent, can enable researchers and administrators alike to come closer to assessing, measuring, evaluating, comparing, and sustaining a caring philosophical, value-guided empirical foundation in the midst of external healthcare reforms. By assessing caring empirically, nursing and other health sciences can uncover more caring science practice, affirming its basic relational–ethical–ontological assumptions. In addition to the development of a more formal researching of caring, the conceptual–theoretical caring values and philosophies may more clearly emerge, thereby more distinctively informing, if not transforming, the biophysical–technological–cure model of medical care.

There are still rhetorical questions about nursing's tendency to jump to methods and models of measurement before addressing the meaningful philosophical questions that inform knowledge as well as method and measurement. While these questions and debates will and should continue, this updated collection of caring instruments is a means to bridge opposing viewpoints, dualisms, and conflicting paradigms. Researching caring does not guarantee a caring ideology, values, theories, attitudes, and manifestations in practices but leads closer to putting caring into the formula.

Moreover, it is a time to expand or even change our models of research in this era of shifting and emergent paradigms, time to move between and among worldviews and dualisms; it is a time for openness, for exploration, a time of pragmatics and heuristic means to move forward. Contemporary debates and dualistic mind-sets about caring in nursing–healthcare science will probably not go away. However, it is a global moment in nursing and healthcare history to reconcile dualisms and either-or positions, whether they are about caring/noncaring in the disciplinary matrix or about measuring or not measuring caring itself.

Compromises can and are made, and assumptions can be purposefully violated, if one can remain mindful and conscious of what compromises are made, and when they are made, and for what goals. This work acknowledges that deep philosophical ethical–ontological–subjective dimensions of caring cannot be fully measured, but some forms of measurement, derived theoretically, can elucidate the manifest field of caring practice, while still pointing toward the nonmanifest whole.

In addition, it is important to honor human caring's central and significant place in nursing science and patient healing. Caring offers philosophical ethical values foundation for the profession, as well as grounds for the development of additional knowledge to guide clinical practice and research. The whole realm of human relationships and health and healing may be tied back to caring and compassion, agape, and universal love—*caritas* (Brewer & Watson, 2015; Watson, 2008, 2012, 2018)—as the basis of any and all authentic caring–healing relationships and measures. Thus the ability to capture the phenomenon of caring and its effects on health and healing may provide new knowledge and insights as well as new mind-sets about caring in both education and practice. Caring-based models that affect and honor integrity of relations and purpose with costs and empirical outcomes are needed to further develop disciplinary knowledge, as well as improve working environments for practitioners and patients alike.

The acknowledgment of some aspects of these positions and debates opens up a horizon of possibilities that can be informed by the dialectical dance, rather than polarized in an either-or position. While caring may never be truly measured, this evolving collection of extant measurement instruments, gleaned from existing reliable nursing literature, is one way forward. This third edition points toward a partial end of assessing and capturing the theoretical, subjective, intersubjective phenomenon of human caring and its relationship to objective patient experiences as well as hospital outcomes.

SUMMARY

If more evidence can be offered in the form of quality indicators of caring, then nursing and healthcare will be positioned to more clearly manifest that which is often taken for granted or dismissed. In addition, empirical evidence of caring captured in an elusive practice world that is unstable, unseen, chaotic, and changing can provide a tangible grasp and glimpse of nursing's relational contribution to both science and public health welfare. Human caring, glimpsed through empirical measurement, whether qualitative or quantitative, may help us see, through an expanded epistemological lens, what has long been hidden from the profession, the healthcare system, the public consciousness, as well as science.

More specifically, some purposes for the use of formal measurement tools on human caring include:

■ Continuing improvement of human caring practices and healing systems through the use of outcomes and more mindful interventions to improve relational caring

■ Obtaining reliable data of patient's experience of caring

■ Benchmarking of structures, culture, settings, and environments in which caring is more manifest

■ Tracing levels and models of caring in care settings against routine care practices

■ Evaluating the consequences of caring versus noncaring for both nurses and patients

■ Creating a "report care" model for a unit or an institution in a critical area of practice

■ Identifying areas of weakness and strength in caring processes and interventions in order to stimulate self-correction and models of excellence in practice

■ Increasing our knowledge and understanding of the human-to-human relationship between caring, health, and healing

■ Validating empirically extant caring theories, as well as generating new theories of caring, caring relationships, and healing–health practices

■ Motivating new directions for caring science curricula, expanded pedagogies in nursing and health sciences, including interdisciplinary/transdisciplinary education and research

Measuring caring? In my view, human caring may never be "measured" in our conventional Western objective model of science. These measures, however, point toward the subjective, illusive, relational, authentic hidden aspects of caring. They provide us with objective indicators that are guided by philosophical–theoretical premises underlying the empirical forms. This coherent integration helps the discipline and public to honor the otherwise neglected and unexamined core aspect of health and healing. As such, this work offers multiple lenses to view and to measure caring, while still acknowledging that any measurement is only a manifestation, a way-finder toward something deeper. The something deeper remains in the world of the human–environmental–universal field of life processes. Such Unitary Caring science phenomena may never be fully known in totality, but point toward it. These instruments serve as pointers along the way.

THEORETICAL CONTEXT OF INSTRUMENTS

The measurement tools of caring included in this work are presented chronologically. They have not developed in any systematic way, but rather through the theoretical–philosophical interests of individuals and their foci of concern, be it patients, care systems, education, research, and so on. While some are informed by shared theories of caring, others draw upon diverse nursing theories of caring; in some other instances, theories have stimulated development of specific tools for assessing caring. Some of the measurement tools here have evolved to capture significant indicators of caring, based on general information and the literature of both nursing and related fields, such as psychology and philosophy. Others have been devised to address a specific area of focus, such as environment, learning environments, pedagogy, and so on, while making implicit philosophical assumptions about what caring is. Thus there is a connection between the choice of the caring measures to be assessed and the prevailing theoretical philosophy of caring.

Taken together, they represent the major measurements tools on caring that have been reported in the nursing literature since the early 1980s; for example, Larson, 1984 through 2018 and Sitzman (2018). This third edition includes the latest updates to earlier tools and offers a matrix structure and framework for all these tools. The matrix includes the following information:

- Identity of each of the measurements, and when each was developed
- The authors and their contact information
- The year the tool was published and key source citations in the literature
- What the tool was developed to measure
- A description of the instrument
- The nature and number of participants used in tool development
- Reported reliability/validity of the tool, if available
- Whether the tool was theory derived or atheoretical (conceptual basis of the measure)
- The latest citations in the nursing literature for instrument use

In addition to the matrix format for each of the caring measurement tools, when possible information as to specific requirements for each instrument's use is included in the appendix. This collection and compilation of the measurements of caring allow nursing and healthcare research to move forward in the areas of quality, outcomes, and evidence. They allow for consideration of relationships between caring-based interventions, patient–student experiences of caring, faculty–student data, and other variables such as cost and barometers of caring relationships.

New instruments and processes will have to continue to develop and evolve. The future is already identifying hard science criteria, and even the possibility of biological instrumentation, to capture the soft science experience and expression such as human caring. For example, some of the continuous developments at HeartMath (www.heartmath.org), the Institute for Research in Unlimited Love, the Heart-Brain Center of Cleveland Clinic, the Center for Compassion at Stanford Health, the research of the Institute of Noetic Sciences, and the special projects of the Fetzer Institute represent this shift toward researching phenomena such as love, gratitude, forgiveness, compassion, peaceful feelings, and loving kindness—all connected with the vicissitudes, phenomenon, and experience of human caring.

It is anticipated that even more sophistication will be forthcoming in the next generation of design, method, measurement, and analysis of data. As measurement evolves in harmony with shifts in scientific worldviews and new precision possibilities, it is inevitable that creative new options and approaches to measuring will increase.

At best these measurements serve as quality empirical indicators of theoretical caring assumptions, and point back toward the deeper aspects behind the measurements. Nevertheless, the fact that caring is a complex human phenomenon does not mean we should not try to capture as much of its depth as possible. As we do so, clarification of assumptions can be made and reconciliations identified between and among ontological, ethical, philosophical, epistemological, and even practical assumptions, within the various theoretical–conceptual systems of caring. Finally, the result may lead to a better fit between and among research traditions, design methods, and processes as well as a better interface between theory, research, and practice. All of these dimensions are vital if we are to develop knowledge, understanding, and appreciation of the human health–human caring experience (Chinn, 2016). This collection stands as a foundation for extant as well as new forms of caring inquiry, and serves as a background for the development of creative new empirical measurements.

REFERENCES

Benner, P., & Wrubel, J. (1989). *The primacy of caring*. Menlo Park, CA: Addison-Wesley.

Bowden, P. (1997). *Caring, gender sensitive ethics*. London: Routledge.

Brewer, B., & Watson, J. (2015). Evaluation of authentic human caring professional practices. *Journal of Nursing Administration, 45*(12), 622–627. doi:10.1097/NNA.0000000000000275

Brilowski, G. A., & Wendler, M. C. (2005). An evolutionary concept analysis of caring. *Journal of Advanced Nursing, 50*(6), 641–650. doi:10.1111/j.1365-2648.2005.03449.x

Brody, J. (1988). Virtue ethics, caring and nursing. *Scholarly Journal for Nursing Practice, 2,* 87–101.

Brown, J., Kitson, A., & McKnight, T. (1992). *Challenges in caring, explorations in nursing and ethics.* London: Chapman and Hall. Fry, 1989

Chinn, P. (2016). Acknowledging theoretical, philosophical and empiric linkages. Editorial. *Advances in Nursing Science, 39*(4), 291. doi: 10.1097/ANS.0000000000000154

Cowling, W. R., Smith, M. C., & Watson, J. (2008). The power of wholeness, consciousness and caring. A dialogue on nursing science, art, and healing. *Advances in Nursing Science, 31*(1), E41–E51. doi:10.1097/01.ANS.0000311535.11683.d1

Duffy, J. (2002). Caring assessment tools. In J. Watson (Ed.), *Instruments for assessing and measuring caring in nursing and health science* (pp. 120–150). New York, NY: Springer Publishing.

Duffy, J. (2009). *Quality caring in nursing: Applying theory to clinical practice, education and leadership.* New York, NY: Springer Publishing.

Fry, S. (1989). Towards a theory of nursing ethics. *Advances in Nursing Science, 11,* 9–22. doi:10.1097/00012272-198907000-00005

Kuhse, H. (1993). Caring is not enough: Reflections on a nursing ethics of care. *Australian Journal of Advanced Nursing, 11,* 32–41.

Larson, P. (1984). Important nurse caring behaviors perceived by patients with cancer. *Oncology Nursing Forum, 11*(6), 46–50.

Lee, M. H., Larson, P. J., & Holzemer, W. L. (2006). Psychometric evaluation of the modified CARE-Q among Chinese nurses in Taiwan. *International Journal for Human Caring, 10*(4), 8–13. doi:10.20467/1091-5710.10.4.8

Nelson, J., Watson, J., & Inova Health. (2009). Caring factor survey. In J. Watson (Ed.), *Assessing and measuring caring in nursing and health sciences* (2nd ed., pp. 253–260). New York, NY: Springer Publishing.

Newman, M. A., Smith, M. C., Pharris, M., Dexheimer, M., & Jones, D. (2008). The focus of the discipline revisited. *Advances in Nursing Science, 31*(1), E16–E27. doi:10.1097/01.ANS.0000311533.65941.f1

Nyman, A., & Sivonen, K. (2005). The concept of meaning of life in caring science. *Nursing Science and Research in Nordic Countries, 25*(4), 20–24.

Persky, G., Nelson, J., Watson, J., & Bent, K. (2008). Creating a profile of a nurse effective in caring. *Nursing Administrative Quarterly, 32*(1), 15–20. doi:10.1097/01.naq.0000305943.46440.77

Ray, M., Turkel, M., & Marino, F. (2002). The transformative process for nursing in workforce redevelopment. *Nursing Administration Quarterly, 26*(2), 1–14. doi:10.1097/00006216 -200201000-00003

Rosa, W., Horton-Deutsch, S., & Watson, J. (Eds.). (2018). *Handbook for caring science: Expanding the paradigm.* New York, NY: Springer Publishing.

Sitzman, K. (2018). The evolution of knowledge development related to caring in Online Classrooms and Beyond. In W. Rosa, S. Horton-Deutsch, & J. Watson, J. (eds.) *Handbook for Caring Science: Expanding the Paradigm* (pp. 327–340). New York, NY: Springer Publishing.

Smith, M. (1999). Caring and the science of unitary human beings. *Advances in Nursing Science, 21*(4), 14–28.

Smith, M., & Reeder, F. (1998). Clinical outcomes research and Rogerian science: Strange or emergent bedfellows? *Visions, 6*(1), 27–38.

Stockdale, M., & Warelow, P. J. (2000). Is the complexity of care a paradox? *Journal of Advanced Nursing, 31*(5), 1258–1264.

Swanson, K. (1999). What is known about caring in nursing science. In A. S. Hinshaw, S. Fleetham, & J. Shaver (Eds.), *Handbook of clinical nursing research* (pp. 31–60). Thousand Oaks, CA: Sage.

Valentine, K. (1991). Comprehensive assessment of caring and its relationship to outcome measures. *Journal of Nursing Quality Assurance, 5*(2), 59–68.

Van der Wal, D. M. (2006). Factors erosive to caring. *African Journal of Nursing and Midwifery, 8*(1), 55–75.

Watson, J. (1999). *Postmodern nursing and beyond.* Edinburgh, Scotland: Churchill Livingstone.

Watson, J. (2005a). *Caring science as sacred science.* Philadelphia, PA: F. A. Davis.

Watson, J. (2005b). Caring science: Belonging before being as ethical cosmology. *Nursing Science Quarterly, 18*(4), 4–5. doi:10.1177/0894318405280395

Watson, J. (2008). *Nursing: The philosophy and science of caring* (2nd ed.). Boulder: University Press of Colorado.

Watson, J. (2012). *Human caring science* (2nd ed.). Boston, MA: Jones & Bartlett.

Watson, J. (2018). *Unitary caring science. The philosophy and praxis of nursing.* Boulder: University Press of Colorado.

Watson, J., & Brewer, B. (2015). Caring science research criteria, evidence and measurement. *Journal of Nursing Administration, 45*(5), 235–236. doi:10.1097/NNA.0000000000000190

Watson, J., & Smith, M. C. (2002). Caring science and the science of unitary human beings: A trans-theoretical discourse for nursing knowledge development. *Journal of Advanced Nursing, 37*(5), 452–461. doi:10.1046/j.1365-2648.2002.02112.x

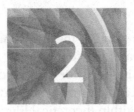

Caring and Nursing Science: Contemporary Discourse

Jean Watson

STATE OF CARING KNOWLEDGE IN NURSING SCIENCE

In addition to the debate about measuring caring and ambiguity around the concept of caring itself, there is uncertainty about the state of caring knowledge in nursing. While this debate is not as dynamic or even pertinent as it was in past years, there remains a lack of consensus about the nature of caring as well as its location within nursing's disciplinary matrix. It seems clear that further development of knowledge of caring through research and measurement approaches is one way to ensure that caring remains a seminal aspect of nursing's distinction as a discipline and profession, fulfilling its global covenant to its public.

Indeed, while the academic debates may linger, clinical care issues and new professional models of caring practice are accelerating the development of nursing practices that demonstrate new professional practice models designed to sustain caring. With the proliferation of the nursing shortage and clinical systems' despair over patient care and outcomes, this focus on human caring and outcomes of patients' experiences of caring becomes more critical than ever.

Further, with the expansion of and additional research among Magnet® hospitals throughout the United States and other parts of the world, there is growing evidence of the essential benefits of theory-guided professional caring practices. Such informed practices are showing that improvements and advancements in nursing can and are making important differences in the lives of patients and nursing colleagues as well. Therefore, it is important to point out some of the converging developments that position caring and caring knowledge more clearly within nursing's domain of concern.

© Springer Publishing Company DOI:10.1891/9780826195425.0002 **13**

The classic attempt to reconcile the dissonance around caring in nursing was the Newman, Sime, and Corcoran-Perry (1991) critique of the existing metaparadigm. They noted the need for a more explicit relationship between caring and the social relevance to describe the field of study. They asserted that caring and health are linked within theoretical literature in nursing, and that the quality of the relationship is what facilitates health and makes it possible for the nurse and patient to connect in a way that is transforming. Thus they presented a unifying statement for the disciplinary focus by framing nursing as "the study of caring in the human health experience" (Newman et al., 1991, p. 3).

Smith (1999) later made a strong case for the concept of caring, critiquing and then offering counterpoints against the arguments for why caring is not a central concept. For example, she made a case for how none of the concerns for not including caring hold merit, overturning arguments relating to ambiguity, a limiting perspective, ubiquitousness, nonsubstantiveness, nongeneralizability, and femininity. She went on to identify five constitutive meanings of caring from the perspective of Rogerian science of unitary human beings: manifesting intentions, appreciating patterns, attuning oneself to dynamic flow, experiencing the infinite, and inviting creative emergence.

Each of these constitutive meanings is present in the extant nursing literature on caring. Semantic expressions of each of these meanings were explicated by Smith.

Even though there remains a latent lack of formal disciplinary consensus about caring as part of the meta-paradigm of nursing, caring has emerged during the past 3 to 4 decades as a central component and paradigm feature of nursing. Newman et al. (1991), Smith (1999), and others (Rosa, Horton-Deutsch, & Watson, 2019; Swanson, 1999; Watson, 2018; Watson & Smith, 2002) help to make this explicit and demonstrate its validity at this point in time.

RECENT EVIDENCE OF THE PRESENCE OF CARING IN NURSING

In addition to the aforementioned developments, some other major events attest to the centrality of caring as part of nursing's focus. For example, the following evidence attesting to the relevance and presence of caring knowledge as a focus in nursing has accumulated in the past few years:

- In academic nursing structures and academic departments in Scandinavian countries named "Caring Science"

- Two international journals in nursing with focus on caring: the *Scandinavian Journal of Caring Sciences* and the *International Journal of Human Caring; Nordic Journal of Caring Sciences*

- The International Professional Nursing Organization and the International Association for Human Caring, which is more than 40 years old

- Over 30 years of the publication of *Science of Caring Research* from the University of California, San Francisco
- Key recommendations for caring as a core concept in nursing in national reports from the American Academy Nursing Wingspread Conference
- The National League for Nursing's curriculum standards
- Special monographs, conferences, and journal issues devoted to caring

The year 2019 will be the 40-year anniversary of Watson's first book on Caring Science: *Nursing. The Philosophy and Science of Caring* (1979). Boston, MA: Little Brown & Co.

The American Nurses Association's *Agenda for the Future* (2002), which extends to 2020, acknowledges that nursing is "the pivotal health care profession, highly valued for its specialized knowledge, skill and caring in improving the health status of the public and ensuring safe, effective, quality care" (p. 3). Further, of the 10 domains the American Nurses Association identified as key for nursing's agenda, at least five have direct relevance to the need for knowledge of caring and its effects. These are delivery systems/nursing models, a professional nursing culture, a work environment, economic recruitment/retention, and leadership. Each of these categories is associated with a need for attention to knowledge, skills, and research related to caring.

In addition, the case for the necessity of more knowledge of caring to nurses and patients is bolstered by Halldorsdottir's (1999) classic research on the ethical and clinical consequences of caring and noncaring, as well as Swanson's (1999) meta-analysis of 130 empirical nursing studies; new caring theory-guided practice Magnet hospital and educational initiatives; the recent implementation of the International Caring Comparative Database; and the founding of the International Caritas Consortium (www.watsoncaringscience.org/intl-caritas-consortium), the Caring International Research Collaborative (www.hcenvironment.com), and the Watson Caring Science Institute (WCSI) (www.watsoncaringscience.org). More recently, items from Watson Caritas Patient Score derived from 10 Caritas Processes of Watson Theory of Human Caring were shown to be highly correlated with overall hospital outcomes in a 2016 Pilot with Press Ganey Corporation (Watson, 2018 Press, Ganey-WCSI Project).

This accumulation of converging developments helps to resolve the dissonance about caring and its place in nursing science and the importance of assessing caring to make new connections with outcomes of care. Regardless of whether one considers the discourse to be unresolved or believes caring is a central and unifying concept for the discipline, the need to grasp the phenomenon in diverse ways is one of the responsibilities for nursing's maturing as a distinct discipline. The fact that new international multisite research projects have emerged is additional evidence of the need to increase the knowledge, research, study, and application of caring as a critical variable in professional practice and quality healthcare.

MEASURING CARING AND OUTCOMES—NURSING KNOWLEDGE AND INTERNATIONAL RESEARCH PRIORITIES

Hinshaw's (2000) review of trends of nursing knowledge pointed out Sigma Theta Tau International's Strategic Plan for 2005, which is "To create a global community of nurses who lead in using scholarship, knowledge, and technology to improve the health of the world's people" (p. 117). As part of her review, Hinshaw provided three perspectives for generating nursing knowledge trends and identifying priorities for the 21st century:

- Via an analysis of the top five nursing research priorities evident in the American nursing literature of the past 5 years
- Via future directions for nursing research outlined by 60 American investigators
- Via identified international nursing research priorities from a number of countries

It is interesting to note from Hinshaw's review that priority areas identified by both American nursing scholars and relevant U.S. nursing publications include "quality of care outcomes and their measurements, impact or effectives of nursing interventions." In other words, as Hinshaw (2000) noted, "The emphasis on quality of care outcomes indicates the profession's commitment to identify and measure nursing sensitive outcomes as both clinical measures and research tools" (p. 118).

What is perhaps even more interesting than the general consensus regarding American nursing research priorities is the fact that similar priorities related to concern for care issues, quality of care outcomes, and nursing interventions have been identified in international nursing circles. For example, in Great Britain, "research into patients' perspectives of care and 'how they are assessed' and 'nursing interventions' were named as priorities; in the Nordic countries "quality of care balanced with cost outcomes, along with theoretical and philosophical perspectives of developing knowledge in nursing practice," was identified as their top issue; and in Thailand and Africa, priorities for nursing research included an improvement in nursing interventions and care of individuals with specific conditions. Similarly, the European work group representing 19 European countries included "effective care and continuity" of care across settings and "effect of variations . . . on quality and costs of care and patient outcomes" in their list of challenges for generating knowledge for the discipline of nursing (Hinshaw, 2000, p. 121).

As reflected by the international work on caring assessment by Arthur and Randle (2007) throughout Hong Kong, China, Singapore, and other nearby countries, caring continues to be a seminal universal element in defining and researching nursing and patient care worldwide.

In all these international nursing circles, care issues and outcomes of care, along with measurement of such, looms as the top priorities for nursing research. Hence, a collection of tools or measurements of caring as indicators of sensitive nursing approaches to these global nursing priorities is relevant to the facilitation of the development of further knowledge and research. Researching the phenomenon of caring more specifically and intentionally within the context of "quality of caring outcomes" as well as the "impact or effectiveness of nursing interventions" can help inform and strengthen both the discipline and the practice of nursing for this 21st century.

While Smith and others have made a theoretical and philosophical case for caring in nursing, this discussion highlights broader international professional activities, priorities, safety, structures, organizations, position statements, and definitions. Taken together, these intellectual and professional developments attest to the placement of caring within the discipline and priorities for researching and measuring caring and its outcomes as almost a universal mandate in nursing circles.

The consequences of both caring and noncaring for both nurses and patients are dramatic messages for nursing research and practice. At a time when nursing is declining and its survival threatened, nurses' satisfaction is enhanced when the practice of caring is enabled. When caring is not present in nursing practices or settings, the research indicates that nurses become depressed, robotic, hardened, oblivious, and worn down. These empirical data invite much more research into and attention to the emotional and physical healing consequences for patients when caring is present, including cost savings. The same is true from the other side of the equation, in that nurses are much more satisfied, fulfilled, purposeful, and knowledge seeking when caring is present.

In addition to empirical evidence of the importance of caring in the profession, there is growing attention to caring within the disciplinary matrix as it has evolved. More recently, Cowling et al. (2008) made a case for caring along with wholeness and consciousness as critical concepts to distinguish the discipline of nursing from other disciplines. They posit a unitary caring science praxis focus as evidence of a "mature caring-healing-health discipline and profession, helping affirm and sustain humanity, caring and wholeness in our daily work and in the world" (p. E41). More recently, Watson has published: *Unitary Caring Science, Philosophy and Praxis of Nursing* (2018), making a case for not only caring as a core metaparadigm concept, but unitary caring as the evolved paradigmatic context for wholeness, caring, quantum, nonlocal consciousness thinking. Moreover, a newly released *Handbook for Caring Science* (2019), edited by Rosa, Horton-Deutsch, and Watson, provides a state of the art and science of caring science and the importance of human caring as a serious epistemic, ontological, philosophical, concrete-ethical and concrete-practical endeavor. This work serves as a foundation to maturing the discipline, practice, education, and research and policy of human caring in nursing and health sciences.

The instruments in this text have been developed to empirically assess caring, and offer one pathway toward more focused research and inquiry into the nursing and caring phenomenon. When evidence and language of caring is made more manifest, more explicit, it can then be more systematically explored for models of practice excellence. By continuing to explore the phenomenon of caring through empirical measures as well as nonempirical means, nursing continues to build its nursing science disciplinary foundation for a new century of nursing practice.

Development and research of caring knowledge and practices have another contribution to make at this turn in nursing's history. For example, nursing scholars have addressed the unsettled state of nursing knowledge. As early as 1999, Fawcett noted a concern for the continued existence of the discipline of nursing in critiquing the hallmarks of 20th- and 21st-century nursing theory and knowledge development. She acknowledged some major accomplishments: specification of a metaparadigm for nursing knowledge, explication of conceptual models, explication of unique nursing theories, and theories shared with other disciplines. Elizabeth Barrett (2017) issued a perennial call to nursing in her seminal article in *Nursing Science Quarterly*: Again: What Is Nursing. Who Knows? Who Cares. She calls for nursing to honor its phenomenon of human-universe and health. These foci require knowledge and research of human caring, healing, and health.

In spite of these accomplishments, Cowling, Smith, Barrett, Watson, and others such as Kim (1996) suggest that issues of fragmentation, arbitrariness, and lack of nursing research that truly advances nursing science (in contrast to other disciplines and medical science) are all lingering dilemmas that nursing must resolve if it is to survive as a distinct discipline and mature profession. These theoretical positions about nursing phenomena continue to make a case for nursing's maturation within a unitary caring science model for this turn in its history as a distinct discipline.

This work on instruments for assessing and measuring caring assists nursing in more specifically theorizing, attending to, and researching the caring phenomenon in the discipline and practice of nursing; it can be explored as structure, process, and outcome. Moreover, when caring relationships are considered as part of the nature of specific intervention models for practice, nursing knowledge is generated that can strengthen the distinct nature of nursing's role and importance in clinical care and nursing science, informing other disciplines as well as maturing.

However, nursing is not alone in identifying care issues and outcomes. Indeed, other disciplines are now also recognizing and incorporating caring into their disciplinary foci. Renewed attention to caring allows nursing and its development to further inform such transdisciplinary interests as caring therapeutics in health practices among a range of diverse practitioners; relationship-centered caring (e.g., the Fetzer Institute project on relationship-centered care); and the fields of feminist studies, women's health, ethics, and philosophy, as well as the emergence of caring science and an evolved unitary caring science focus

(Cowling et al., 2008; Eriksson & Lindstrm, 1999; Rosa et al., 2019; Watson, 2005a, 2008, 2018).

Indeed, in the field of medicine, some empirical research findings related to caring relationships and communication between physicians and patients reinforce the early empirical findings of Swanson's (1999) analysis in the nursing science field. It is common knowledge that the absence of a caring relationship and patient dissatisfaction are tied to low patient scores and even lawsuits. Such convergence of outcomes of caring research in nursing science and medical research attests to the importance of more research in the field and the need for empirical indicators for measuring caring. Nursing science and nursing researchers offer an array of empirical measurements as a background and foundation for additional nursing and interdisciplinary research on caring outcomes, as well as a basis for addressing caring measurement issues.

REFERENCES

American Nurses Association. (2002). *Nursing's agenda for the future: A call to the nation.* Retrieved from http://ana.nursingworld.org/mods/archive/mod725/cedecfull.htm

American Nurses Association. (2002). *Nursing's agenda for the future: Future vision.* Retrieved from http://nursingworld.org/MainMenuCategories/HealthcareandPolicyIssues/Reports/AgendafortheFuture.aspx

Arthur, D., & Randle, J. (2007). The professional self concept of nurses: A review of the literature from 1992–2006. *Australian Journal of Advanced Nursing, 24*(3), 60–64.

Barrett, E. (2017). Again. What is nursing science? Who knows? Who care? *Nursing Science Quarterly, 30*(2), 129–133. doi:10.1177/0894318417693313

Cowling, R., Smith, M., & Watson, J. (2008). The power of wholeness, consciousness and caring. A dialogue on nursing science, art, and healing. *Advances in Nursing Science, 31*(1), E41–E51. doi:10.1097/01.ans.0000311535.11683.d1

Eriksson, K., & Lindstrom, U. (1999). A theory of science for caring science. *Hoitotiede, 11*(6), 358–364.

Fawcett, J. (1999). The state of nursing science: Hallmarks of the 20th and 21st centuries. *Nursing Science Quarterly, 12*(4), 311–318. doi:10.1177/08943189922107025

Halldorsdottir, S. (1991). Five basic modes of being with another. In D. A. Gaut & M. M. Leininger (Eds.), *Caring: The compassionate healer* (pp. 37–49). New York, NY: National League for Nursing.

Hinshaw, A. (2000). Nursing knowledge for the 21st century: Opportunities and challenges. *Journal of Nursing Scholarship, 32*(2), 117–123. doi:10.1111/j.1547-5069.2000.00117.x

Kim, H. S. (1996). *Challenges of new perspectives.* Paper presented at Nursing Knowledge Impact Conference, Boston.

Newman, M. A., Sime, A. M., & Corcoran-Perry, S. A. (1991). The focus of the discipline of nursing. *Advances in Nursing Science, 14*(1), 1–6.

Rosa, W., Horton-Deutsch, S., & Watson, J. (2019). *Handbook for caring science.* New York, NY: Springer Publishing.

Smith, M. (1999). Caring and the science of unitary human beings. *Advances in Nursing Science, 21*(4), 14–28. doi:10.1097/00012272-199906000-00006

Swanson, K. (1999). What is known about caring in nursing science. In A. S. Hinshaw, S. Fleetham, & J. Shaver (Eds.), *Handbook of clinical nursing research* (pp. 31–60). Thousand Oaks, CA: Sage.

Watson, J. (1979). *Nursing: The philosophy and science of caring.* Boston, MA: Little, Brown.

Watson, J. (2005a). *Caring science as sacred science.* Philadelphia, PA: F. A. Davis.

Watson, J. (2008). *Nursing: The philosophy and science of caring* (2nd ed.). Boulder: University Press of Colorado.

Watson, J. (2018). *Unitary caring science. Philosophy and praxis of nursing.* Boulder: University Press of Colorado.

Watson, J., & Smith, M. (2000, October). *Re-visioning caring science and Rogerian science of unitary human beings.* Paper presented at Boston Knowledge Development Conference.

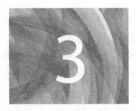

Background and Selection of Caring Instruments

Jean Watson

The original project for this book began in the early 1990s as an initiative of what was then the Center for Human Caring at the University of Colorado. The project was initiated under the guidance of Center director Dr. Jean Watson. It had the special administration leadership of Karen Holland, the executive director of the Center at the time. Due to some life and system changes, the project was interrupted between 1997 and 1999. It was reactivated in 1999 with the special research and tracking-skill assistance of Jeannie Zuk, a doctoral student research assistant at that time.

The first edition project was guided by an extensive review of the Cumulative Index to Nursing and Allied Health Literature (CINAHL) database, which was used to identify all empirical caring measurements that were published in the nursing literature. The earliest one detected was published in 1984. The search continued until December 2000, during which time each doctoral student cohort engaged in intensive and extensive follow-up of the use of the specific measurements, as well as locating the origin of the tools and the names of the developers of the tools and other studies that used the measurement. Over these past few years, there continues to be a cadre of devoted doctoral nursing students and caring science colleagues who have engaged in intensive research to identify and update any empirical measurement tools of caring.

This second edition benefited from the special research assistance of the late Kathryn Lynch, who dedicated time and effort to updating and tracking new instruments in the nursing literature. It has followed the general extensive review from the first edition through the CINAHL database from 2000 to the present. In addition, personal contact was initiated with the authors of the instruments regarding any updates about their instruments, any new revised forms, and general use of the tools. Authors of tools included in the first and second editions were invited to update their descriptions and instruments, their contact information, and information regarding the latest use of the instruments, and provide information on any other uses or new versions since 2000 and into 2018. The search for each of these tools and their use has been continued through diverse approaches and an extensive literature review for any recent citations to capture information on the latest use of any of the identified instruments.

A range of extant empirical measurements that includes caring attributes, caring behaviors, patients' perceptions, and satisfaction with nurses' caring exists. As a result of the diversity of approaches, caring is treated in different ways, and there are varying conceptual notions that underline their developments. Likewise, varying degrees of reliability and validity exist for each tool. Most all of the measurements included here have reports of reliability and validity, and there is an attempt to note the conceptual-theoretical developmental origin of the instruments.

Both the second and third editions have introduced new instruments that capture deeper dimensions of caring, even though some remain in exploratory stages. Nevertheless, they have promise as innovative approaches or focus on a unique population, for example, family caring (by Goff, developer of tool), organizational caring (Ray & Turkel, 2000), and the *caritas* nurse profile (Persky et al., 2008; Watson, 2008). These new instruments continue to be actively tested and used to establish further validation and reliability data.

Additional instruments specific to the third edition include both revisions of previous instruments as well as new ones such as the New Versions Caring Assessment Tool (e.g., Version V; administrative and educational version). Others included in this third edition are Relational Caring Questionnaire and Questionnaire on Instructor Behavior. New instruments included in this edition are Student Perceptions of Caring Online, and Relationship-Based Care Environment Scale.

In the new edition we made no attempt to include an extensive psychometric critique of each instrument. Rather, we chose to report the face value about each of the measurements. Some of the major background facts about each tool's development and the latest source citations for research using the tool are presented. Final compilation of each measurement and its update resulted in the final matrix.

To the best of my knowledge, the ordering of the instruments is chronological. In some instances there is ambiguity as to which instruments were developed first, since the date of publication—not the dates of developmental efforts—was the date selected for chronological ordering. However, earlier developmental dates are noted in the summary and matrix of each instrument when available.

The final section of the book provides a comprehensive blueprint matrix of all the instruments. Where possible, the specific instruments and the author's information and contact are included in the Appendix. The matrix blueprint and copies of selected measurements make this compendium a useful and functional resource for anyone wishing to obtain information, summary data, and access to empirical instruments that measure caring.

REFERENCES

Persky, G., Nelson, J., Watson, J., & Bent, K. (2008). Creating a profile of a nurse effective in caring. *Nursing Administrative Quarterly, 32*(1), 15–20. doi:10.1097/01.naq.0000305943.46440.77

Ray, M., & Turkel, M. (2000, August). *Economic and patient outcomes of the nurse-patient relationship.* Grant funded by the Department of Defense, Washington DC, Tri-Service Nursing Research Council.

Watson, J. (2008). *Nursing: The philosophy and science of caring* (2nd ed.). Boulder: University Press of Colorado.

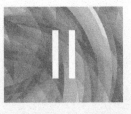

Compilation and Summary Data of Each Instrument for Measuring Caring

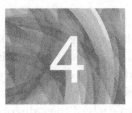

CARE-Q and CARE/SAT and Modified CARE-Q

Patricia Larson

The Caring Assessment Report Evaluation Q-Sort, commonly known as CARE-Q (Larson, 1984), is the first quantitative caring tool cited in the nursing literature and is the most frequently used instrument for assessing caring. It has the longest-standing reputation for repeated use and has generated additional empirical research in different settings with different patient populations, as well as cross-cultural versions of the tool. Larson and Ferketich (1993) developed the CARE-Q into a caring satisfaction instrument to attempt to measure patients' satisfaction with the nursing care they received. In 2006, Lee, Larson, and Holzemer modified the CARE-Q from the Q-methodology approach into a 7-point Likert scale questionnaire with 50 items. The Modified CARE-Q measures the frequency, perceived by the patients, with which nurses enact caring behaviors while providing care to patients (Lee et al., 2006).

The original CARE-Q tool was developed from a somewhat a priori orientation to caring assumptions. The authors acknowledged some of the early writers in the field of caring theory and philosophies at the time but developed the CARE-Q items from the ground up with special concern about the caring needs and perceptions of cancer patients. The view of nurse caring used to inform the instrument development was the nurse's "intent . . . to create a subjective sense of feeling cared for in the patient. Feeling cared for is a sensation of well-being and safety resulting from enacted behaviors of another" (Larson, 1986, p. 86).

In developing the tool itself, Larson used a Delphi survey of practicing nurses on caring behaviors and a study of patients' perceptions of nurse-caring behaviors, which resulted in the identification of 69 nurse-caring behaviors and was later reduced to 50 items, each printed on an individual card. The 50 behavioral items were then ordered in six subscales of caring: is accessible (6 items); comforts (9 items); anticipates (5 items); develops a trusting relationship (16 items); monitors and follows through (8 items); and explains and facilitates (6 items).

© Springer Publishing Company DOI:10.1891/9780826195425.0004 **27**

The CARE-Q uses Q-methodology to identify the most important nurse-caring behaviors, as perceived by patients. With this methodology, only a certain number of cards can be placed in each designated pile. Thus, each participant is faced with a forced-choice distribution. The participant is asked to rank a predetermined number of items in each of the categories from "most important" to "least important." Once the items are selected, the CARE-Q Sort of each participant is then numerically coded for statistical analysis.

The content validity was obtained from an expert nurse panel of graduate nursing students, who agreed upon 60 items. These items were verified by a panel of nurses and patients in an oncology unit. As a result, the final version of the CARE-Q comprised 50 items. Larson (1987) then attempted to establish reliability and validity. Face and content validity were identified from samples of both nurses and patients. The test-retest reliability of the CARE-Q was obtained from a sample of 82 oncology nurses randomly selected from a national oncology organization. The most important caring item had a test-retest reliability of 79%, and for the least important caring items the result was 63% (Andrews, Daniels, & Hall, 1996; Beck, 1999; Kyle, 1995).

Larson (1984, 1986) identified some limitations of the Q-methodology and the forced-choice format of the CARE-Q. Respondents have had difficulties designating one item the most important over others. Some commented they would have liked to respond a second time to the selection, while others reported that they wished they had done the Q-Sort the way they wanted to, as opposed to the way it was expected for them to report (Kyle, 1995). Others have criticized the length of time necessary to complete the CARE-Q (reported to be 26 minutes) and problems related to the fact that some participants did not sort the cards according to directions (Beck, 1999). Kyle notes these shortcomings and questions the validity of the instrument.

In spite of these limitations, numerous other studies have reported use of the original CARE-Q and culturally derived versions of it. Beck identified several studies that report reliabilities for the CARE-Q (see Table 4.1).

To date, no new reliability or validity work on the CARE-Q has been found. Researchers have relied largely upon Larson's original developmental work, although other researchers using the tool have noted some problems in its use, such as the use of nonspecific and vague items, which lead to a variety of interpretations; the instrument's length and the time required to complete it; and respondents' difficulty understanding all the instrument statements (Kyle, 1995).

Nevertheless, studies using the CARE-Q have agreed on the most important caring behaviors perceived by nurses and patients; however, a difference between patients' perceptions of caring and those of nurses has been reported, with nurses focusing on psychosocial skills, and patients on those skills that demonstrate professional competency (Kyle, 1995). Various interpretations of these findings have been attempted, but these differences have not been resolved, even with additional research and new explanatory models. As a result of these findings, use of the CARE-Q has stimulated additional research and continued use, often as a part of nurses' master thesis projects.

TABLE 4.1 CARE-Q		
STUDY	SAMPLE	RELIABILITY
Komorita, Koehring, and Hirchert (1991)	110 master's-prepared nurses	64.4% for five most important and five least important caring behaviors with nine nurses
von Essen and Sjödén (1991a)	86 medical-surgical patients and 73 nursing staff in Sweden	Cronbach's alpha = .95 Subscales: ■ explains and facilitates = .59 ■ comforts = .86 ■ trusting relationship = .86 ■ anticipates = .72 ■ monitors and follows through = .79 ■ accessible = .76
Widmark-Petersson et al. (1996)	72 cancer patients and 63 nurses	Total Cronbach's alpha = .94 Subscales: ■ explains and facilitates = .60 ■ comforts = .78 ■ trusting relationship = .86 ■ anticipates = .60 ■ monitors and follows through = .59 ■ is accessible = .59

It has been recommended that further tests of the psychometric properties of the CARE-Q address the length and ambiguity of the sorting process and the possibility of the use of a Likert format to make the CARE-Q more user friendly (Andrews et al., 1996). Further refinement and evolution of this important and widely used empirical measurement of caring is necessary to strengthen the reliability of the findings with ease of use (Figure 4.1).

The matrix in Table 4.2 provides background information on the original CARE-Q (Tool 4.1), along with all the research studies that have been generated using the CARE-Q, including the Swedish version. The matrix also provides information about the Modified CARE-Q developed by Lee and her associates (2006).

CARE SATISFACTION QUESTIONNAIRE: CARE/SAT

This scale was developed as an extension of the CARE-Q by Larson and Ferketich (1993). They incorporated all 50 items of the CARE-Q into a visual analog scale and renamed it the CARE Satisfaction Questionnaire (CARE/SAT). Some additional items were developed and added in order to assess overall patient satisfaction with nurse-caring behaviors. The final version consists of 29 behaviors (Tool 4.2). The initial testing of the CARE/SAT included 268 hospitalized adult

FIGURE 4.1 3″ × 5″ cards.

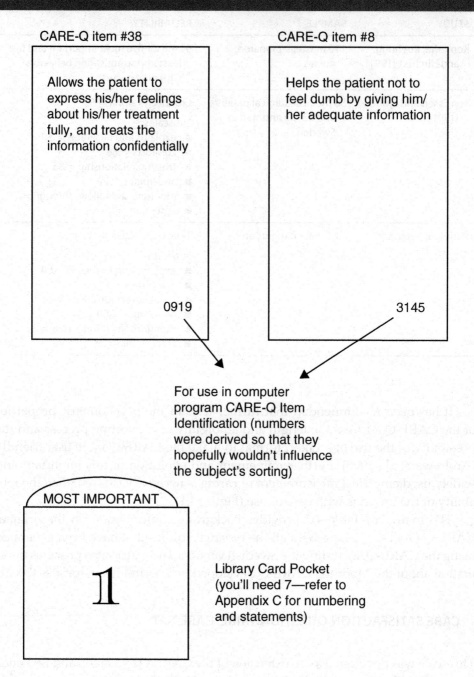

CARE-Q item #38

Allows the patient to express his/her feelings about his/her treatment fully, and treats the information confidentially

0919

CARE-Q item #8

Helps the patient not to feel dumb by giving him/her adequate information

3145

For use in computer program CARE-Q Item Identification (numbers were derived so that they hopefully wouldn't influence the subject's sorting)

MOST IMPORTANT

1

Library Card Pocket (you'll need 7—refer to Appendix C for numbering and statements)

TABLE 4.2 Matrix of Caring Assessment Instruments

INSTRUMENT	AUTHOR CONTACT INFORMATION	PUBLICATION SOURCE	DEVELOPED TO MEASURE	INSTRUMENT DESCRIPTION	PARTICIPANTS	REPORTED VALIDITY/ RELIABILITY	CONCEPTUAL-THEORETICAL BASIS OF MEASUREMENT	LATEST CITATION IN NURSING LITERATURE
Caring Assessment Instrument (1984)	Patricia Larson, DNS, RN University of California, San Francisco School of Nursing Department of Physiology Nursing Box 0610 N 611Y San Francisco, CA 94143-0610 Email: pattwkw@msn.com	Larson (1984)	Perceptions of nurse-caring behaviors	Q-Sort 50 cards into 7 piles/7-point scale to prioritize perceptions of nurse-caring behaviors. The most commonly used instrument, both nationally and internationally, although it is noted to be confusing, ambiguous, and time consuming.	N = 57 oncology patients	Expert panel test-retest Content and face validity	General references to nursing theories of caring A priori development Guided by care needs of cancer patients	Chinese version of CARE-Q Holroyd, Yue-kuen, Sau-wai, Fung-shan, and Wai-wan (1998)
CARE-Q	Patricia Larson, DNS, RN University of California, San Francisco School of Nursing Department of Physiology Nursing Box 0610 N 611Y San Francisco, CA 94143-0610 Email: pattwkw@msn.com	Larson (1986)	Perceptions of nurse-caring behaviors	Q-Sort	N = 57 oncology nurses	Extension of Larson (1984) See Larson (1984)	See Larson (1984)	See Larson (1984)

(continued)

TABLE 4.2 Matrix of Caring Assessment Instruments (*continued*)

INSTRUMENT	AUTHOR CONTACT INFORMATION	PUBLICATION SOURCE	DEVELOPED TO MEASURE	INSTRUMENT DESCRIPTION	PARTICIPANTS	REPORTED VALIDITY/ RELIABILITY	CONCEPTUAL-THEORETICAL BASIS OF MEASUREMENT	LATEST CITATION IN NURSING LITERATURE
CARE-Q	Patricia Larson, DNS, RN University of California, San Francisco School of Nursing Department of Physiology Nursing Box 0610N 611Y San Francisco, CA 94143-0610 Email: pattwkw@msn.com	Larson (1987)	Identifies nurse-caring behaviors	Q-Sort	*n* = 57 oncology nurses *n* = 57 oncology patients	See Larson (1984)	See Larson (1984)	See Larson (1984)
CARE-Q Replication study and use	D. Mayer, PhD, RN Clinical Specialist Massachusetts General Hospital	Mayer (1987)	Evaluate nurse-caring behaviors	Q-Sort	*n* = 28 oncology nurses *n* = 54 oncology patients	Content and face validity Test-retest reliability (refers to Larson, 1984, original testing)	Replication of instrument plus extension of conceptual foundation of original Larson version of CARE-Q	See Larson (1984)
CARE-Q	Nori Komorita, PhD, RN; Kathleen Doehring, MS, RN; and Phyllis Hirchert, MS, RN Urbana Regional Program College of Nursing University of Illinois, Urbana	Komorita et al. (1991)	Nurse educators' perceptions of caring behaviors	Q-Sort	*N* = 110 nurse educators	Refers to Larson's (1984) original work	Caring in relation to nursing education No new reliability or validity reported for nursing educational use	See Larson (1984)

Instrument	Author/Contact	Citation	Purpose	Type	Sample	Reliability/Validity	Conceptual Basis	References
CARE-Q	Antonia Mangold, MSN, RN Oncology Clinical Staff Nurse Thomas Jefferson University Hospital Philadelphia, PA	Mangold (1991)	Identifies and compares nursing students' and RNs' perceptions of caring behaviors	Q-Sort	N = 30 nursing students	See Larson (1984) Original citation for test-retest reliability	Larson's original conceptual basis Informed by Watson's 10 carative factors	See Larson (1984)
CARE-Q Original	—	—	—	—	—	—	—	Hulela, Seboni, and Akinsola (2000); Gardner et al. (2001)
CARE-Q	Louise von Essen, MS, and Per-Olow Sjödén, PhD Center for Caring Sciences Uppsala University Akademiska Hospital S-751 85 Uppsala, Sweden Email: Louise-von.essen@ccs.uu.se	von Essen and Sjödén (1991a)	Perceived caring behaviors by nurses and patients	Q-Sort International Swedish version	n = 81 oncology, general surgery, and orthopedic patients n = 105 nurses	No reliability or validity reported for Swedish version Refers to information reported by Larson (1981, 1984)	Affective components of care and a caring relationship	Chang, Lin, Chang, and Lin (2005); Larsson, Peterson, Lampic, von Essen, and Sjödén (1998)

(continued)

TABLE 4.2 Matrix of Caring Assessment Instruments (*continued*)

INSTRUMENT	AUTHOR CONTACT INFORMATION	PUBLICATION SOURCE	DEVELOPED TO MEASURE	INSTRUMENT DESCRIPTION	PARTICIPANTS	REPORTED VALIDITY/ RELIABILITY	CONCEPTUAL-THEORETICAL BASIS OF MEASUREMENT	LATEST CITATION IN NURSING LITERATURE
CARE-Q	Louise von Essen, MS, and PhD, Per-Olow Sjödén, PhD Center for Caring Sciences Uppsala University Akademiska Hospital S-751 85 Uppsala, Sweden Email: Louise-von.essen@ ccs.uu.se	von Essen and Sjödén (1991b)	Perceived caring behaviors by nurses and patients (Swedish population)	International version Q-Sort of same items of 7-point scale (Swedish version) Replication of 1991 study Questionnaires with items of Q-Sort	n = 73 nurses n = 86 medical patients	See von Essen and Sjödén (1991a)		Larsson et al. (1998)
CARE-Q	Kathryn Rosenthal, MS, RN University of Colorado	Rosenthal (1992)	Examines the relationship of patient-perceived and nurse-perceived caring behaviors	Q-Sort	n = 30 coronary nurses n = 30 coronary patients	See Larson (1984, 1987)	General nursing caring literature (Larson, 1984, 1987, for tool) Watson et al. included in background of study	None to date

Tool	Author	Citation	Purpose	Description	Sample	Reliability/Validity	Theoretical Framework
CARE-Q	Louise von Essen, MS, and Per-Olow Sjödén, PhD Center for Caring Sciences Uppsala University Akademiska Hospital S-751 85 Uppsala, Sweden Email: Louise-von-essen@ccs.uu.se	von Essen and Sjödén (1993)	Nurse-caring behaviors as perceived by psychiatric patients compared with somatically ill patients	Q-Sort Comparative study with different patient populations International Swedish version of tool Modified for psychiatric patients (Used free response format)	$n = 63$ psychiatric nurses, RNs, and students $n = 61$ mental health patients	Discussion of difficulty with Q-Sort Found to be unreliable due to forced distribution Discusses internal consistency using a free response format	General nursing caring literature (Larson, 1984, 1987, for tool) Watson et al. included in background of study Perception of caring relationship and caring behaviors
CARE-Q	Margaret K. Smith, MSN, RN Assistant Nurse Manager Nursing Home Care Unit VA Palo Alto Health Care System Menlo Park, CA	Smith and Sullivan (1997)	Compare rankings of caring behaviors as perceived by patients and nurses	50 items with six subscales Q-Sort	$n = 12$ men and 2 women patients $n = 15$ RNs from a nursing home care unit at Veterans Affairs Medical Center	Content validity addressed Reliability and validity not addressed	No theoretical/conceptual model mentioned

Larsson et al. (1998)

(continued)

TABLE 4.2 Matrix of Caring Assessment Instruments (*continued*)

INSTRUMENT	AUTHOR CONTACT INFORMATION	PUBLICATION SOURCE	DEVELOPED TO MEASURE	INSTRUMENT DESCRIPTION	PARTICIPANTS	REPORTED VALIDITY/ RELIABILITY	CONCEPTUAL-THEORETICAL BASIS OF MEASUREMENT	LATEST CITATION IN NURSING LITERATURE
CARE/SAT Questionnaire (1993)	Patricia Larson, DNS, RN, and Sandra Ferketick, PhD, RN College of Nursing University of Arizona, Tucson, AZ	Larson and Ferketich (1993)	Patient satisfaction with nursing care	Descriptive correlational study Visual analog scale adapted from CARE-Q; 29 items	$n = 268$ patients	Cronbach's alpha Construct and concurrent validity reported Factor analysis = 3 factors to account for variance	Caring Behaviors Original	Manojlovich (2005)
Modified CARE-Q (2006)	Mei-Hua Lee, P. Larson, and W. L. Holzemer Mei-Hua Lee 8250 Hardester Drive Sacramento, CA 95828 Email: mefalee@yahoo .com	Lee et al. (2006)	Modified for Chinese nurses in Taiwan	Adapted from original CARE-Q into a 7-point Likert scale	$n = 770$ nurses	Test-retest reliability .0803 between Chinese version and original English version Internal consistency coefficient alpha .97 for total modified CARE-Q; .82–.92 subscales	Original work of Larson, with adaptation. Also available in Chinese version upon request	Lee et al. (2006)

A Chinese version of the Modified CARE-Q is available from the tool authors.

medical-surgical patients ready for discharge within 48 hours. Cronbach's alpha for the total scale was reported as 0.94. The authors reported a Pearson's correlation coefficient of $r = 0.80$ between the CARE/SAT and the Risser Patient Questionnaire (Hinshaw & Atwood, 1982). This correlation provided evidence of construct validity.

Limited use of this instrument has occurred to date due to difficulties related to a mix of negatively and positively worded statements. Each patient is asked to place an X on a 100-mm visual analog line to indicate his or her degree of agreement or disagreement. Because the behaviors are worded both positively and negatively, it has been reported to be difficult and tedious to analyze, which also suggests that the total scores are unreliable for use in a correlation design study (Andrews et al., 1996). This instrument is in its first generation of development and use. However, Andrews and associates reported in 1996 that the CARE/SAT had one of the shortest mean times to complete (6 minutes) and the instrument specifically addresses caring actions and perceives caring as a therapeutic intervention.

MODIFIED CARE-Q

The Modified CARE-Q (Holroyd, Yue-kuen, Sau-wai, Fung-shan, & Wai-wan, 1998) is a new addition to this edition and illustrates the continued use and refinement of the original CARE-Q scale. It is based on the CARE-Q, but instead of using a Q-methodology approach, it utilizes a 7-point Likert scale, which is designed to measure the perceived frequency with which nurses are able to perform caring behaviors while providing care. Response categories for each item are never (1), almost never (2), rarely (3), sometimes (4), usually (5), almost always (6), and always (7). Internal consistency, reliability, and factor analysis were conducted with 770 nurses from 65 inpatient units at a medical center in Taiwan. The English version of the Modified CARE-Q was translated into Chinese; the accuracy of meaning for the 50 items was rated at 96% by five bilingual nurses (Lee et al., 2006). The modified CARE-Q is more user friendly, with increased variability of responses, and results are easier to analyze. Further testing with both nurses and patients in other settings is needed; there is also a need to address the consequences of caring, such as patients' satisfaction with care, nurses' job satisfaction, and the relationship between perceptions of experiencing caring and varied healthcare outcomes.

TOOL 4.1

CARE-Q and CARE/SAT[a]

DIRECTIONS
THE NURSE-CARING BEHAVIOR STUDY

To participate in the study you will be required to sort cards containing statements about nurse-caring behaviors, ranking them from most important to least important. See the enclosed directions for the specific details. This will require about 45 to 60 minutes of your time. When you have completed this first phase of the study and mailed it to me (no postage is required) within 30 days, I will mail a second CARE-Q (the retest) and have you do the sort again. Individual responses will be kept confidential and every effort will be made to protect your anonymity. Your participation indicates your consent.

> *The purpose of the Nurse-Caring Behavior Study is to identify the nurse-caring behaviors that are perceived as important in making patients feel cared for.*

The Caring Assessment Report Evaluation Q-Sort (CARE-Q) packet contains seven pockets, each labeled with a number (1, 4, 10, 20, 10, 4, 1). Included in the packet are a deck of 50 cards, each with a different caring nurse behavior typed on it.

To identify the nurse-caring behaviors that are perceived as most important, sort the deck of 50 cards from most important to least important, placing each card into one of the pockets—on a range of most important to least important.

It is essential that only the designated number of cards be placed in each pocket, with the numbers (1, 4, 10, 20, etc.) on the pocket indicating the number of cards which can be placed in each pocket. When you have completed the sorting, please count the number of cards in each pocket to make sure that the right number of cards is in each pocket.

Please answer the questions on the Nurse Demographic Information Sheet.

When you have completed the study, place the seven pockets containing the sorted cards and the Nurse Demographic Sheet into the enclosed envelope and mail. No postage is required.

Thank you so much for your help.

(Below is an example of how to place the pockets to aid in the sorting. They are placed from your left to your right.)

1	**4**	**10**	**20**	**10**	**4**	**1**
Most Important	Fairly Important	Somewhat Important	Neither Important or Unimportant	Somewhat Unimportant	Unimportant	Not Important

[a]© Dr. Patricia Lawson. Reprinted with permission of author.

TOOL 4.2

Caring Satisfaction (CARE/SAT)[a]

THE PURPOSE OF THIS QUESTIONNAIRE IS TO HAVE PATIENTS ASSESS THEIR NURSING CARE. YOUR IMPRESSIONS, ALONG WITH THOSE OF OTHER PATIENTS, WILL HELP NURSES IN DECIDING WAYS TO IMPROVE PATIENT CARE.

EACH STATEMENT REFERS TO A SPECIFIC NURSING ACTION. BASED ON YOUR EXPERIENCE, DECIDE HOW MUCH YOU AGREE OR DISAGREE WITH THE VIEW EXPRESSED. ON THE LINE NEXT TO THE STATEMENT PLACE AN "X" AT THE POINT ALONG THE LINE THAT BEST DESCRIBES HOW MUCH YOU AGREE OR DISAGREE WITH THE STATEMENT. THERE ARE NO RIGHT OR WRONG ANSWERS. YOUR RESPONSE IS A MATTER OF YOUR PERSONAL OPINION. YOUR INDIVIDUAL RESPONSE WILL NOT BE SHARED WITH ANYONE. ONLY GROUP DATA WILL BE REPORTED.

BELOW ARE EXAMPLES WHICH MAY HELP YOU IN RESPONDING TO THE QUESTIONNAIRE.

A. DURING MY HOSPITAL STAY THE NURSES ON THE UNIT:

TAUGHT ME HOW TO TAKE
MY TEMPERATURE.

          X
_____
STRONGLY   STRONGLY
DISAGREE   AGREE

THE PLACEMENT OF THE "X" ON THE LINE FOR QUESTION A INDICATES THAT YOU DISAGREE BUT NOT TOTALLY, THAT THE NURSES TAUGHT YOU HOW TO TAKE YOUR TEMPERATURE.

B. DURING MY HOSPITAL STAY THE NURSES ON THE UNIT:

DID NOT GIVE MY BATH ON TIME.

                          X
_____
STRONGLY   STRONGLY
DISAGREE   AGREE

THE PLACEMENT OF THE "X" FOR QUESTION B IS AN EXAMPLE OF WHERE YOU CANNOT QUITE DECIDE IF YOU AGREE OR DISAGREE BECAUSE AT TIMES YOUR BATH WAS ON TIME AND AT OTHER TIMES IT WAS NOT.

PLACE AN "X" AT THE POINT ON THE LINE THAT BEST DESCRIBES HOW MUCH YOU AGREE OR DISAGREE WITH EACH STATEMENT.

DURING THE PAST WEEK THE NURSES:

1. TOLD ME OF SUPPORT SYSTEMS
   AVAILABLE TO ME, SUCH AS
   SELF-HELP GROUPS.

_____
STRONGLY   STRONGLY
DISAGREE   AGREE

2. PROVIDED BASIC COMFORT
   MEASURES, SUCH AS APPROPRIATE
   LIGHTING, CONTROL OF NOISE,
   BLANKETS, ETC.

_____
STRONGLY   STRONGLY
DISAGREE   AGREE

(continued)

TOOL 4.2

Caring Satisfaction (CARE/SAT) (*continued*)

3. ENCOURAGED ME TO CALL IF I HAD ANY PROBLEMS.

STRONGLY DISAGREE   STRONGLY AGREE

4. DID NOT GIVE A QUICK RESPONSE TO MY CALL.

STRONGLY DISAGREE   STRONGLY AGREE

5. MADE ME FEEL DUMB BY GIVING ME INADEQUATE INFORMATION.

STRONGLY DISAGREE   STRONGLY AGREE

6. DID NOT WANT TO TALK ABOUT MY FEELINGS ABOUT MY DISEASE AND TREATMENT.

STRONGLY DISAGREE   STRONGLY AGREE

7. APPEARED BUSY AND UPSET.

STRONGLY DISAGREE   STRONGLY AGREE

8. KNEW WHEN TO CALL THE DOCTOR.

STRONGLY DISAGREE   STRONGLY AGREE

9. CREATED A SENSE OF TRUST FOR ME AND MY FAMILY.

STRONGLY DISAGREE   STRONGLY AGREE

10. PROVIDED ENCOURAGEMENT BY IDENTIFYING THE POSITIVE ASPECTS RELATED TO MY CONDITION AND TREATMENT.

STRONGLY DISAGREE   STRONGLY AGREE

(continued)

TOOL 4.2
Caring Satisfaction (CARE/SAT) (*continued*)

11. DID NOT TEACH ME HOW TO CARE FOR MYSELF.

STRONGLY DISAGREE   STRONGLY AGREE

12. ANTICIPATED MY FAMILY'S AND MY SHOCK OVER MY DIAGNOSIS AND PLANNED OPPORTUNITIES, INDIVIDUALLY OR AS A GROUP, TO TALK ABOUT IT.

STRONGLY DISAGREE   STRONGLY AGREE

13. PUT ME FIRST, NO MATTER WHAT ELSE HAPPENED.

STRONGLY DISAGREE   STRONGLY AGREE

14. DID NOT MAKE SURE OTHERS KNEW HOW TO CARE FOR ME.

STRONGLY DISAGREE   STRONGLY AGREE

15. GAVE ME GOOD PHYSICAL CARE.

STRONGLY DISAGREE   STRONGLY AGREE

16. DID NOT HELP ME FIGURE OUT QUESTIONS FOR ME TO ASK MY DOCTOR.

STRONGLY DISAGREE   STRONGLY AGREE

17. VOLUNTEERED TO DO "LITTLE" THINGS SUCH AS BRINGING ME A CUP OF COFFEE, PAPER, ETC.

STRONGLY DISAGREE   STRONGLY AGREE

18. DID *NOT* KNOW MY NEEDS WITHOUT ME HAVING TO ASK.

STRONGLY DISAGREE   STRONGLY AGREE

(*continued*)

TOOL 4.2

Caring Satisfaction (CARE/SAT) (*continued*)

19. EXPLAINED THINGS IMPORTANT TO MY CARE.

STRONGLY DISAGREE   STRONGLY AGREE

20. CHECKED ON ME FREQUENTLY.

STRONGLY DISAGREE   STRONGLY AGREE

21. DID NOT GIVE MY MEDICATIONS OR TREATMENTS ON TIME.

STRONGLY DISAGREE   STRONGLY AGREE

22. ENCOURAGED ME TO ASK ANY QUESTIONS I MIGHT HAVE.

STRONGLY DISAGREE   STRONGLY AGREE

23. WERE PROFESSIONAL IN APPEARANCE.

STRONGLY DISAGREE   STRONGLY AGREE

24. KNEW HOW TO GIVE SHOTS, I.V.s, ETC., AND HOW TO MANAGE THE EQUIPMENT LIKE THE I.V.s, SUCTION MACHINES.

STRONGLY DISAGREE   STRONGLY AGREE

25. WERE DISORGANIZED.

STRONGLY DISAGREE   STRONGLY AGREE

26. WERE INCONSISTENT IN HOW THEY TREATED ME.

STRONGLY DISAGREE   STRONGLY AGREE

(*continued*)

TOOL 4.2

Caring Satisfaction (CARE/SAT) *(continued)*

27. DID NOT SEEM TO KNOW ME AS A
    PERSON.

    STRONGLY   STRONGLY
    DISAGREE   AGREE

28. CHECKED WITH ME AS TO THE BEST
    TIME TO TALK ABOUT CHANGES IN
    MY CONDITION.

    STRONGLY   STRONGLY
    DISAGREE   AGREE

29. HELPED ME TO CLARIFY MY
    THINKING IN REGARD TO MY
    DISEASE AND TREATMENTS.

    STRONGLY   STRONGLY
    DISAGREE   AGREE

[a]© Dr. Patricia Lawson. Reprinted with permission of author.

REFERENCES

Andrews, L. W., Daniels, P., & Hall, A. G. (1996). Nurse caring behaviors: Comparing five tools to define perceptions. *Ostomy/Wound Management, 42*(5), 28–37. doi:10.1111/j.1745-7599.2004.b00451.x

Beck, C. T. (1999). Quantitative measurement of caring. *Journal of Advanced Nursing, 30*(1), 24–32. doi:10.1046/j.1365-2648.1999.01045.x

Chang, Y., Lin, Y., Chang, H., & Lin, C. (2005). Cancer patient and staff ratings of caring behaviors: Relationship to level of pain intensity. *Cancer Nursing, 28*(5), 331–319. doi:10.1097/00002820-200509000-00001

Gardner, A., Goodsell, J., Duggan, T., Murtha, B., Peck, C., & Williams, J. (2001). "Don't call me Sweetie!" Patients differ from nurses in their perceptions of caring. *Collegian, 8*(3), 32–38. doi:10.1016/S1322-7696(08)60020-7

Hinshaw, A., & Atwood, J. (1982). A patient satisfaction instrument: Precision by replication. *Nursing Research, 31*, 170–175. doi:10.1097/00006199-198205000-00011

Holroyd, E., Yue-kuen, C., Sau-wai, C., Fung-shan, L., & Wai-wan, W. (1998). A Chinese cultural perspective of nursing care behaviors in an acute setting. *Journal of Advanced Nursing, 28*(6), 1289–1294. doi:10.1046/j.1365-2648.1998.00849.x

Hulela, E. B., Seboni, N. M., & Akinsola, H. A. (2000). The perception of acutely ill patients about the caring behaviors of nurses in Botswana. *West African Journal of Nursing, 11*(2), 24–30.

Komorita, N., Doehring, K., & Hirchert, P. (1991). Perceptions of caring by nurse educators. *Journal of Nursing Education, 30*(1), 23–29.

Kyle, T. V. (1995). The concept of caring: A review of the literature. *Journal of Advanced Nursing, 21*, 506–514. doi:10.1111/j.1365-2648.1995.tb02734.x

Larson, P. (1981). Oncology patients' and professional nurses' perceptions of important nurse caring behaviors. *Dissertation Abstracts International, 42*(3), 0528B. (UMI No. 8116511)

Larson, P. (1984). Important nurse caring behaviors perceived by patients with cancer. *Oncology Nursing Forum, 11*(6), 46–50.

Larson, P. (1986). Cancer nurses' perceptions of caring. *Cancer Nursing, 9*(2), 86–91.

Larson, P. (1987). Comparison of cancer patients' & professional nurses' perceptions of important nurse caring behaviors. *Heart and Lung, 16*(2), 187–193.

Larson, P., & Ferketich, S. (1993). Patients' satisfaction with nurses' caring during hospitalization. *Western Journal of Nursing Research, 15*(6), 690–707. doi:10.1177/019394599301500603

Larsson, G., Peterson, V. W., Lampic, C., von Essen, L., & Sjödén, P. (1998). Cancer patient and staff ratings of the importance of caring behaviors and their relations to patient anxiety and depression. *Journal of Advanced Nursing, 27*, 855–864. doi:10.1046/j.1365-2648.1998.00583.x

Lee, M. H., Larson, P. J., & Holzemer, W. L. (2006). Psychometric evaluation of the modified CARE-Q among Chinese nurses in Taiwan. *International Journal for Human Caring, 10*(4), 8–13. doi:10.20467/1091-5710.10.4.8

Mangold, A. (1991). Senior nursing students' & professional nurses' perceptions of effective caring behaviors: A comparative study. *Journal of Nursing Education, 30*(3), 134–139.

Manojlovich, M. (2005). The effect of nursing leadership on hospital nurses' professional practice behaviors. *Journal of Nursing Administration, 35*(7/8), 366–374. doi:10.1097/00005110-200507000-00009

Mayer, D. (1987). Oncology nurses' vs cancer patients' perceptions of nurse caring behaviors: A replication study. *Oncology Nursing Forum, 14*(3), 48–52.

Rosenthal, K. (1992). Coronary care patients' and nurses' perceptions of important nurse caring behaviors. *Heart and Lung, 21*(6), 536–539.

Smith, M., & Sullivan, J. M. (1997). Nurses' and patients' perceptions of most important caring behaviors in a long-term care setting. *Geriatric Nursing, 18*(2), 70–73. doi:10.1016/s0197-4572(97)90060-4

von Essen, L., & Sjödén, P. (1991a). The importance of nurse caring behaviors as perceived by Swedish hospital patients and nursing staff. *International Journal of Nursing Studies, 28*(3), 267–281. doi:10.1016/0020-7489(91)90020-4

von Essen, L., & Sjödén, P. (1991b). Patient & staff perceptions of caring: Review and replication. *Journal of Advanced Nursing, 16*(11), 1363–1374. doi:10.1111/j.1365-2648.1991.tb01566.x

von Essen, L., & Sjödén, P. (1993). Perceived importance of caring behaviors to Swedish psychiatric inpatients and staff, with comparisons to somatically-ill samples. *Research in Nursing and Health, 16*, 293–303. doi:10.1002/nur.4770160408

Widmark-Petersson, V., von Essen, L., Lindman, E., & Sjoden, P. (1996). Cancer patient and staff perceptions of caring vs clinical care. *Scandinavian Journal of Caring Sciences, 10*(4), 227–233.

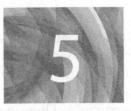

5

Caring Behaviors Inventory and Caring Behaviors Inventory for Elders

Zane Robinson Wolf

CARING BEHAVIORS INVENTORY

The Caring Behaviors Inventory (CBI), developed by Wolf and colleagues (Wolf, 1981, 1986; Wolf, Dillon, Townsend, & Glasofer, 2017; Wolf, Giardino, Osborne, & Ambrose, 1994), was the second empirical measurement instrument of caring to be reported in the nursing literature (following Larson's publication of the CARE-Q). The conceptual and theoretical basis was derived from caring literature, in general, and Watson's (1985, 1988) Transpersonal Caring Theory, in particular. The conceptual definition reported nurse caring as an "interactive and inter-subjective process that occurs during moments of shared vulnerability between nurse and patient, and that is both both-and other-directed" (Wolf et al., 1994, p. 107).

The first version of the CBI was a Likert-scaled instrument with total scores ranging from 42 to 168. Subjects are asked to rate caring words and phrases on a 4-point scale: 1 = strongly disagree; 2 = disagree; 3 = agree; 4 = strongly agree. The instrument was originally developed with 75 items, and was later revised through psychometric processes, resulting in 43 items and finally 42 (Beck, 1999; Kyle, 1995; Wolf et al., 1994).

At first, the CBI's 43 items were tested on 541 subjects: 278 nursing staff and 263 patients. The internal consistency reliability was reported as .96 (Wolf et al., 1994). The highest ranked caring behavior phrase was identified as "attentive listening," comparable with findings in studies using the CARE-Q instrument (Kyle, 1995). One item did not load during exploratory factor analysis and was eliminated from the CBI.

There are five correlated subscales within the 42-item version of the CBI: respectful deference to the other; assurance of human presence; positive connectedness; professional knowledge and skill; and attentiveness to the other's experience. Each of the five subscales had a Cronbach's alpha range of .81 (attentiveness to the other's experience) to .92 (assurance of human presence; Wolf et al., 1994).

After the 1994 study, the Likert scale of the CBI was revised immediately. The second version uses a 6-point scale: 1 = never; 2 = almost never; 3 = occasionally; 4 = usually; 5 = almost always; 6 = always. Later, overall internal consistency reliability coefficients for the CBI were reported, $\alpha = .98$ for previously hospitalized adults ($N = 335$) and $\alpha = .95$ for hospitalized interventional cardiac patients ($N = 73$; Wolf et al., 1998; Wolf, Miller, & Devine, 2003). Cronbach's alpha coefficient was also reported on patient-perceived nurse caring ($\alpha = .98$; Larrabee et al., 2004). Additional internal reliability coefficients have been reported by other authors; for example, in the study in a cancer hospital, the alpha was .96 for the CBI-24 (Keeley, Wolf, Regul, & Jadwin, 2015), a reduced-item version (Wu, Larrabee, & Putnam, 2006).

Factorial validity has been established sequentially (Wolf et al., 1994, 2017; Wu et al., 2006). The latest version of the instrument, CBI-16, was tested on adult, hospitalized patients ($N = 303$). Principal components analysis revealed that a 1-factor solution had merit as a result of item-reduction methods. Other types of construct validity, including convergent and known groups, have been tested.

The CBI is one of the earliest to be developed with clarity of conceptual–theoretical basis, along with ongoing testing and refinement of the instrument. It is one of the few instruments in caring that provides supporting evidence for empirical validation of Watson's Transpersonal Caring Theory. The instrument has been reported to be among those with the shortest length of time; it has consistent language, with easy to understand instructions, and easy to analyze results, which have been used in descriptive, correlational, cross-sectional, predictive, comparative descriptive, and mixed methods design studies. A total score is calculated by summing item responses. Some studies have tested the effect of a caring protocol (Wolf, Bailey, & Keeley, 2014) on patient satisfaction and measured perceived caring of patients immediately before their discharge from a cancer hospital in a program evaluation study (Wolf, Keeley, Regul, Cobb, & Jadwin, 2016). See Table 5.1 for examples of studies in which the CBI was administered.

The CBI has been described as useful in determining perceptions of nurse caring in patients and nurses in hospitals (Andrews, Daniels, & Hall, 1996) and nurse practitioners. Versions have also been completed by nursing students (Murphy, Jones, Edwards, James, & Mayer, 2009). Alternate scoring, using composite means, has been used in some studies (Wu et al., 2006). Wu et al. (2006) tested the CBI with the intent of deriving a shorter CBI. They administered the CBI-42 to hospitalized patients ($N = 362$) and registered nurses ($N = 90$). In the same study, the factor structure of the CBI-24 was tested using patients' responses. Four subscales were identified: assurance, knowledge and skill, respectful, and connectedness. The newest English version of the instrument, CBI-16 (Figure 5.1),

TABLE 5.1 Caring Behaviors Inventory: Selected Studies

CITATION	CONCEPTUAL–THEORETICAL BASIS IN CARING	SCALING	RELIABILITY	VALIDITY	PARTICIPANTS
Wolf (1986)	Strongly informed by Watson's theory (1988); refers to transpersonal and 10 carative factors; attitudes and actions	Phrases 4-point Likert scale		Content validity: literature sources, theoretical	N = 108 nurses N = 43 patients
Wolf et al. (1994)	Watson's theory, transpersonal dimensions	4-point Likert (suggested to use 6-point Likert scale; scale modified)	Test–retest reliability = .96	Content (expert) and construct validity (factor analysis 5 factors; 42 items)	N = 278 nurses N = 263 patients
Plowden (1997)	General Systems Theory	42-item CBI with 6-point scale		Construct validity factorial	N = 43 patients N = 108 nurses
Swan (1998)	Donabedian Quality Care Model	42-item CBI with 6-point scale	Cronbach's alpha = .96		N = 100 ambulatory surgical adult patients
Coogan (1998)		42-item CBI with 6-point Likert scale	Cronbach's alpha = .94		N = 104 perioperative nurses

(continued)

TABLE 5.1 Caring Behaviors Inventory: Selected Studies (*continued*)

CITATION	CONCEPTUAL–THEORETICAL BASIS IN CARING	SCALING	RELIABILITY	VALIDITY	PARTICIPANTS
Wolf et al. (1998)	Watson's Transpersonal Caring Theory	42-item CBI with 6-point Likert scale	Overall Cronbach's alpha = .98; reading level reported at 5.9 and reading ease at 60.7		N = 335 adult patients
Brunton and Beaman (2000)	Caring concept of nurse practitioners in primary care				N = 140 nurse practitioners
Green and Davis (2002)	Watson's Theory of Caring, Dunphy's satisfaction model	42-item CBI with 6-point Likert scale	Cronbach's alpha = .95		N = 817 patients, 30 nurse practitioners selected patients
Wolf et al. (2003)	Watson's Transpersonal Caring Theory	42-item CBI with 6-point Likert scale	Overall Cronbach's alpha = .95		N = 73 adult patients cardiac
Coulombe, Yeakel, Maljanian, and Bohannon (2002)	Nurse caring behavior	6-item CBI with 6-point Likert scale	Cronbach's alpha for 6 items = .89		N = 316 patients
Yeakel, Maljanian, Bohannon, and Coulombe (2003)		6-item CBI with 6-point Likert scale	Cronbach's alpha for 6 items = .86		Preintervention N = 172, postintervention N = 181

Author (Year)	Theory/Model	Instrument	Reliability	Validity	Sample
Larrabee et al. (2004)	Nursing Systems Outcomes Research (NSOR) model (Mark, Sayler, & Smith, 1996)	CBI-42	Cronbach's alpha for 42 items = .98		$N = 360$ hospitalized patients
Green (2004)			Cronbach's alpha for 42 items = .94	Construct validity, known groups	$N = 348$ nurse practitioners
Wu et al. (2006)		CBI-42 and CBI-24 6-point scale	Cronbach's alpha for 24 items = .96 patients, .95 ($N = 64$); .96 nurses ($N = 42$) Test–retest reliability $r = .88$ patients ($N = 64$); $r = .82$ nurses ($N = 42$)	Four-factor solution; Construct validity, convergent	$N = 362$ patients
Rafii, Hajinezhad, and Haghani (2007)	Watson Human Caring Theory; Donabedian: structure, process, outcome	CBI-42 Persian alpha = .97			$N = 250$ patients
Hayes and Tyler-Ball (2007)		CBI-42 with 6-point Likert scale	Cronbach's alpha = .985	Construct validity, convergent	$N = 70$ patients

(continued)

TABLE 5.1 Caring Behaviors Inventory: Selected Studies *(continued)*

CITATION	CONCEPTUAL–THEORETICAL BASIS IN CARING	SCALING	RELIABILITY	VALIDITY	PARTICIPANTS
Murphy et al. (2009)	Caring and nurse education literature Nursing curriculum over 3 years	CBI-42 with 4-point Likert scale (1 = strongly disagree, 2 = disagree, 3 = agree, 4 = strongly agree)		Construct validity, known groups (implied)	N = 80 first year students N = 94 third year students
Mlinar (2010)	Nursing education program Relational caring behaviors	CBI-42 with 4-point scale			N = 117 first year students N = 49 third year students
Palese et al. (2011)	Perceived caring and outcomes	CBI-24 Cyprus, Czech Republic, Greece, Finland, Hungary, Italy	Cronbach's alpha = .96 (pooled). (.87 = .97 for countries)		N = 1,565 patients
Papastavrou, Efstathiou, et al. (2011)		Cyprus, Czech Republic, Finland, Greece, Hungary, Italy CBI-24 translated into language of countries 6-point scale	Cronbach's alpha pooled = .94 Patients α = .87–.97 Nurses α = .94–.97		N = 1,659 patients N = 1,195 nurses
Papastavrou, Karlou, et al. (2011)		CBI-GR 24	Cronbach's alpha = .92	Construct validity, factorial	N = 245 Greek & Cypriot nurses

Study	Theory/Purpose	Instrument	Validity/Reliability	Sample
Palese et al. (2011)	Watson's Transpersonal Caring Theory (1985)	Czech Republic, Cyprus, Finland, Greece, Hungary, Italy; CBI-24; 6-point Likert scale		N = 1,565 patients
Papastavrou et al. (2012)	Perceptions of respect, human presence, and caring behaviors	Czech Republic, Cyprus, Finland, Greece, Hungary, Italy; CBI-24; 6-point Likert scale	Patients' Cronbach's alpha = .96; Nurses' Cronbach's alpha = .94	N = 1,537 patients; N = 1,148 nurses
Merrill, Hayes, Clukey, and Curtis (2012)		CBI-42; 6-point scale	Cronbach's alpha = .974; Construct validity, factorial and known groups	N = 103 patients
Patiraki et al. (2014)	Patient and nurse characteristics in relation to their perceptions of care	CBI-24 with 6-point scale	Patients' Cronbach's alpha = .96; Nurses' Cronbach's alpha = .94	N = 1,659 patients; N = 1,195 nurses
Porter, Cortese, Vezina, and Fitzpatrick (2014)	Professional practice model implementation and nurse caring behaviors	CBI-24 with 6-point scale		Nurses = 538

(continued)

TABLE 5.1 Caring Behaviors Inventory: Selected Studies (*continued*)

CITATION	CONCEPTUAL–THEORETICAL BASIS IN CARING	SCALING	RELIABILITY	VALIDITY	PARTICIPANTS
Labraque et al. (2015)	Watson's Theory of Human Caring (2002)	CBI-24 English version or language of country with 6-point scale	Overall Cronbach's alpha = .96	Content validity, expert for translated versions	*N* = 467 student nurses
Bucco (2015)	Watson's Theory of Human Caring	CBI-24 Nurse version and Patient version	Cronbach's alpha = .94		*N* = 86 nurses *N* = 86 patients
Chana, Kennedy, and Chessell (2015)	Structural factors (work-related stressors), individual factors (personal resources), transactional factors (coping responses), nurse outcomes (burnout, anxiety and depression, caring behaviors)	CBI-42 with 6-point scale			*N* = 102 nursing staff
Loke, Lee, Lee, and Noor (2015)	Pre-registration nursing education curriculum Instrumental and expressive caring	CBI-42 with 4-point Likert scale	Cronbach's alpha = .922		*N* = 240 first year students *N* = 417 fourth year students *N* = 55 nurse lecturers *N* = 33 nurses

Author (Year)	Theory/Framework	Instrument	Reliability	Validity	Sample
Edvardsson et al. (2015)		CBI-6	Cronbach's alpha = .89	Construct validity, factorial	N = 210 patients
Nantz and Hines (2015)	Watson's Theory of Human Caring	CBI-24 with 6-point scale			N = 9 family members
Sarafis et al. (2016)	Occupational stress caring behaviors, quality of life	Greek Version Caring Behaviors Inventory (CBI-GR) 24 items			N = 246 nurses
Boiman (2017)	Experiential learning (Kolb, 1984), transformative adult learning theories (Mezirow, 1990), theory of transpersonal caring (Watson, 2008)	CBI-24 with 6-point scale	Cronbach's alpha = .94		N = 65 students
Wolf et al. (2017)	Watson	CBI-24R CBI-16 6-point scale	Cronbach's alpha = .97 for CBI-24R Cronbach's alpha = .95 CBI-16	Construct validity, factorial, contrasted groups, discriminant, convergent reported	N = 303 patients

Source: From Poirier, P., & Sossong, A. (2010). Oncology patients' and nurses' perceptions of caring. Canadian Oncology Nursing Journal, 20(2), 62–65. doi:10.5737/1181912x2026265

available as a one-dimensional instrument, was tested with a patient sample (Wolf et al., 2017). The CBI has been shared with all nurses and others who have requested it. Examples of studies are found in the references and in Table 5.1.

Coulombe, Yeakel, Maljanian, and Bohannon (2002) tested the 42-item CBI to determine its completeness and to derive a shorter version. They identified six items to explain most of the variance in the CBI score ($N = 316$, $R = .979$, adjusted $R^2 = .958$, $\alpha = .893$); consequently, the CBI-6 was described. The Adult Primary Care Practices Caring Behaviors Inventory or CBI-5, a modification of the CBI-6, was used in a primary care practice study.

New and experienced investigators request and obtain the CBI-42 and the CBI-24. They complete a release form. The instrument has been shared with nurses in Australia, Cambodia (Khmer), Canada, Chile, China, Colombia, Cyprus, Czech Republic, Egypt, Estonia, India, Indonesia, Iran, Ireland, Israel, Italy, Japan, Malaysia, Mexico, Nepal, Nigeria, Pakistan, Philippines, Saudi Arabia, Singapore, Slovenia, South Korea, Sweden, Tanzania, Tunisia, Turkey, United Kingdom (England, Scotland), and the United States. Permission has been given to translate the CBI-42 or the CBI-24 and to change directions and minor wording of items. If a translation from English to another language is available, the email of the investigator involved in the translation may be sent to a researcher in the same country who requests the CBI. The CBI has been translated into various languages and back translated into English. An Excel spreadsheet tracks requestor details.

The author retains copyright of the CBI and requests that anyone wishing to use it contact her for permission, further advice, and follow-up testing. There is no charge for use. A release form is found in this chapter. Once the CBI is translated, researchers own the copyright.

Selected studies are found in a matrix whereby versions of the CBI have been administered (see Table 5.1).

TOOL 5.1

Caring Behaviors Inventory

Directions

Please read the list of items that describe nurse caring. For each item, please *circle* the answer that stands for the extent that a nurse or nurses made caring visible during your last hospitalization.

Remember, *you* are the patient.

1. Attentively listening to the patient.					
never	almost never	occasionally	usually	almost always	always
2. Giving instructions or teaching the patient.					
never	almost never	occasionally	usually	almost always	always

(continued)

TOOL 5.1

Caring Behaviors Inventory (*continued*)

3. Treating the patient as an individual.

| never | almost never | occasionally | usually | almost always | always |

4. Spending time with the patient.

| never | almost never | occasionally | usually | almost always | always |

5. Touching the patient to communicate caring.

| never | almost never | occasionally | usually | almost always | always |

6. Being hopeful for the patient.

| never | almost never | occasionally | usually | almost always | always |

7. Giving the patient information so that he or she can make a decision.

| never | almost never | occasionally | usually | almost always | always |

8. Showing respect for the patient.

| never | almost never | occasionally | usually | almost always | always |

9. Supporting the patient.

| never | almost never | occasionally | usually | almost always | always |

10. Calling the patient by his/her preferred name.

| never | almost never | occasionally | usually | almost always | always |

11. Being honest with the patient.

| never | almost never | occasionally | usually | almost always | always |

12. Trusting the patient.

| never | almost never | occasionally | usually | almost always | always |

13. Being empathetic or identifying with the patient.

| never | almost never | occasionally | usually | almost always | always |

14. Helping the patient grow.

| never | almost never | occasionally | usually | almost always | always |

15. Making the patient physically or emotionally comfortable.

| never | almost never | occasionally | usually | almost always | always |

16. Being sensitive to the patient.

| never | almost never | occasionally | usually | almost always | always |

(*continued*)

TOOL 5.1

Caring Behaviors Inventory (*continued*)

17. Being patient or tireless with the patient.

never	almost never	occasionally	usually	almost always	always

18. Helping the patient.

never	almost never	occasionally	usually	almost always	always

19. Knowing how to give shots, IVs, etc.

never	almost never	occasionally	usually	almost always	always

20. Being confident with the patient.

never	almost never	occasionally	usually	almost always	always

21. Using a soft, gentle voice with the patient.

never	almost never	occasionally	usually	almost always	always

22. Demonstrating professional knowledge and skill.

never	almost never	occasionally	usually	almost always	always

23. Watching over the patient.

never	almost never	occasionally	usually	almost always	always

24. Managing equipment skillfully.

never	almost never	occasionally	usually	almost always	always

25. Being cheerful with the patient.

never	almost never	occasionally	usually	almost always	always

26. Allowing the patient to express feelings about his or her disease and treatment.

never	almost never	occasionally	usually	almost always	always

27. Including the patient in planning his or her care.

never	almost never	occasionally	usually	almost always	always

28. Treating patient information confidentially.

never	almost never	occasionally	usually	almost always	always

29. Providing a reassuring presence.

never	almost never	occasionally	usually	almost always	always

(*continued*)

TOOL 5.1

Caring Behaviors Inventory (*continued*)

30. Returning to the patient voluntarily.

never	almost never	occasionally	usually	almost always	always

31. Talking with the patient.

never	almost never	occasionally	usually	almost always	always

32. Encouraging the patient to call if there are problems.

never	almost never	occasionally	usually	almost always	always

33. Meeting the patient's stated and unstated needs.

never	almost never	occasionally	usually	almost always	always

34. Responding quickly to the patient's call.

never	almost never	occasionally	usually	almost always	always

35. Appreciating the patient as a human being.

never	almost never	occasionally	usually	almost always	always

36. Helping to reduce the patient's pain.

never	almost never	occasionally	usually	almost always	always

37. Showing concern for the patient.

never	almost never	occasionally	usually	almost always	always

38. Giving the patient's treatments and medications on time.

never	almost never	occasionally	usually	almost always	always

39. Paying special attention to the patient during first time, as hospitalization, treatments.

never	almost never	occasionally	usually	almost always	always

40. Relieving the patient's symptoms.

never	almost never	occasionally	usually	almost always	always

41. Putting the patient first.

never	almost never	occasionally	usually	almost always	always

42. Giving good physical care.

never	almost never	occasionally	usually	almost always	always

Source: Wolf, Z.R., Giardino, E.R., Osborne, P.A., & Ambrose, M.S. (1994). Dimensions of nurse caring. *Image: Journal of Nursing Scholarship, 26*(2), 107–111. doi:10.1111/j.1547-5069.1994. tb00927.x

TOOL 5.2

Patients and Former Patients Form

Directions for Patients and Former Patients:

Please complete the following information. Kindly circle or write in your answer:

1. Sex: 1. female   2. male

2. Age: _____

3. Marital Status:
   1. Single
   2. Married
   3. Divorced
   4. Widowed
   5. Separated

4. Race:
   1. African American
   2. Asian
   3. Caucasian
   4. Hispanic
   5. Native American Indian
   6. Other, please specify _____

5. Educational Level:
   1. 1 to 8 grade
   2. 9 to 12 grade
   3. 1 to 2 years college
   4. 3 to 4 years college
   5. 5 years college and over

6. Highest degree earned _____

7. Type of hospital or healthcare setting where you were cared for by nurses:
   1. University hospital
   2. Community hospital
   3. Other, please specify _____

8. Number of admissions to hospital or other healthcare setting in the last 5 years _____

9. Reason for last admission or need for healthcare services of nurse _____

10. Number of days in hospital during the last admission _____

11. Unit where nurses cared for you:
    1. Intensive Care Unit
    2. Cardiac Care Unit
    3. Medical Unit
    4. Surgical Unit
    5. Other, please specify _____

TOOL 5.3

Caring Behaviors Inventory-24

Directions

Please read the list of items that describe nurse caring. For each item, please circle the answer that stands for the extent that a nurse or nurses made caring visible during your last hospitalization.

Remember, you are the patient.

1. Attentively listening to the patient.

| never | almost never | occasionally | usually | almost always | always |

2. Giving instructions or teaching the patient.

| never | almost never | occasionally | usually | almost always | always |

3. Treating the patient as an individual.

| never | almost never | occasionally | usually | almost always | always |

4. Spending time with the patient.

| never | almost never | occasionally | usually | almost always | always |

5. Supporting the patient.

| never | almost never | occasionally | usually | almost always | always |

6. Being empathetic or identifying with the patient.

| never | almost never | occasionally | usually | almost always | always |

7. Helping the patient grow.

| never | almost never | occasionally | usually | almost always | always |

8. Being patient or tireless with the patient.

| never | almost never | occasionally | usually | almost always | always |

9. Knowing how to give shots, IVs, etc.

| never | almost never | occasionally | usually | almost always | always |

10. Being confident with the patient.

| never | almost never | occasionally | usually | almost always | always |

11. Demonstrating professional knowledge and skill.

| never | almost never | occasionally | usually | almost always | always |

12. Managing equipment skillfully.

| never | almost never | occasionally | usually | almost always | always |

(continued)

TOOL 5.3

Caring Behaviors Inventory-24 (*continued*)

13. Allowing the patient to express feelings about his or her disease and treatment.

| never | almost never | occasionally | usually | almost always | always |

14. Including the patient in planning his or her care.

| never | almost never | occasionally | usually | almost always | always |

15. Treating patient information confidentially.

| never | almost never | occasionally | usually | almost always | always |

16. Returning to the patient voluntarily.

| never | almost never | occasionally | usually | almost always | always |

17. Talking with the patient.

| never | almost never | occasionally | usually | almost always | always |

18. Encouraging the patient to call if there are problems.

| never | almost never | occasionally | usually | almost always | always |

19. Meeting the patient's stated and unstated needs.

| never | almost never | occasionally | usually | almost always | always |

20. Responding quickly to the patient's call.

| never | almost never | occasionally | usually | almost always | always |

21. Helping to reduce the patient's pain.

| never | almost never | occasionally | usually | almost always | always |

22. Showing concern for the patient.

| never | almost never | occasionally | usually | almost always | always |

23. Giving the patient's treatments and medications on time.

| never | almost never | occasionally | usually | almost always | always |

24. Relieving the patient's symptoms.

| never | almost never | occasionally | usually | almost always | always |

Source: From Wu, Y., Larrabee, J. H., & Putman, H. P. (2006). Caring Behaviors Inventory: A reduction of the 42-item instrument. *Nursing Research, 55*(1), 18–25. doi:10.1097/00006199-200601000-00003. Copyright ©Zane Robinson Wolf. 1981, 1990, 1991, 10/91, 1/92, 3/92, 8/94, 12/95.

TOOL 5.4

Caring Behaviors Inventory-16 Revised

Directions: Please read the list of items that describe nurse caring. For each item, please *mark an X or circle* the answer that stands for the extent that a nurse or nurses demonstrated caring during your hospitalization.

1. Attentively listening to you.

| never | almost never | occasionally | usually | almost always | always |

2. Giving instructions or teaching you.

| never | almost never | occasionally | usually | almost always | always |

3. Treating you as an individual.

| never | almost never | occasionally | usually | almost always | always |

4. Spending time with you.

| never | almost never | occasionally | usually | almost always | always |

5. Supporting you.

| never | almost never | occasionally | usually | almost always | always |

6. Being empathetic or identifying with you.

| never | almost never | occasionally | usually | almost always | always |

7. Being confident with you.

| never | almost never | occasionally | usually | almost always | always |

8. Demonstrating professional knowledge and skill.

| never | almost never | occasionally | usually | almost always | always |

9. Including you in planning your care.

| never | almost never | occasionally | usually | almost always | always |

10. Treating your information confidentially.

| never | almost never | occasionally | usually | almost always | always |

11. Returning to you voluntarily.

| never | almost never | occasionally | usually | almost always | always |

12. Talking with you.

| never | almost never | occasionally | usually | almost always | always |

13. Meeting your stated and unstated needs.

| never | almost never | occasionally | usually | almost always | always |

(continued)

TOOL 5.4

Caring Behaviors Inventory-16 Revised (*continued*)

14. Responding quickly when you call.

never	almost never	occasionally	usually	almost always	always

15. Giving your treatments and medications on time.

never	almost never	occasionally	usually	almost always	always

16. Relieving your symptoms.

never	almost never	occasionally	usually	almost always	always

Biographical Information

Directions: Please complete the following information. Kindly circle or write in your answer:

1. Gender:
   1. female
   2. male
   3. other

2. Age: _____

3. Marital status:
   1. single
   2. married
   3. divorced
   4. widowed
   5. separated
   6. partner

4. Race:
   1. Asian
   2. Black
   3. Hispanic
   4. Native American Indian
   5. White
   6. Other, please specify _____

5. Educational level:
   1. 1 to 8 grade
   2. 9 to 12 grade
   3. 1 to 2 years college
   4. 3 to 4 years college
   5. 5 years college and over

6. Employment status:
   1. employed
   2. unemployed
   3. work at home
   4. retired
   5. disabled

(continued)

TOOL 5.4

Biographical Information (*continued*)

7. Type of hospital or healthcare setting where you were cared for by nurses:	1. university hospital 2. community hospital 3. other, please specify _____
8. Reason for this current admission or need for healthcare services of healthcare team	1. medical condition 2. surgery 3. diagnostic study 4. other, please specify _____

TOOL 5.5

Caring Behaviors Inventory-6 (CBI-6)

Please read the list of items that describe nurse caring. For each item, please *circle* the answer that stands for the extent that a nurse or nurses made caring visible during your last hospitalization.

Remember, *you* are the patient.

1. Being hopeful for you.

never	almost never	occasionally	usually	almost always	always

2. Being sensitive to you.

never	almost never	occasionally	usually	almost always	always

3. Demonstrating professional knowledge and skill.

never	almost never	occasionally	usually	almost always	always

4. Allowing you to express feelings about your disease and treatment.

never	almost never	occasionally	usually	almost always	always

5. Showing concern for you.

never	almost never	Occasionally	usually	almost always	always

6. Giving your treatments and medications on time.[a]

never	almost never	occasionally	usually	almost always	always

[a]Item eliminated by Yavinsky et al. (2006).

Source: From Coulombe, K. H., Yeakel, D., Maljanian, R., & Bohannon, R. W. (2002). Caring Behaviors Inventory: Analysis of responses by hospitalized patients. *Outcomes Management, 6*(3), 138–141.

CARING BEHAVIORS INVENTORY FOR ELDERS (WOLF, 2004, 2006)

The Caring Behaviors Inventory for Elders (CBI-E) was developed by Wolf and colleagues (Wolf, Zuzelo, Goldberg, Crothers, & Jacobson, 2006; Wolf et al., 2004) so that an instrument would be available to measure perceptions of the nurse-caring process reported by elderly people and their caregivers. The items originated in the Caring Behaviors Inventory (Wolf et al., 1994) and emerged following efforts to establish construct validity. The CBI-E is framed in Watson's theory (1979, 1988, 1998, 1999) and stresses the interaction and intersubjective responses of nurses, other caregivers, and patients in relationship. The instrument is consistent with the position that caring takes place in moments and the caring process, as directed to the good of patients, incorporates a moral commitment to the care recipient, and acknowledges the vulnerability that nurses, other caregivers, and patients share as humans. Table 5.2 compares CBI-E items with Swanson's (1991) and Watson's (2005) formulations.

The first phase of the CBI-E's development generated 29 items (Wolf et al., 2004). The items of the CBI-E used a 3-point Likert scale (1 = never, 2 = occasionally, 3 = always), rather than a 6-point scale to elicit responses. Investigators hoped that the instrument would be a better fit with elderly residents and patients and their caregivers (Lockett, Aminzadeh, Faranak, & Edwards, 2002; Streiner & Norman, 1995). The CBI-E is printed on yellow paper (Gueldner & Hanner, 1989) with Times New Roman type style, 14-font type size, and sufficient open space (Vanderplas & Vanderplas, 1980). The readability level of the overall instrument, including directions, individual items, and demographic profile, was 4.5 according to the Flesch-Kincaid grade level.

Content validity of the expert type (Burns & Grove, 2005) was established for the CBI-E. Items were revised based on expert reviews and one item was eliminated from the 29-item draft (Wolf et al., 2004). This item had the lowest mean. Several items were modified. Twenty-eight items were retained to reduce measurement error during the next phase of instrument development (Brink & Wood, 1998).

Pilot subjects ($N = 46$) included elderly home dwellers or seniors who lived in independent living facilities. Cronbach's internal consistency, reliability coefficient was .94 for the overall CBI-E. The total score of summed responses of two groups of elders, ages 70 to 79 and 80 to 94, revealed no statistically significant difference when construct validity of the known groups type was tested. There was great variability in the amount of time answering the instrument that older persons reported (Wolf et al., 2004).

Phase II included the development, specification, and application of the 28-item CBI-E for the elderly population and nursing staff caregivers. Construct validity of the convergent, factorial, and contrasted-group types was established as was test–retest and internal consistency reliability (Wolf et al., 2006).

TABLE 5.2 Comparison of CBI-E Items with Watson's Carative Factors (Processes) and Swanson's Carative Processes

CARATIVE FACTORS (WATSON, 1979)	CARING PROCESSES AND SUBDIMENSIONS (SWANSON, 1991)	CARING BEHAVIORS INVENTORY FOR ELDERS ITEMS
W1: Formation of a humanistic–altruistic system of values	S1: Knowing: striving to understand the event as it has meaning in the life of the other	1. Carefully listening to you. (W3, S1)
W2: Instillation of faith–hope	Avoiding assumptions	2. Helping you to feel at home. (W8, S4)
W3: Cultivation of sensitivity to one's self and to others	Centering on the one cared for	3. Helping you and your family make decisions. (W5, S1, S2, S4)
W4: Development of a helping–trust relationship	Assessing thoroughly	4. Calling you by your preferred name. (W4, S2)
W5: Promotion and acceptance of the expression of positive and negative feelings	Seeking cues	5. Being honest with you. (W1, W2, W4, W5, W8, S3, S5)
W6: Systematic use of scientific problem-solving method for decision making	Engaging the self of both	6. Assisting you to meet your religious or spiritual needs. (W1, W8, W9, W10, S1, S3, S4, S5)
W7: Promotion of interpersonal teaching–learning	S2: Being with: being emotionally present to the other	7. Helping you feel comfortable. (W3, W4, W5, W8, W9, S1, S2, S3, S4)
W8: Provision for supportive, protective, and/ or corrective mental, physical, sociocultural, and spiritual environment	Being there	8. Recognizing how you feel. (W1, W3, W5, W8, W9, W10, S1, S2, S4, S5)
W9: Assistance with gratification of human needs	Conveying ability	9. Being patient with you. (W3. W5, W7, W9, W10, S1, S2, S3, S4, S5)
W10: Allowance for existential–phenomenological forces	Sharing feelings	10. Knowing how to give you needles, enemas, treatments, etc. (W6, W8, W9, S3)
	Not-burdening	11. Adjusting to your limitations. (W3, W7, W8, W9, S1, S2, S3, S4, S5)
	S3: Doing for: doing for the other as he/she would do for the self if it were at all possible	12. Appreciating your life story. (W3, W4, W5, W8, W10, S1, S2)
	Comforting	13. Speaking to you with a clear, friendly voice. (W4, S2, S3)
	Anticipating	14. Knowing your likes, dislikes, and routines. (W3, W4, W8, S1, S2, S3)
	Performing competently/skillfully	15. Checking on you. (W4, W9, S2)
	Protecting	
	Preserving dignity	

(continued)

TABLE 5.2 Comparison of CBI-E Items with Watson's Carative Factors (Processes) and Swanson's Carative Processes *(continued)*

CARATIVE FACTORS (WATSON, 1979)	CARING PROCESSES AND SUBDIMENSIONS (SWANSON, 1991)	CARING BEHAVIORS INVENTORY FOR ELDERS ITEMS
	S4: Enabling: facilitating the other's passages through life transitions and unfamiliar events	16. Being pleasant with you. (W4, W8, S2)
	Informing/explaining	17. Including you when planning your care. (W3, W6, W9, S2, S3, S4)
	Supporting/allowing	18. Protecting your privacy. (W1, W3, W4, W8, S1, S2)
	Focusing	19. Watching out for your safety. (W1, W4, W8, W9, S3, S4)
	Generating alternatives/thinking it through	20. Meeting your needs whether or not you ask. (W3, W5, W8, S3)
	Validating/giving feedback	21. Responding quickly to your call. (W4, W8, S2)
	S5: Maintaining belief: sustaining faith in the other's capacity to get through an event or transition and face a future with meaning.	22. Appreciating you as a unique person. (W1, W3 W10, S1, S2, S3)
		23. Managing your pain.
	Believing in/holding in esteem	24. Showing concern for you.
	Maintaining a hope-filled attitude	25. Giving your treatments and medicines on time. (W8, W9, S3)
	Offering realistic optimism	26. Trying to relieve your ailments. (W6 W8, W9, S3)
	"Going the distance"	27. Standing up for your interests. (W1, W3, W8, W9, W10, S1, SS2, S3)
		28. Giving you a hand when you need it. (W1, S1, S3, S4)

S, Swanson; W, Watson.

Source: Reprinted with permission Wolf, Z. R., Zuzelo, P. R., Goldberg, E., Crothers, R., & Jacobson, N. (2006). The Caring Behaviors Inventory of elders: Development and psychometric characteristics. *International Journal for Human Caring, 10*(1), 49–59. doi:10.20467/1091-5710.10.1.49

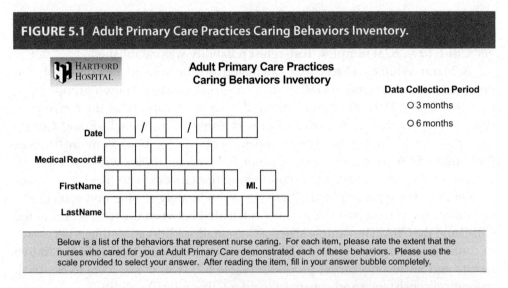

FIGURE 5.1 Adult Primary Care Practices Caring Behaviors Inventory.

Source: Reprinted with permission from The Institute for Outcomes Research & Evaluation @ Hartford Hospital, Hartford, CT. This form should not be used, distributed, or copied without prior written permission. Caring Behaviors Inventory modified and used with permission of author Zane Robinson Wolf, PhD, RN.

The revised CBI-E (Wolf et al., 2006) includes 28 items and is scaled with a 3-point Likert-like scale (1 = rarely, 2 = sometimes, 3 = often). Total scores may range from 28 to 84. The CBI-E is self-administered. Elder and caregiver versions differ by directions and by role as recipient of care versus giver of care. Items of both versions correspond item by item. For example, Item 1 for the elder version was "Carefully listening to you." Item 1 for the caregiver version was "Carefully listening to a resident" (Wolf et al., 2006).

Elderly residents (*N* = 215), from assisted living and independent living agencies, responded to CBI-E items by indicating how often they experienced nurse caring during nursing care moments. Nursing staff (*N* = 138) from the same institutions rated how often they cared for residents on the staff version of the CBI-E.

Cronbach's internal consistency, reliability coefficient was calculated for overall, combined CBI-E ($\alpha = .936$), the elders' CBI-E ($\alpha = .941$), and the caregivers' CBI-E ($\alpha = .823$) samples. Test–retest reliability was established.

A Mann–Whitney U-test was calculated on the ranked responses of two groups, elders and nursing staff, to test construct validity, known groups' type ($U = 4,612$, $p < .001$); the groups differed. Construct validity of the convergent type (Waltz, Strickland, & Lenz, 1984) was tested using the CBI-E and Cronin and Harrison's Caring Behaviors Assessment (CBA), a 62-item instrument (Baldursdottir & Jonsdottir, 2002; Cronin & Harrison, 1988) with the authors' (Cronin & Harrison) permission. Fourteen senior citizens who lived in an independent residence participated. There was a moderately strong, non-statistically significant correlation ($r = .50$, $p = .06$) calculated between the total scores of the CBI-E and the CBA. The sample size was too small; additional testing is necessary to confirm convergent validity. CBI-E items are compared to Watson's carative factors and Swanson's caring processes (Table 5.2; Wolf et al., 2006) to establish theoretical consistency and construct (content, theoretical) validity.

Construct validity of the factorial type was tested on the responses of the combined sample. The scree plot confirmed a 5-factor solution that explained a cumulative 61.90% of the variance. Five factors with eigenvalues greater than 1 were extracted initially and subsequently. Items 19, 11, 9, 7, and 2 loaded on two factors and were retained in Factor I. Item 16 loaded on two factors and was retained in Factor II; Item 3 loaded on two factors and was retained in Factor IV. Factor V is item 6. Communalities for all items, with the exception of item 17 (.464), exceeded .50 at an acceptable level of explanation (Hair, Anderson, Tatham, & Black, 1998). Factors were named by investigators: Factor I, Attending to Individual Needs; Factor II, Showing Respect; Factor III, Practicing Knowledgeably and Skillfully; Factor IV, Respecting Autonomy; and Factor V, Supporting Religious/ Spiritual Needs. Subscales, corresponding items, and factor loadings were noted (Wolf et al., 2006).

The CBI-E has been shared with a nurse and social science researchers at this beginning point in its development. Ongoing testing of the CBI-E's reliability and validity is necessary. Address requests to wolf@lasalle.edu to obtain elder and caregiver versions electronically and for permission to use them. See Table 5.3 for studies in which the CBI-E was administered.

TABLE 5.3 Caring Behaviors Inventory for Elders' Citations

CITATION	CONCEPTUAL–THEORETICAL BASIS; CONCEPTUAL DEFINITION	SCALING	RELIABILITY	VALIDITY	PARTICIPANTS
Wolf et al. (2004)	Watson's Theory of Caring Nurse caring emphasizes the interaction and intersubjective responses of humans, nurses, and patients in relationship. Nurses and patient cocreate caring and caring takes place in moments. The caring process, as directed to the good of patients, reflects a moral commitment to the person and acknowledges the vulnerability that nurses and patients share as humans.	3-point Likert scale (1 = rarely, 2 = sometimes, 3 = often)	Cronbach's alpha = .94	Content validity, expert	$N = 36$ older persons living at home or in independent living facilities

(continued)

TABLE 5.3 Caring Behaviors Inventory for Elders' Citations (continued)

CITATION	CONCEPTUAL–THEORETICAL BASIS; CONCEPTUAL DEFINITION	SCALING	RELIABILITY	VALIDITY	PARTICIPANTS
Wolf et al. (2006)	Watson's theory of human care	3-point scale	Cronbach's alpha = .936 (overall) Older persons = .941 Nursing staff = .823 Test–retest reliability (p = .752)	Construct validity, known groups, convergent (more testing required), factorial Content validity, theoretical	N = 215 older residents of assisted living, independent living settings N = 138 nursing staff of the facilities
Poirier and Sossong (2010)	Watson's Theory of Human Caring		Cronbach's alpha = .89 combined sample, .087, oncology nurses, .89, oncology patients		N = 19 patients N = 15 nurses
Jordan (2010)	Watson's (1979) Theory of Human Care	28 items 3-point scale (Rarely = 1, Sometimes = 2, Often = 3)	Cronbach's alpha = .913		N = 51 adults
Burt (2011)	Watson's Theory of Human Care (1985)	28 items 3-point scale (Rarely = 1, Sometimes = 2, Often = 3)	Cronbach's alpha = .87		N = 85 hospitalized adults

Author (Year)	Theory/Framework	Items/Scale	Reliability	Validity	Sample
Wolf and Goldberg (2011)	Watson's (1979) Theory of Human Care	28 items 3-point scale (Rarely = 1, Some-times = 2, Of-ten = 3)	Cronbach's alpha = .93	Construct validity, known groups (gender, ethnic group)	$N = 232$ community dwelling older persons
Asadi and Najafabadi (2014)		24 items	Cronbach's alpha = .71	Translation: Persian Face and content validity	$N = 140$
Dey (2016)		26 items	Cronbach's alpha = .91		$N = 180$ Acute care elder and telemetry units

TOOL 5.6

Caring Behaviors Inventory for Elders: Older Person Version

Please read the list of items that describe "nurse caring." For each item, please *circle* the answer that shows how **often** you felt that a nurse or nurses cared for you during your experience.

Rating scale: Consider "rarely" as compared to **never**; consider "frequently" as compared to **always**. Consider the degree or extent that the subject **felt** (perceived) nurse caring.

1. Listening carefully to you.	Never	Sometimes	Always
2. Helping you to feel at home.	Never	Sometimes	Always
3. Helping you and your family make decisions.	Never	Sometimes	Always
4. Calling you by your preferred name.	Never	Sometimes	Always
5. Being honest with you.	Never	Sometimes	Always
6. Assisting you to meet your religious or spiritual needs.	Never	Sometimes	Always
7. Helping you feel comfortable.	Never	Sometimes	Always
8. Recognizing how you feel.	Never	Sometimes	Always
9. Being patient with you.	Never	Sometimes	Always
10. Knowing how to give you needles, enemas, treatments, etc.	Never	Sometimes	Always
11. Adjusting to your limitations.	Never	Sometimes	Always
12. Appreciating your life story.	Never	Sometimes	Always
13. Speaking to you with a clear, friendly voice.	Never	Sometimes	Always
14. Knowing your likes, dislikes, and routines.	Never	Sometimes	Always
15. Checking on you frequently.	Never	Sometimes	Always
16. Being pleasant with you.	Never	Sometimes	Always
17. Including you when planning your care.	Never	Sometimes	Always
18. Protecting your privacy.	Never	Sometimes	Always
19. Watching out for your safety.	Never	Sometimes	Always
20. Meeting your needs whether or not you ask.	Never	Sometimes	Always
21. Responding quickly to your call.	Never	Sometimes	Always
22. Appreciating you as a unique person.	Never	Sometimes	Always
23. Managing your pain.	Never	Sometimes	Always
24. Showing concern for you.	Never	Sometimes	Always
25. Giving your treatments and medicines on time.	Never	Sometimes	Always
26. Trying to relieve your ailments.	Never	Sometimes	Always
27. Standing up for your interests.	Never	Sometimes	Always
28. Giving you a hand when you need it.	Never	Sometimes	Always

Profile Form

Participant Number: _____
State of residence: _____

Age: _____
Gender:
        1. Female
        2. Male

Ethnicity:
        1. African American
        2. Asian
        3. White
        4. Latino
        5. Other _____

Marital Status:
        1. Married
        2. Single
        3. Separated
        4. Divorced
        5. Widowed
        6. Partner
        7. Other _____

Religion:
        1. Catholic
        2. Jewish
        3. Muslim
        4. Protestant
        5. Other _____

Schooling:
        1. 1st grade to 5th grade
        2. 6th grade to 8th grade
        3. 9th grade to 12th grade
        4. Graduated from high school
        5. Some college classes without a degree
        6. College degree

Caring Behaviors Inventory for Elders: Caregivers' Version

Please read the list of items that describe "nurse caring." For each item, please *circle* the answer that shows how **often** you felt that you cared for residents where you are employed.

1. Listening carefully to a resident.	Rarely	Sometimes	Often
2. Helping a resident to feel at home.	Rarely	Sometimes	Often
3. Helping a resident and his or her family make decisions.	Rarely	Sometimes	Often
4. Calling a resident by his or her preferred name.	Rarely	Sometimes	Often
5. Being honest with a resident.	Rarely	Sometimes	Often
6. Assisting a resident to meet his or her religious or spiritual needs.	Rarely	Sometimes	Often
7. Helping a resident feel comfortable.	Rarely	Sometimes	Often
8. Recognizing how a resident feels.	Rarely	Sometimes	Often
9. Being patient with a resident.	Rarely	Sometimes	Often
10. Knowing how to give a resident treatments, needles, enemas, etc.	Rarely	Sometimes	Often
11. Adjusting to a resident's limitations.	Rarely	Sometimes	Often
12. Appreciating a resident's life story.	Rarely	Sometimes	Often
13. Speaking to a resident with a clear, friendly voice.	Rarely	Sometimes	Often
14. Knowing a resident's likes, dislikes, and routines.	Rarely	Sometimes	Often
15. Checking on a resident.	Rarely	Sometimes	Often
16. Being pleasant with a resident.	Rarely	Sometimes	Often
17. Including a resident when planning his or her care.	Rarely	Sometimes	Often
18. Protecting a resident's privacy.	Rarely	Sometimes	Often
19. Watching out for a resident's safety.	Rarely	Sometimes	Often
20. Meeting a resident's needs whether or not he or she asks.	Rarely	Sometimes	Often
21. Responding quickly to a resident's call.	Rarely	Sometimes	Often
22. Appreciating a resident as a unique person.	Rarely	Sometimes	Often
23. Managing a resident's pain.	Rarely	Sometimes	Often
24. Showing concern for a resident.	Rarely	Sometimes	Often
25. Giving a resident's treatments and medicines on time.	Rarely	Sometimes	Often
26. Trying to relieve a resident's ailments.	Rarely	Sometimes	Often
27. Standing up for a resident's interests.	Rarely	Sometimes	Often
28. Giving a resident a hand when a he or she needs it.	Rarely	Sometimes	Often

Please identify how many minutes it took to complete this instrument: _____ minutes.

Personal Information Form: Nursing Staff

Participant Number: _____
State of residence: _____
Work Setting: 1. Nursing Home
               2. Medical Center
               3. Other, please specify _____

Age: _____   Job Title: _____

Gender:
    1. Female
    2. Male

Ethnicity:
    1. African American
    2. Asian
    3. White
    4. Latino
    5. Other _____

Marital Status:
    1. Married
    2. Single
    3. Separated
    4. Divorced
    5. Widowed
    6. Partner
    7. Other _____

Religion:
    1. Catholic
    2. Jewish
    3. Muslim
    4. Protestant
    5. Other _____

Education:
    1. 1st grade to 5th grade
    2. 6th grade to 8th grade
    3. 9th grade to 12th grade
    4. Graduated from high school
    5. Some college classes without a degree
    6. Diploma registered nurse program
    7. LPN nurse program
    8. College degree: please specify _____

Release Form	
Caring Behaviors Inventory: CBI 42, 24, 16, and 6	
Caring Behaviors Inventory for Elders: CBI-E	
Zane Robinson Wolf	
©1981, 1994, 2017 CBI	
©2006 CBI-E	

You have my permission to use a version of the Caring Behaviors Inventory or Caring Behaviors for Elders in your research or project. Completing, signing, scanning, and returning this form grants permission.

Please complete the items on the form and return by email. I am also asking your permission to share your name and email address with future colleagues interested in using a translated version of the instrument.

Name:	Degrees and Certifications:
Address:	
Employer:	
University:	
Phone-Cell:	Phone-Work:
Phone-Home, Land:	Other Phone:
Email Address:	Second Email Address:

Version of the CBI that you are interested in administering:

Version	☐ Please check
CBI-42	
CBI-24	
CBI-16	
CBI-6	
CBI-E	

1. Very briefly describe your use of the CBI:

2. Estimate how many subjects/participants/students, and others will be involved in your use of the CBI.

3. If you translate the instrument, please identify the language of the translation: _____. If you translate the instrument, you own the copyright and will cite the CBI research literature.

4. If your research study involves a thesis or dissertation, identify the major advisor's name and address:

Name:	Degrees and Certifications:
Address	
Email:	

5. I plan to modify the instrument; please circle: Yes   No

6. I will translate and reverse translate the instrument; please circle: Yes   No

I will email the version that I administer to Dr. Wolf and will notify Zane Robinson Wolf when a publication results from administration of the CBI. I will send current postal and email addresses.

_____   _____
             Signature   **Date**

_____
                     Print

Please retain one copy of this form for your records and send the original back as a scanned pdf.

Thank you for your interest in the Caring Behaviors Inventory. I own the copyright for the instrument.

Zane Robinson Wolf

Zane Robinson Wolf
_____

Zane Robinson Wolf, PhD, RN, FAAN

27 Haverford Road

Ardmore, PA 19003 USA

REFERENCES

Andrews, L. W., Daniels, P., & Hall, A. G. (1996). Nurse caring behaviors: Comparing five tools to define perceptions. _Ostomy/Wound Management, 42_(5), 28–30, 32–34, 36–37.

Asadi, S. E., & Najafabadi, R. S. (2014). Nurses' perception of caring behaviors in intensive care units in hospitals of Lorestan University of Medical Sciences, Iran. _Medical-Surgical Nursing Journal, 3_, 170–175.

Baldursdottir, G., & Jonsdottir, H. (2002). The importance of nurse caring behaviors as perceived by patients receiving care at an emergency department. _Heart and Lung, 31_(1), 67–75. doi:10.1067/mhl.2002.119835

Beck, C. T. (1999). Quantitative measurement of caring. _Journal of Advanced Nursing, 30_(1), 24–32. doi:10.1046/j.1365-2648.1999.01045.x

Boiman, C. (2017). _Teaching caring behaviors to ADN students: A quasi-experimental study_ (Doctoral dissertation). Available from ProQuest Dissertations and Theses database. (UMI No. 10690861)

Brink, P. J., & Wood, M. J. (1998). _Advanced design in nursing research_ (2nd ed.). Thousand Oaks, CA: Sage.

Brunton, B., & Beaman, M. (2000). Nurse practitioners' perceptions of their caring behaviors. _Journal of the American Academy of Nurse Practitioners, 12_, 451–456. doi:10.1111/j.1745-7599.2000.tb00153.x

Bucco, T. (2015). *The relationships between patients' perceptions of nurse caring behaviors, nurses' perceptions of nurse caring behaviors and patient satisfaction in the emergency department* (Doctoral dissertation). Available from ProQuest Dissertations and Theses database. (UMI No. 3689885)

Burns, N., & Grove, S. K. (2005). *The practice of nursing research: Conduct, critique, & utilization* (5th ed.). Philadelphia, PA: W. B. Saunders.

Burt, K. M. (2011). *The relationship between nurse caring and selected outcomes of care in hospitalized older adults* (Doctoral dissertation, Catholic University of America, Washington, DC). Available from ProQuest Dissertations and Theses database. (UMI No. 3257620)

Chana, N., Kennedy, P., & Chessell, Z. J. (2015). Nursing staffs' emotional well-being and caring behaviours. *Journal of Clinical Nursing, 24*, 2835–2848. doi:10.1111/jocn.12891

Coogan, R. S. (1998). *Caring behaviors of perioperative nurses* (Master's thesis, Florida Atlantic University, Boca Raton, FL/Ann Arbor, MI). Available from ProQuest Dissertations and Theses database.

Coulombe, K. H. (2003). Nurse caring behaviors and patient satisfaction: Improvement after a multifaceted staff intervention. *Journal of Nursing Administration, 33*(9), 434–436. doi:10.1097/00005110-200309000-00002

Coulombe, K. H., Yeakel, S., Maljanian, R., & Bohannon, R. W. (2002). Caring Behaviors Inventory: Analysis of responses by hospitalized surgical patients. *Outcomes Management, 6*(3), 138–141.

Cronin, S. N., & Harrison, B. (1988). Importance of nurse caring behaviors as perceived by patients after myocardial infarction. *Heart & Lung, 17*(4), 374–380.

Dey, M. M. (2016). Relationship of hospitalized elders' perceptions of nurse caring behaviors, type of care unit, satisfaction with nursing care, and the health outcome of functional status. *International Journal for Human Caring, 20*, 134–141. doi:10.20467/1091-5710-20.3.134

Edvardsson, D., Mahoney, A.-M., Hardy, J., McGillion, T., McLean, A., Pearce, F., . . . Wart, E. (2015). Psychometric performance of the English language six-item Caring Behaviours Inventory in an acute care context. *Journal of Clinical Nursing, 24*, 2538–2544. doi:10.1111/jocn.12849

Green, A. (2004). Caring behaviors as perceived by nurse practitioners. *Journal of the American Academy of Nurse Practitioners, 16*, 283–290. doi:10.1111/j.1745-7599.2004.tb00451.x

Green, L. A. E., & Davis, S. P. (2002). *Toward a predictive model of patient satisfaction with nurse practitioner care* (Doctoral dissertation, University of Mississippi Medical Center, Lafayette Center, Lafayette County, MS). Available from ProQuest Dissertations and Theses database. (UMI No. 3091788)

Gueldner, S. H., & Hanner, M. B. (1989). Methodological issues related to gerontological nursing research. *Nursing Research, 38*(3), 183–184. doi:10.1097/00006199-198905000-00022

Hair, J. F., Anderson, R. E., Tatham, R. L., & Black, W. C. (1998). *Multivariate data analysis* (5th ed.). Upper Saddle River, NJ: Prentice Hall.

Hayes, J. S., & Tyler-Ball, S. (2007). Perceptions of nurses' caring behaviors by trauma patients. *Trauma Nursing, 14*, 187–190. doi:10.1097/01.JTN.0000318920.83003.a2

Jordan, L. G. (2010). *The perceptions of nursing team caring behaviors among residents of an assisted living facility for retired veterans* (Doctoral dissertation). Available from ProQuest Dissertations and Theses databases. (UMI No. 3391247)

Keeley, P., Wolf, Z., Regul, L., & Jadwin, A. (2015). Effectiveness of standard of care protocol on patient satisfaction and perceived staff caring. *Clinical Journal of Oncology Nursing, 19*, 352–360. doi:10.1188/15.CJON.352-360

Kolb, D. (1984). *Experiential learning: Experience as the source of learning and development.* Englewood Cliffs, NJ: Prentice-Hall.

Kyle, T. V. (1995). The concept of caring: A review of the literature. *Journal of Advanced Nursing, 21*, 506–514. doi:10.1111/j.1365-2648.1995.tb02734.x

Labraque, L. L., McEnroe-Petitte, D. M., Papathanasiou, J. V., Edet, O. B., Arulappan, J., & Tsaras, K. (2015). Nursing students' perceptions of their own caring behaviors: A multicountry study. *International Journal of Nursing Knowledge, 28*, 225–232. doi:10.1111/2047-3095.12108

Larrabee, J. H., Ostrow, C. L., Withrow, M. L., Janney, M. A., Hobbs, G. R., & Burant, C. (2004). Predictors of patient satisfaction with inpatient hospital nursing care. *Research in Nursing & Health, 27*, 254–268. doi:10.1002/nur.20021

Lockett, D., Aminzadeh, F., & Edwards, N. (2002). Development of an instrument to measure seniors' attitudes toward the use of bathroom bars. *Public Health Nursing, 19*(5), 390–397. doi:10.1046/j.1525-1446.2002.19508.x

Loke, J. C. F., Lee, K. W., Lee, B. K., & Noor, A. M. (2015). Caring behaviours of student nurses: Effects of pre-registration nursing education. *Nurse Education in Practice, 15*, 421–429. doi:10.1016/j.nepr.2015.05.005

Mark, B. A., Sayler, J., & Smith, C. S. (1996). A theoretical model for nursing systems outcomes research. *Nursing Administration Quarterly, 20*(4), 12–27. doi:10.1097/00006216-199602040-00004

Merrill, A. S., Hayes, J. S., Clukey, L., & Curtis, D. (2012). Do they really care? How trauma patients perceive nurses' caring behaviors. *Journal of Trauma Nursing, 19*, 33–37. doi:10.1097/JTN.0b013e318249fcac

Mezirow, J., & Associates (Eds.). (1990). *Fostering critical reflection in adulthood*. San Francisco, CA: Jossey-Bass.

Mlinar, S. (2010) First- and third-year student nurses' perceptions of caring behaviours. *Nursing Ethics, 17*, 491–500. doi:10.1177/0969733010364903

Murphy, F., Jones, S., Edwards, M., James, J., & Mayer, A. (2009). The impact of nurse education on the caring behaviors of nursing students. *Nurse Education Today, 29*, 254–264. doi:10.1016/j.nedt.2008.08.016

Nantz, S., & Hines, A. (2015). Trauma patients' family members' perceptions of nurses' caring behaviors. *Journal of Trauma Nursing, 22*, 249–254 doi:10.1097/JTN.0000000000000149

Palese, A., Tomietto, M., Suhonen, R., Efstathiou, G., Tsangari, H. Merkouris, A., . . . Papastavrou, E. (2011). Surgical patient satisfaction as an outcome of nurses' caring behaviors: A descriptive and correlational study in six European countries. *Journal of Nursing Scholarship, 43*(4), 341–350. doi:10.1111/j.1547-5069.2011.01413.x

Papastavrou, E., Efstathiou, G., Tsangari, H., Suhonen, R., Leino-Kilpi, H., Patiraki, E., . . . Merkouris, A. (2011). A cross-cultural study of the concept of caring through behaviours: Patients' and nurses' perspectives in six different EU countries. *Journal of Advanced Nursing, 68*, 1026–1037. doi:10.1111/j.1365-2648.2011.05807.x

Papastavrou, E., Efstathiou, G., Tsangari, H., Suhonen, R., Leino-Kilpi, H., Patiraki, E., . . . Merkouris, A. (2012). Patients' and nurses' perceptions of respect and human presence through caring behaviours: A comparative study. *Nursing Ethics, 19*, 369–379. doi:10.1177/0969733011436027

Papastavrou, E., Karlou, C., Tsangari, H., Efstathiou, G., Souse, V. D., Merkouris, A., & Patiraki, E. (2011). Cross-cultural validation and psychometric properties of the Greek version of the caring behaviours inventory: A methodological study. *Journal of Evaluation in Clinical Practice, 17*, 435–443. doi:10.1111/j.1365-2753.2010.01445.x

Patiraki, E., Karlou, C., Efstathiou, G., Tsangari, H., Merkouris, A., Jarosova, D., . . . Papastavrou, E. (2014). The relationship between surgical patients and nurses characteristics with their perceptions of caring behaviors: A European survey. *Clinical Nursing Research, 23*, 132–152. doi:10.1177/1054773812468447

Plowden, K. O. (1997). *Caring Behavior Inventory: An exploration of dimensions of nurse caring at the Department of Veterans Affairs Medical Center*. (Doctoral dissertation, Walden University, Atlanta, GA).

Poirier, P., & Sossong, A. (2010). Oncology patients' and nurses' perceptions of caring. *Canadian Journal of Oncology Nursing, 20*(2), 62–65. doi:10.5737/1181912x2026265

Porter, C. A., Cortese, M., Vezina, M., & Fitzpatrick, J. J. (2014). Nurse caring behaviors following implementation of a relationship centered care professional practice model. *International Journal of Caring Sciences, 7*, 818–822.

Rafii, F., Hajinezhad, M. E., & Haghani, H. (2007). Nurse caring and patient satisfaction in Iran. *International Journal for Human Caring, 12*(3), 14–23. doi:10.20467/1091-5710.12.3.14

Sarafis, P., Rousaki, E., Tsounis, A., Malliarou, M., Lahana, L., Barnidis, P., . . . Papastavrou, E. (2016). The impact of occupational stress on nurses' caring behaviors and their health-related quality of life. *BMC Nursing, 15*, 56. doi:10.1186/s12912-016-0178-y

Streiner, D. L. (1993). *Health measurement scales: A practical guide to their development* (3rd ed.). Oxford, UK: Oxford University Press.

Streiner, D. L., & Norman, G. R. (1995). *Health measurement scales: A practical guide to their development* (3rd ed.). Oxford, UK: Oxford University Press.

Swanson, K. (1991). Empirical development of a middle range theory of caring. *Nursing Research, 40*, 161–166. doi:10.1097/00006199-199105000-00008

Vanderplas, J. M., & Vanderplas, J. H. (1980). Some factors affecting legibility of printed materials for older adults. *Perceptual and Motor Skills, 50*, 923–932. doi:10.2466/pms.1980.50.3.923

Waltz, C. F., Strickland, O. L., & Lenz, E. R. (1984). *Measurement in nursing research*. Philadelphia, PA: F. A. Davis.

Watson, J. (1979). *Nursing: The philosophy and science of caring*. Boston, MA: Little, Brown.

Watson, J., Burckhardt, C., Brown, L., Bloch, D., & Hester, N. (1979). *A model of caring: An alternative health care model for nursing practice and research*. Kansas City, KS: ANA Clinical and Scientific Sessions.

Watson, J. (1985). *Nursing: Human science and human care*. Norwalk, CT: Appleton-Century-Crofts.

Watson, J. (1988). *Nursing: Human science and human care*. New York, NY: National League for Nursing.

Watson, J. (1998). New dimensions of human caring theory. *Nursing Science Quarterly, 1*(4), 175–181.

Watson, J. (1999). *Postmodern nursing and beyond*. Edinburgh, Scotland: Churchill Livingstone.

Watson, J. (2005). *Caring science as sacred science*. Philadelphia, PA: F. A. Davis.

Watson, J. (2008). *Nursing: The philosophy and science of caring* (2nd ed.). Boulder: University Press of Colorado.

Wolf, Z. R. (1981). *The concept of caring: Beginning exploration*. Candidacy Paper, University of Pennsylvania School of Nursing, Philadelphia, PA.

Wolf, Z. R. (1986). The caring concept and nurse identified caring behaviors. *Topics in Clinical Nursing, 8*, 84–93.

Wolf, Z. R., Bailey, D. N., & Keeley, P. A. (2014). Caring protocol creation: Activities and dissemination strategies in caring research and instruments. *International Journal for Human Caring, 18*(1), 66–82. doi:10.20467/1091-5710.18.1.66

Wolf, Z. R., Colahan, M., Costello, A., Warwick, F., Ambrose, M. S., & Giardino, E. R. (1998). Relationship between nurse caring and patient satisfaction. *MEDSURG Nursing, 7*(2), 99–105.

Wolf, Z. R., Dillon, P. M., Townsend, A. B., & Glasofer, A. (2017). Caring Behaviors Inventory-24 Revised: CBI-16 validation and psychometric properties. *International Journal for Human Caring, 21*, 185–192. doi:10.20467/1091-5710.21.4.185

Wolf, Z. R., Giardino, E. R., Osborne, P. A., & Ambrose, M. S. (1994). Dimensions of nurse caring. *Image: Journal of Nursing Scholarship, 26*(2), 107–111. doi:10.1111/j.1547-5069.1994.tb00927.x

Wolf, Z. R., & Goldberg, E. (2011). Community-dwelling elders' perceptions of LIFE staff caring: A comparative descriptive study. *International Journal for Human Caring, 15*(2), 35–41. doi:10.20467/1091-5710.15.2.35

Wolf, Z. R., Keeley, P. A., Regul, L., Cobb, S. C., & Jadwin, A. (2016). Strategies to implement the Standard of Care/Caring Protocol in an acute care oncology hospital setting: A focus group study. *International Journal for Human Caring, 20*(1), 48–57. doi:10.20467/1091-5710-20.1.48

Wolf, Z. R., Miller, P. A., & Devine, M. (2003). Relationship between nurse caring and patient satisfaction in patients undergoing invasive cardiac procedures. *MEDSURG Nursing, 12*(6), 391–396.

Wolf, Z. R., Zuzelo, P. R., Goldberg, E., Crothers, R., & Jacobson, N. (2006). The Caring Behaviors Inventory of elders: Development and psychometric characteristics. *International Journal for Human Caring, 10*(1), 49–59. doi:10.20467/1091-5710.10.1.49

Wolf, Z. R., Zuzelo, R. R., Costello, R., Cattilico, D., Cooper, K. A., Crothers, R., & Karbach, H. (2004). Development of the Caring Behaviors Inventory for elders. *International Journal for Human Caring, 8*(1), 48–54. doi:10.20467/1091-5710.8.1.49

Wu, Y., Larrabee, J. H., & Putman, H. P. (2006). Caring Behaviors Inventory: A reduction of the 42-item instrument. *Nursing Research, 55*(1), 18–25. doi:10.1097/00006199-200601000-00003

Yeakel, S., Maljanian, R., Bohannon, R. W., & Coulombe, K. H. (2003). Nurse caring behaviors and patient satisfaction: Improvement after a multifaceted staff intervention. *Journal of Nursing Administration, 33*(9), 434–436. doi:10.1097/00005110-200309000-00002

Caring Behaviors
Assessment Tool

Sherill N. Cronin and Barbara H. Lee

The Caring Behaviors Assessment (CBA) is one of the early tools developed to assess caring. It was the first one reported in the nursing literature to have an explicit theoretical-conceptual basis from which specific items were derived. It is based on Watson's (1985, 1988) theory and the 10 carative factors identified in her original work. The tool was developed by Cronin and Harrison (1988) to identify nursing behaviors perceived by patients to indicate caring. There have been no substantive changes to the scale itself since the first edition of this book.

Since its development and original publication, the CBA has been used in a number of published and unpublished studies and has been translated into several languages, including Arabic, Chinese, Croatian, Dutch, Filipino, Icelandic, Japanese, Spanish, and Yoruba (Nigeria). Ayala and Calvo (2017) also took the CBA through the process of translation, cultural adaptation, and validation in Chile, resulting in a version in a Latin American variation of the Spanish language.

The CBA has been modified in order to identify patients' perceptions of the degree to which caring behaviors are demonstrated by healthcare providers; that is, their satisfaction with caring. In addition, adapted versions have been used to measure nurses' and other caregivers' perceptions of caring, family members' perceptions, and nursing students' perceptions of, and competencies in, caring behaviors. Findings from the use of these adapted versions of the tool suggest that, beyond validating a set of actions and attitudes that are pertinent to Watson's theoretical framework, reliable theoretically grounded instruments can contribute to enhancements in nursing care quality (Ayala & Calvo, 2017).

The CBA consists of 63 nurse-caring behaviors that are grouped into seven subscales that are congruent with Watson's carative factors. The first three of the 10 carative factors are grouped together into one subscale, which is conceptually congruent with Watson's theory. The sixth carative factor, "Use of a creative,

 DOI:10.1891/9780826195425.0006 **83**

problem-solving, caring process," was assumed by the authors to be inherent in all aspects of nursing care, and thus imperceptible to patients. Therefore, this factor was omitted as a subscale. The tool uses sixth-grade-level language. Respondents are asked to rate items on a 5-point Likert scale to reflect the degree to which each nursing behavior reflects caring.

The tool was first used with a sample of 22 patients who had experienced a myocardial infarction. Content validity was assessed by four experts familiar with Watson's caring theory. Cronin and Harrison (1988) took into account readability and reliability, as well as face and content validity. They reported the following internal consistency reliabilities, tested with Cronbach's alpha, on each of the subscales:

Humanism/faith-hope-sensitivity	.84
Helping/trust	.76
Expression of positive/negative	.67
Teaching/learning	.90
Supportive/protective/corrective behaviors	.79
Human need/assistance	.89
Existential/phenomenological dimensions	.66

Similar reliability rates have been reported in recent uses of the CBA, including Omari, AbuAlRub, and Ayasreh's (2013) study of adults with coronary artery disease and nurses who cared for them. One of the most recent reports of the instrument's use is by Ayala and Calvo (2017), who tested a culturally adapted and validated version of the CBA with 443 users of a primary care center who had been hospitalized within the previous 6 months. They report Cronbach's alpha reliability of .96 for the entire scale, with subscale reliabilities that ranged from .81 to .88. Both of these studies were conducted outside the United States, in Jordan and Chile, respectively. When taken together with similar results from studies in China (Wu, Chin, & Chen, 2009), Iceland (Baldursdottir & Jonsdottir, 2002), Ireland (O'Connell & Landers, 2008), and Saudi Arabia (Suliman, Welmann, Omer, & Thomas, 2009; Yousseif, Mansour, Ayasreh, & Al-Mawajdeh, 2013), these findings suggest the CBA may demonstrate internal consistency across countries and languages.

In the original research, the two specific items found to be the most important by patients were "Makes me feel someone is there if I need them" and "Knows what they are doing." The least important items were "Visits me when I move to another hospital unit" and "Asks me what I like to be called." These findings have been interpreted as suggesting that the most important caring behaviors, as perceived by patients, were those demonstrating professional competence. However, subsequent uses of the tool suggest that age, illness acuity, care location, and culture may impact the relative importance of various behaviors and subscales (Adereti, Olaogun, Olagunju, & Afolabi, 2014; Gillespie, Hounchell, Pettinichi, Mattei, & Rose, 2012; O'Connell & Landers, 2008; Omari et al., 2013).

   Cronin and Harrison (1988) recognized the limitations of the CBA, including the instrument's length and variability in number of items listed within subscales, as well as the small sample size of this initial testing, and suggested further use and evaluation of the tool. Continued testing of the tool by multiple researchers suggests that its reliability and validity hold up in larger and more varied samples. Length of the tool and the potential burden it places on some patient populations continue to be a concern (Suliman et al., 2009). Efforts to shorten the tool, without negatively affecting its reliability, should be considered. Table 6.1 summarizes published studies that have used the CBA (Tool 6.1).

   This instrument is copyrighted by the authors and developers of the CBA, who request that anyone using the instrument contact them at:

Sherill Nones Cronin, PhD, RN-BC, and
Barbara Harrison Lee, MSN, MEd, RN-BC, CWOCN
Lansing School of Nursing and Health Sciences
Bellarmine University
2001 Newburg Road
Louisville, KY 40205-0671
email: scronin@bellarmine.edu

TABLE 6.1 Matrix of Caring Behavior Assessment Tool (CBA; Cronin & Harrison, 1988)

INSTRUMENT/ YEAR DEVELOPED	YEAR PUBLISHED/ SOURCE CITATION	DEVELOPED TO MEASURE	INSTRUMENT DESCRIPTION	PARTICIPANTS	REPORTED RELIABILITY/VALIDITY	THEORETICAL-CONCEPTUAL BASIS	LATEST CITATION IN NURSING LITERATURE
Caring Behavior Assessment Instrument (CBA) 1988	Cronin and Harrison (1988)	Patients' perceptions of nurse-caring behaviors; explicitly attempts to address process	63 items 7 subscales 5-point Likert rating	Post-myocardial infarction patients $n = 22$	Cronbach's alpha established; face and content validity obtained	Watson's theory of caring and 10 carative factors in theory	Ayala and Calvo (2017)
CBA Original (translated into Spanish)	Ayala and Calvo (2017)	Cultural adaptation and reliability of a CBA translated in a Latin American variation of the Spanish language	63 items 7 subscales 5-point Likert rating	Users of a primary care center who had been hospitalized within the previous 6 months $n = 443$	Translation by a non-nursing translator and two nurses familiar with Watson's theory Cronbach's alpha for entire CBA = .96 Subscale alphas ranged from .81 to .88	Watson's theory of caring and 10 carative factors	

Instrument	Author(s)	Purpose	Items	Sample	Reliability/Validity	Theory	Reference
CBA Modified (translated into Yoruba)	Adereti et al. (2014)	Most important nurse-caring behaviors to pediatric patients and their primary caregivers	44 items 7 subscales 5-point Likert rating	Hospitalized pediatric patients between 7 and 14 years of age; $n = 114$ Primary caregivers of pediatric study participants; $n = 114$	Face and content validity by pediatric nurse and physician Cronbach's alpha for Yoruba translation of the CBA = .82 Alpha for English CBA = .88	Watson's theory of caring and 10 carative factors	Salmani, Hasanvand, Bagheri, and Mandegari (2017)
CBA Original (translated into Arabic)	Omari et al. (2013)	Perceptions of nurse-caring behaviors by Jordanian critical care nurses and patients who suffer from coronary artery disease	63 items 7 subscales 5-point Likert rating	Adults with coronary artery disease; $n = 150$ Critical care unit nurses; $n = 60$	Cronbach's alpha for entire CBA = .80 for patients; .91 for nurses Subscale alphas ranged from .62 to .97 for patients; .70 to .93 for nurses	Watson's theory of caring and 10 carative factors	Ayala and Calvo (2017)
CBA Original (translated into Arabic)	Yousseif et al. (2013)	Medical-surgical nurses' perceptions of caring behaviors	63 items 7 subscales 5-point Likert rating	Medical-surgical nurses in two hospitals $n = 90$	Cronbach's alpha for entire CBA = .91 Subscale alphas ranged from .70 to .93	Watson's theory of caring and 10 carative factors	Bakar et al. (2017)

(continued)

TABLE 6.1 Matrix of Caring Behavior Assessment Tool (CBA; Cronin & Harrison, 1988) *(continued)*

INSTRUMENT/ YEAR DEVELOPED	YEAR PUBLISHED/ SOURCE CITATION	DEVELOPED TO MEASURE	INSTRUMENT DESCRIPTION	PARTICIPANTS	REPORTED RELIABILITY/VALIDITY	THEORETICAL-CONCEPTUAL BASIS	LATEST CITATION IN NURSING LITERATURE
CBA (Modified)	Gillespie et al. (2012)	Perceptions of nurse–caring behaviors by parents of pediatric patients in the emergency room	61 items 7 subscales 5-point Likert rating	Parents of pediatric emergency room patients *n* = 300	Five content experts evaluated content validity of modified CBA Cronbach's alpha for entire CBA = .971 Subscale alphas ranged from .807 to .925	Watson's theory of caring and 10 carative factors	Balboni and Peteet (2017)
CBA (Modified)	Labrague (2012)	Perceptions of nursing students' caring competencies by adult patients and/or parents of pediatric patients	63 items 7 subscales 5-point Likert rating	1) Hospitalized patients over the age of 18, and 2) parents of hospitalized children who responded regarding their child's care *n* = 174	No information provided by author	Watson's theory of caring and 10 carative factors	Bagnall (2017)

CBA (Modified)	Suliman et al. (2009)	Patient perceptions of importance of nurse-caring behaviors and those most frequently attended to by nursing staff	63 items 7 subscales 5-point Likert rating Asked both "Importance" and "Frequency" of each behavior	Hospitalized medical-surgical patients $n = 392$	Cronbach's alpha for total CBA "importance" = .958; for "frequency" = .983	Watson's theory of caring and 10 carative factors	Kwak and Lee (2018)
CBA Original (In Chinese)	Wu et al. (2009)	Examination of efficacy of a caring educational program for nursing students	63 items 7 subscales 5-point Likert rating	Female full-time second-year students in the second year of an RN to BSN program without previous clinical employment $n = 33$ in control group; $n = 35$ in experimental group	Cronbach's alpha for total CBA Pretest = .97 Posttest = .98 Subscale alphas Pretest = .81–.91 Posttest = .87–.91	Watson's theory of caring and 10 carative factors	Ayala and Calvo (2017)

(continued)

TABLE 6.1 Matrix of Caring Behavior Assessment Tool (CBA; Cronin & Harrison, 1988) *(continued)*

INSTRUMENT/ YEAR DEVELOPED	YEAR PUBLISHED/ SOURCE CITATION	DEVELOPED TO MEASURE	INSTRUMENT DESCRIPTION	PARTICIPANTS	REPORTED RELIABILITY/VALIDITY	THEORETICAL-CONCEPTUAL BASIS	LATEST CITATION IN NURSING LITERATURE
CBA (Modified)	O'Connell and Landers (2008)	Perceptions of nurse-caring behaviors by nurses and relatives of critically ill patients	62 items 7 subscales 5-point Likert rating	Critical care nurses $n = 40$ Relatives of critically ill patients $n = 30$	Face validity by an expert on Watson's work and by an expert in critical care nursing Cronbach's alpha for subscales ranged from .747 to .896 for nurses; Alphas for relatives ranged from .358 to .858	Watson's theory of caring and 10 carative factors	Sunaryo, Nirwanto, and Manan (2017)
CBA Original	Wolf, Zuzelo, Goldberg, Crothers, and Jacobsen (2006)	To evaluate construct validity of the convergent type with the CBI-E	CBA 63 items; 7 subscales, 5-point Likert scale	Senior citizens in an independent living residence $n = 14$	None reported for CBA	Watson's Theory of Human Caring	Ayala and Calvo (2017)
CBA Original and Spanish translation	Brown et al. (2005)	Importance of role of patient care facilitator in making patients feel cared for and about	CBA 63 items; 7 subscales, 5-point Likert scale	Hospitalized patients from three nursing units $n = 559$	Reliability and validity as reported by Cronin and Harrison (1988)	Watson's theory of caring; Carative factors	Fishman (2018)

CBA Original	Baldursdottirand Jonsdottir (2002)	Patients' perceptions of the relative importance of nurse-caring behaviors	CBA 63 items; 7 subscales, 5-point Likert scale	Convenience sample; adult patients who had received care in an emergency department $n = 182$	Subscale reliabilities, tested with Cronbach's alphas, ranged from .69 to .89	Watson's theory of caring; Carative factors	Ayala and Calvo (2017)
CBA (Modified) 2001	Dorsey, Phillips, and Williams (2001)	Patients' perceptions of the degree of caring behaviors demonstrated by healthcare providers	CBA 63 items; 7 subscales, 5-point Likert scale	Convenience sample; $n = 63; 29$ adult patients with sickle cell disease and 34 adults with other medical conditions	Subscale reliabilities, tested with Cronbach's alphas, ranged from .81 to .94	Watson's theory of caring; Carative factors	Ruta and Ballas (2016)
CBA Original 2000	Manogin, Bechtel, and Rami (2000)	Perception of nurse-caring behaviors by women during childbirth	CBA 63 items; 7 subscales, 5-point Likert scale	Convenience sample; $n = 31$ women hospitalized for uncomplicated labor and delivery birth	Expert panel for content validity; Cronbach's alpha for each of 7 subscales ranged from .66 to .90	Watson's theory of caring and Carative Factors; earlier work of Cronin and Harrison	Drake (2016)

(continued)

91

TABLE 6.1 Matrix of Caring Behavior Assessment Tool (CBA; Cronin & Harrison, 1988) *(continued)*

INSTRUMENT/ YEAR DEVELOPED	YEAR PUBLISHED/ SOURCE CITATION	DEVELOPED TO MEASURE	INSTRUMENT DESCRIPTION	PARTICIPANTS	REPORTED RELIABILITY/VALIDITY	THEORETICAL-CONCEPTUAL BASIS	LATEST CITATION IN NURSING LITERATURE
CBA Original 1999	Marini (1999)	Perceptions of caring from older adults, institutionalized	CBA with 64 nurse-caring behaviors, with 7 subscales; plus 1 open-ended question: "Is there anything else that nurses do to make you feel cared for or about?"	Residents in long term care, assisted living facility $N = 21$	Additional correlations established on subscales by gender; highest range .89 for women; .85 for men	Watson's theory; Carative factors	Shinan-Altman and Ayalon (2017)
CBA Original 1999	Gay (1999)	Importance of caring to cardiac patients	CBA 63 items; 7 subscales, 5-point Likert scale	Hospitalized cardiac patients $n = 18$	Report content and face validity with use of panel of experts familiar with Watson's theory; Reliability Cronbach's alpha .66–.90	Watson's caring theory; Carative factors	Mercer (2013)

CBA Original 1998	Schultz, Bridgham, Smith, and Higgins (1998)	Describe and compare similarities and differences in the perceptions of caring behaviors between antepartum patients and short-term postpartum patients	CBA as developed by Cronin and Harrison (1988) 63 items; 7 subscales, 5-point Likert scale	Convenience sample of antepartum and short term post-partum patients; $n = 42$	Reports additional test of reliability: .71–.88 for subscales; alpha of .93 for total scale	Watson's theory; Carative factors	Ross-Davie and Cheyne (2014)
CBA Original 1996	Mullins (1996)	Identify caring behaviors desired by patients with AIDS/HIV	63 nurse-caring behaviors, opened-ended question at end of CBA	Individuals from AIDS outreach groups and AIDS support groups; four geographical areas in SE USA $n = 46$	Reliability and validity as reported by Cronin & Harrison (1988)	Watson theory and carative factors as rationale for selecting CBA	Hogan (2015)
CBA (Revised) 1993	Parson, Kee, and Gray (1993)	Patients' perceptions of nurse-caring behaviors	63 items 7 subscales 5-point Likert (revised original CBA)	Post surgery patients (short stay) $n = 19$	Reliability and validity as reported by Cronin and Harrison (1988)	Watson theory of caring and 10 carative factors	Gillespie et al. (2012)

(continued)

TABLE 6.1 Matrix of Caring Behavior Assessment Tool (CBA; Cronin & Harrison, 1988) *(continued)*

INSTRUMENT/ YEAR DEVELOPED	YEAR PUBLISHED/ SOURCE CITATION	DEVELOPED TO MEASURE	INSTRUMENT DESCRIPTION	PARTICIPANTS	REPORTED RELIABILITY/VALIDITY	THEORETICAL- CONCEPTUAL BASIS	LATEST CITATION IN NURSING LITERATURE
CBA (Revised) 1993	Huggins, Gandy, and Kohut (1993)	Patients' perceptions of nurse-caring behaviors	Modified for phone survey and emergency patients 65 items; 4 point ordinal; 6 subscales	Emergency patients n = 288	Reliability and validity as reported by Cronin and Harrison (1988)	Watson theory and 10 carative factors	Mahmoudi, Mohmmadi, and Ebadi (2017)
CBA (Further Testing) 1991	Stanfield (1991)	Patients' perceptions of caring	63 items 7 subscales, based on Watson's carative factors	Adult patients hospitalized on medical-surgical units n = 104	Alpha for entire instrument .9566; subscale alphas ranged from .7825 to .8867; construct validity established with factor analysis	Watson's theory of caring and 10 carative factors	Kuis, Hesselink, and Goossensen (2014)

TOOL 6.1
Caring Behaviors Assessment Tool

Listed below are things nurses might do or say to make you feel cared for and about. Please decide how important each of these would be in making you feel cared for and about. For each item, indicate if it would be of:

Much Importance							Little Importance
5		4		3		2	1

Please circle the number that tells you how important each item would be to you.

		5	4	3	2	1
1.	Treat me as an individual.	5	4	3	2	1
2.	Try to see things from my point of view.	5	4	3	2	1
3.	Know what they're doing.	5	4	3	2	1
4.	Reassure me.	5	4	3	2	1
5.	Make me feel someone is there if I need them.	5	4	3	2	1
6.	Encourage me to believe in myself.	5	4	3	2	1
7.	Point out positive things about me and my condition.	5	4	3	2	1
8.	Praise my efforts.	5	4	3	2	1
9.	Understand me.	5	4	3	2	1
10.	Ask me how I like things done.	5	4	3	2	1
11.	Accept me the way I am.	5	4	3	2	1
12.	Be sensitive to my feelings and moods.	5	4	3	2	1
13.	Be kind and considerate.	5	4	3	2	1
14.	Know when I've "had enough" and act accordingly (e.g., limiting visitors).	5	4	3	2	1
15.	Maintain a calm manner.	5	4	3	2	1
16.	Treat me with respect.	5	4	3	2	1
17.	Really listen to me when I talk.	5	4	3	2	1
18.	Accept my feelings without judging them.	5	4	3	2	1
19.	Come into my room just to check on me.	5	4	3	2	1
20.	Talk to me about my life outside the hospital.	5	4	3	2	1
21.	Ask me what I like to be called.	5	4	3	2	1
22.	Introduce themselves to me.	5	4	3	2	1

(continued)

TOOL 6.1

Caring Behaviors Assessment Tool (*continued*)

23.	Answer quickly when I call for them.	5	4	3	2	1
24.	Give me their full attention when with me.	5	4	3	2	1
25.	Visit me if I move to another hospital unit.	5	4	3	2	1
26.	Touch me when I need it for comfort.	5	4	3	2	1
27.	Do what they say they will do.	5	4	3	2	1
28.	Encourage me to talk about how I feel.	5	4	3	2	1
29.	Don't become upset when I'm angry.	5	4	3	2	1
30.	Help me understand my feelings.	5	4	3	2	1
31.	Don't give up on me when I'm difficult to get along with.	5	4	3	2	1
32.	Encourage me to ask questions about my illness and treatment.	5	4	3	2	1
33.	Answer my questions clearly.	5	4	3	2	1
34.	Teach me about my illness.	5	4	3	2	1
35.	Ask me questions to be sure I understand.	5	4	3	2	1
36.	Ask me what I want to know about my health/illness.	5	4	3	2	1
37.	Help me set realistic goals for my health.	5	4	3	2	1
38.	Help me plan ways to meet those goals.	5	4	3	2	1
39.	Help me plan for my discharge from the hospital.	5	4	3	2	1
40.	Tell me what to expect during the day.	5	4	3	2	1
41.	Understand when I need to be alone.	5	4	3	2	1
42.	Offer things (position changes, blankets, backrub, lighting, etc.) to make me more comfortable.	5	4	3	2	1
43.	Leave my room neat after working with me.	5	4	3	2	1
44.	Explain safety precautions to me and my family.	5	4	3	2	1
45.	Give me pain medication when I need it.	5	4	3	2	1
46.	Encourage me to do what I can for myself.	5	4	3	2	1

(*continued*)

TOOL 6.1

Caring Behaviors Assessment Tool (*continued*)

47.	Respect my modesty (e.g., keeping me covered).	5	4	3	2	1
48.	Check with me before leaving the room to be sure I have everything I need within reach.	5	4	3	2	1
49.	Consider my spiritual needs.	5	4	3	2	1
50.	Are gentle with me.	5	4	3	2	1
51.	Are cheerful.	5	4	3	2	1
52.	Help me with my care until I'm able to do it for myself.	5	4	3	2	1
53.	Know how to give shots, IVs, etc.	5	4	3	2	1
54.	Know how to handle equipment (e.g., monitors).	5	4	3	2	1
55.	Give me treatments and medications on time.	5	4	3	2	1
56.	Keep my family informed of my progress.	5	4	3	2	1
57.	Let my family visit as much as possible.	5	4	3	2	1
58.	Check my condition very closely.	5	4	3	2	1
59.	Help me feel like I have some control.	5	4	3	2	1
60.	Know when it's necessary to call the doctor.	5	4	3	2	1
61.	Seem to know how I feel.	5	4	3	2	1
62.	Help me see that my past experiences are important.	5	4	3	2	1
63.	Help me feel good about myself.	5	4	3	2	1

Is there anything else that nurses could do or say to make you feel cared for and about? If so, what?

Source: Cronin, S., & Harrison, B. (1988). Importance of nurse caring behaviors as perceived by patients after myocardial infarction. *Heart and Lung, 17*(4), 374–380. Users who wish to reproduce this tool must request permission from authors. Copyright © 1988 Cronin & Harrison. Reprinted with permission of authors.

REFERENCES

Adereti, S. C., Olaogun, A. A., Olagunju, E. O., & Afolabi, K. E. (2014). Paediatric patients and primary care givers' perception of nurse-caring behavior in south western Nigeria. *International Journal of Caring Sciences, 7*(2), 610–620.

Ayala, R. A., & Calvo, M. J. (2017). Cultural adaptation and validation of the Caring Behaviors Assessment tool in Chile. *Nursing & Health Science, 19*(4), 459–466. doi:10.1111/nhs.12364

Bagnall, L. A. (2017). *A quantitative analysis of BSN and ASN nursing students' caring attributes.* Available from ProQuest Dissertations Publishing. (UMI No. 10288579)

Bakar, A., Nursalam, Adriani, M., Kusnanto, Qomariah, S. N., Hidayati, L., . . . Ni'mah, L. (2017). Nurses' spirituality improves caring behavior. *International Journal of Evaluation and Research in Education, 6*(1), 23–30. doi:10.11591/ijere.v6i1.6343

Balboni, M., & Peteet, J. (Eds.). (2017). *Spirituality and religion within the culture of medicine: From evidence to practice*. New York, NY: Oxford University Press.

Baldursdottir, G., & Jonsdottir, H. (2002). The importance of nurse caring behaviors as perceived by patients receiving care at an emergency department. *Heart & Lung, 31*(1), 67–75. doi:10.1067/mhl.2002.119835

Brown, C., Holcomb, L., Maloney, J., Naranjo, J., Gibson, C., & Russell, P. (2005). Caring in action: The patient care facilitator role. *International Journal for Human Caring, 9*(3), 51–58. doi:10.20467/1091-5710.9.3.51

Cronin, S., & Harrison, B. (1988). Importance of nurse caring behaviors as perceived by patients after myocardial infarction. *Heart and Lung, 17*(4), 374–380.

Dorsey, C., Phillips, K. D., & Williams, C. (2001). Adult sickle cell patients' perceptions of nurses' caring behaviors. *The Association of Black Nursing Faculty (ABNF) Journal, 12*(5), 95–100.

Drake, J. (2016). *Tools that measure caring: A systematic literature review of the impact of caring*. Available from ProQuest Dissertations Publishing. (UMI No. 10106266)

Fishman, G. A. (2018). Attending registered nurses: Evolving role perceptions in clinical care teams. *Nursing Economic$, 36*(1), 12–22.

Gay, S. (1999). Meeting cardiac patients' expectations of caring. *Dimensions of Critical Care Nursing, 18*(4), 46–50. doi:10.1097/00003465-199907000-00012

Gillespie, G. L., Hounchell, M., Pettinichi, J., Mattei, J., & Rose, L. (2012). Caring in pediatric emergency nursing. *Research and Theory for Nursing Practice: An International Journal, 26*(3), 216–232. doi:10.1891/1541-6577.26.3.216

Hogan, B. K. (2015). *Professional rationality and the emotional labor of gendered caring in nursing* (Order No. 3739871). Available from Nursing and Allied Health Database; ProQuest Dissertations and Theses Global. (UMI No. 1750068860)

Huggins, K., Gandy, W., & Kohut, C. (1993). Emergency department patient perceptions of nurse caring behaviors. *Heart and Lung, 22*(4), 356–364.

Kuis, E. E., Hesselink, G., & Goossensen, A. (2014). Can quality from a care ethical perspective be assessed? A review. *Nursing Ethics, 21*(7), 774–793. doi:10.1177/0969733013500163

Kwak, S. Y., & Lee, B. S. (2018). Role adaptation process of Hospice nurses. *Journal of Korean Academic Nursing Administration, 24*(2), 149–160. doi:10.11111/jkana.2018.24.2.149

Labrague, L. J. (2012). Caring competencies of baccalaureate nursing students of Samar State University. *Journal of Nursing Education and Practice, 2*(4), 105–113. doi:10.5430/jnep.v2n4p105

Mahmoudi, H., Mohmmadi, E., & Ebadi, A. (2017). The meaning of emergency care in the Iranian Nursing Profession. *Critical Care Nursing Journal, 10*(1), e10073. doi:10.5812/ccn.10073

Manogin, T. W., Bechtel, G., & Rami, R. (2000). Caring behaviors by nurses: Women's perceptions during childbirth. *Journal of Obstetric, Gynecologic, and Neonatal Nursing, 29*(2), 153–157. doi:10.1111/j.1552-6909.2000.tb02035.x

Marini, B. (1999). Institutionalized older adults' perceptions of nurse caring behaviors. *Journal of Gerontological Nursing, 25*(5), 11–16. doi:10.3928/0098-9134-19990501-09

Mercer, C. J. (2013). Cultivating nurses' potential to incorporate assessment and minimisation of the consequences of the effects of illness into presence. *Journal of Nursing Education and Practice, 3*(6), 134–140. doi:10.5430/jnep.v3n6p134

Mullins, I. L. (1996). Nurse caring behaviors for persons with AIDS/HIV. *Applied Nursing Research, 9*(1), 18–23. doi:10.1016/S0897-1897(96)80335-1

O'Connell, E., & Landers, M. (2008). The importance of critical care nurses' caring behaviours as perceived by nurses and relatives. *Intensive and Critical Care Nursing, 24*, 349–358. doi:10.1016/j.iccn.2008.04.002

Omari, F. H., AbuAlRub, R., & Ayasreh, I. R. (2013). Perceptions of patients and nurses towards nurse caring behaviors in coronary care units in Jordan. *Journal of Clinical Nursing, 22,* 3185–3191. doi:10.1111/jocn.12458

Parson, E., Kee, C., & Gray, D. P. (1993). Perioperative nursing caring behaviors. *Association of periOperative Nurses (AORN) Journal, 57*(5), 1106–1114. doi:10.1016/S0001-2092(07)67316-5

Ross-Davie, M., & Cheyne, H. (2014). Intrapartum support: What do women want? *Evidence-Based Midwifery, 12*(2), 52–58.

Ruta, N. S., & Ballas, S. K. (2016). The opioid drug epidemic and sickle cell disease: Guilt by association. *Pain Medicine, 17,* 1793–1798. doi:10.1093/pm/pnw074

Salmani, N., Hasanvand, S., Bagheri, I., & Mandegari, Z. (2017). Nursing care behaviors perceived by parents of hospitalized children: A qualitative study. *International Journal of Pediatrics, 5*(7), 5379–5389. doi:10.22038/IJP.2017.23123.1940

Schultz, A. A., Bridgham, C., Smith, M. E., & Higgins, D. (1998). Perceptions of caring: Comparison of antepartum and postpartum patients. *Clinical Nursing Research, 7,* 363–378. doi:10.1177/105477389800700404

Shinan-Altman, S., & Ayalon, L. (2017). If I am not for myself, who is for me? The experiences of older migrant home care recipients during their hospitalization. *Aging & Mental Health, 21*(2), 182–189. doi:10.1080/13607863.2015.1093604

Stanfield, M. H. (1991). Watson's caring theory and instrument development (Order No. DA 9203096. 158 pp.). *Dissertation Abstracts International, 52*(8), 4128-B.

Suliman, W. A., Welmann, E., Omer, T., & Thomas, L. (2009). Applying Watson's nursing theory to assess patient perceptions of being cared for in a multicultural environment. *Journal of Nursing Research, 17*(4), 295–300. doi:10.1097/JNR.0b013e3181c122a3

Sunaryo, H., Nirwanto, N., & Manan, A. (2017). The effect of emotional and spiritual intelligence on nurses' burnout and caring behavior. *International Journal of Academic Research in Business and Social Sciences, 7*(12), 1211–1227. doi:10.6007/ijarbss/v7-i12/3753

Watson, J. (1985). *Nursing: The philosophy and science of caring* (2nd ed.). Boulder: Associated University Press.

Watson, J. (1988). *Nursing: Human science and human care.* East Norwalk, CT: Appleton-Century-Crofts.

Wolf, Z. R., Zuzelo, P. R., Goldberg, E., Crothers, R., & Jacobsen, N. (2006). The Caring Behaviors Inventory for elders: Development and psychometric characteristics. *International Journal for Human Caring, 10*(1), 50–59. doi:10.20467/1091-5710.10.1.49

Wu, L. M., Chin, C. C., & Chen, C. H. (2009). Evaluation of a caring education program for Taiwanese nursing students: A quasi-experiment with before and after comparison. *Nurse Education Today, 29*(8), 873–878. doi:10.1016/j.nedt.2009.05.006

Yousseif, H. A. M., Mansour, M. A. M., Ayasreh, I., & Al-Mawajdeh, N. A. A. (2013). A medical-surgical nurse's perceptions of caring behavior among hospitals in Taif City. *Life Science Journal, 10*(4), 720–730.

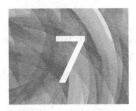

Caring Behaviors of Nurses Scale

Pamela Hinds

The Caring Behaviors of Nurses Scale (CBNS) was developed by Hinds (1988) as a 22-item visual analog scale. The conceptual framework was derived from the existential theory of nursing (humanistic nursing; Paterson & Zderad, 1976). Such a perspective involves the use of an intersubjective nurse–patient relationship to nurture well-being and personal growth of patients (Hinds, 1988). While the theory guiding the tool was existential, the conceptual basis of caring behaviors on the CBNS was designed to detect nursing caring actions as "the composite of purposeful nursing acts and attitudes which seeks to (1) alleviate undue discomforts and meet anticipated needs of patients, (2) convey concern for the well-being of patients, and (3) communicate professional competence to patients" (Hinds, 1988, p. 22).

The tool was developed to explore and describe the relationship of nurses' caring behaviors with hopefulness and healthcare outcomes in a group of adolescents receiving inpatient treatment for substance abuse. One of the unique features of the development of the CBNS was the relationship Hinds established between the abstract existential theory of humanistic (caring) relationship and the middle-range constructs derived from the theory. In her research with adolescents she made explicit the movement from abstract theory to middle-range constructs; she then theorized the relationships among study variables and anticipated findings. The theory and middle-range constructs were translated into specific items. These items ultimately resulted in empirical measurements based on how closely each one indicates that "your thoughts about the actions of the nurse compare with those on the questionnaire," for example: "Nurses try to help me with worries," "Nurses believe I can succeed," and "Nurses give me support when things go bad." Each item has a possible response range of 0 to 100 points. The higher the score is, the more the patient perceives that he or she is being cared for by

© Springer Publishing Company DOI:10.1891/9780826195425.0007

the nurse. Hinds (1985) indicated the CBNS had face and content validity, form equivalence, and internal consistency.

Hind's study testing the tool was a longitudinal descriptive-correlational design using both quantitative and qualitative methods to "systematically study the relationships specified in the conceptual framework, and to elicit information about change in each concept" (Hinds, 1988, p. 23). The study design had three data collection points with 25 adolescents hospitalized in an inpatient substance abuse treatment unit in the Southwest. The first data collection took place 24 to 28 hours after admission (time 1); the second, 96 to 120 hours before discharge (time 2); and the third, 4 to 5 weeks after discharge from the unit (time 3). A Cronbach's alpha of .86 was reported for the CBNS for both time 1 and time 2. In addition to completing the visual analog instruments, study participants responded to a set of open-ended questions indexing the study concepts. The study using the CBNS provided "support for the theorized link between nurse–patient relationships and positive patient change" (Hinds, 1988, p. 22). The instrument is copyrighted, and the author requests that anyone wishing to use it please contact her. The matrix in Table 7.1 shows the most salient features of the CBNS (Tools 7.1 and 7.2).

TABLE 7.1 Matrix of Caring Behaviors of Nurses Scale

INSTRUMENT	AUTHOR CONTACT INFORMATION	PUBLICATION SOURCE	DEVELOPED TO MEASURE	INSTRUMENT DESCRIPTION	PARTICIPANTS	REPORTED VALIDITY/RELIABILITY	CONCEPTUAL-THEORETICAL BASIS OF MEASUREMENT	LATEST CITATION IN NURSING LITERATURE
Caring Behaviors of Nurses Scale (1985, 1988)	Pamela S. Hinds, PhD, RN, CS Director of Nursing Research St. Jude Children's Research Hospital 332 North Lauderdale Memphis, TN 38105 Email: Pam.Hinds@ stjude .org	Hinds (1988)	Caring behaviors of nurses within intersubjective human relationships	Inductively based 22-item visual analog scale, with possible range of 0 to 100 (highest score indicates the respondent feels more cared for by nurse)	N = 25 Inpatient adolescents in substance abuse treatment unit in the Southwest	Reported to have face and content validity, form equivalence, and internal consistency (Hinds, 1985) Cronbach's alpha of .86 for two data collection points for adolescent study (1988) Pragmatic content analysis and semantic content analysis achieved with pre-established criterion levels of .8 or higher across the data collection points Intercoder reliability and stability	Existential-humanistic nursing (Paterson & Zderad, 1976) Intersubjective relationship of caring	Hinds (1988) Dorsey, Phillips, and Williams (2001)

103

TOOL 7.1

Caring Behaviors of Nurses Scale (Form A)

1. **Nurses try to help me with worries.**

   NEVER TRUE FOR ME   ALWAYS TRUE FOR ME

2. **Nurses believe I can succeed.**

   NEVER TRUE FOR ME   ALWAYS TRUE FOR ME

3. **Nurses point out positive things about me.**

   NEVER TRUE FOR ME   ALWAYS TRUE FOR ME

4. **Nurses say I won't have a good future.**

   NEVER TRUE FOR ME   ALWAYS TRUE FOR ME

5. **Nurses give me their suggestions.**

   NEVER TRUE FOR ME   ALWAYS TRUE FOR ME

6. **Nurses are not interested in what I think.**

   NEVER TRUE FOR ME   ALWAYS TRUE FOR ME

7. **Nurses tell me there is a chance if I try.**

   NEVER TRUE FOR ME   ALWAYS TRUE FOR ME

8. **Nurses point out what things could happen to me in the future.**

   NEVER TRUE FOR ME   ALWAYS TRUE FOR ME

9. **Nurses don't try to understand me.**

   NEVER TRUE FOR ME   ALWAYS TRUE FOR ME

10. **When I am upset, nurses help me get my mind off bad things.**

    NEVER TRUE FOR ME   ALWAYS TRUE FOR ME

11. **Nurses do not trust me.**

    NEVER TRUE FOR ME   ALWAYS TRUE FOR ME

12. **Nurses talk to me about things I don't understand.**

    NEVER TRUE FOR ME   ALWAYS TRUE FOR ME

13. **Nurses tell me I can pull myself out of it.**

    NEVER TRUE FOR ME   ALWAYS TRUE FOR ME

14. **Nurses don't point out my progress.**

    NEVER TRUE FOR ME   ALWAYS TRUE FOR ME

15. **Because of the nurses, I know I'm not alone.**

    NEVER TRUE FOR ME   ALWAYS TRUE FOR ME

16. **Nurses don't support my efforts to get better.**

    NEVER TRUE FOR ME   ALWAYS TRUE FOR ME

17. **Nurses are honest with me.**

    NEVER TRUE FOR ME   ALWAYS TRUE FOR ME

18. **Nurses refuse to help me with my problems.**

    NEVER TRUE FOR ME   ALWAYS TRUE FOR ME

(continued)

TOOL 7.1

Caring Behaviors of Nurses Scale (Form A) (*continued*)

19. **If nurses see what I don't see, they point it out to me.**
    NEVER TRUE FOR ME   ALWAYS TRUE FOR ME

20. **Nurses tell me if I work at it, things will get better.**
    NEVER TRUE FOR ME   ALWAYS TRUE FOR ME

21. **Nurses don't seem to care about my getting well.**
    NEVER TRUE FOR ME   ALWAYS TRUE FOR ME

22. **Nurses believe I can change.**
    NEVER TRUE FOR ME   ALWAYS TRUE FOR ME

TOOL 7.2

Caring Behaviors of Nurses Scale (Form B)

1. **Nurses talk with me about my problems.**
   NEVER TRUE FOR ME   ALWAYS TRUE FOR ME

2. **The nurses believe in me.**
   NEVER TRUE FOR ME   ALWAYS TRUE FOR ME

3. **Nurses point out good things about me.**
   NEVER TRUE FOR ME   ALWAYS TRUE FOR ME

4. **Nurses tell me my future won't be good.**
   NEVER TRUE FOR ME   ALWAYS TRUE FOR ME

5. **Nurses give me advice.**
   NEVER TRUE FOR ME   ALWAYS TRUE FOR ME

6. **Nurses are not willing to listen to me.**
   NEVER TRUE FOR ME   ALWAYS TRUE FOR ME

7. **Nurses tell me life is worth it if I try.**
   NEVER TRUE FOR ME   ALWAYS TRUE FOR ME

8. **Nurses point out what my future could be like.**
   NEVER TRUE FOR ME   ALWAYS TRUE FOR ME

9. **Nurses don't show any interest in helping me.**
   NEVER TRUE FOR ME   ALWAYS TRUE FOR ME

10. **Nurses give me support when things go bad.**
    NEVER TRUE FOR ME   ALWAYS TRUE FOR ME

11. **Nurses don't let me make my own decisions.**
    NEVER TRUE FOR ME   ALWAYS TRUE FOR ME

12. **Nurses explain things when I don't see why something happened.**
    NEVER TRUE FOR ME   ALWAYS TRUE FOR ME

(*continued*)

TOOL 7.2

Caring Behaviors of Nurses Scale (Form B) (*continued*)

13. Nurses tell me it's not useless.

NEVER TRUE FOR ME   ALWAYS TRUE FOR ME

14. Nurses don't point out positive change in me.

NEVER TRUE FOR ME   ALWAYS TRUE FOR ME

15. Nurses help by just being around.

NEVER TRUE FOR ME   ALWAYS TRUE FOR ME

16. I don't get help from the nurses.

NEVER TRUE FOR ME   ALWAYS TRUE FOR ME

17. I can believe what the nurses say to me.

NEVER TRUE FOR ME   ALWAYS TRUE FOR ME

18. Nurses won't listen to my problems.

NEVER TRUE FOR ME   ALWAYS TRUE FOR ME

19. Nurses point out things I hadn't thought of.

NEVER TRUE FOR ME   ALWAYS TRUE FOR ME

**20. Nurses tell me something good will happen if
I try to make things better.**

NEVER TRUE FOR ME   ALWAYS TRUE FOR ME

21. Nurses don't seem hopeful for me to do well.

NEVER TRUE FOR ME   ALWAYS TRUE FOR ME

22. Nurses think there is hope for me.

NEVER TRUE FOR ME   ALWAYS TRUE FOR ME

Thank you very much for participating!

Source: ©Pamela S. Hinds, Phd, RN, CS. Reprinted with permission of author.

REFERENCES

Dorsey, C., Phillips, K. D., & Williams, C. (2001). Adult sickle cell patients' perceptions of nurses' caring behaviors. *Association of Black Nursing Faculty (ABNF) Journal, 12*(5), 95–100.

Hinds, P. S. (1985). An investigation of the relationship between adolescent hopefulness, caring behaviors of nurses and adolescent health care outcomes. *Dissertation Abstracts International*, 4012. (UMI No. 8522813)

Hinds, P. S. (1988). The relationship of nurses' caring behaviors with hopefulness and health care outcomes in adolescents. *Archives of Psychiatric Nursing, 2*(1), 21–29.

Paterson, J. G., & Zderad, L. T. (1976). *Humanistic nursing*. New York, NY: Wiley.

Professional Caring Behaviors

Sharon D. Horner

The Professional Caring Behaviors (PCB) is considered a first-generation measurement instrument. A preliminary instrument was developed based on 356 patients' descriptions of caring and noncaring nurse behaviors collected between 1986 and 1988. Ten themes emerged from the patient data and were supplemented by four additional themes identified through a review of literature and content expert review. The themes were use of touch, individualizing practice, listening, interest, explaining, use of time, use of voice, presence, facial expression, level of concern, family involvement, spirituality, managing the environment, and technical proficiency.

Two positive and two negative caring items were generated for each of the 14 themes and used to develop two forms of the PCB instrument (one for patients and one for nurses), each with 28 items. The PCB uses a 4-point Likert scale that ranges from "strongly agree" to "strongly disagree." A panel of four nurse experts reviewed the items to establish content validity. In 1989, Horner conducted pilot tests using the instrument. Test-retest reliability over a 2-week period was assessed by undergraduate nursing students and was found to be strong ($r = .81$). This was followed by a pilot test with a convenience sample of nurses ($N = 31$) and adult patients ($N = 27$) that demonstrated internal consistency of .92 on form A (see Tool 8.1) and .90 on form B of the PCB (see Tool 8.2). There were significant differences between nurses' and patients' assessments of nurse-caring behaviors ($p < .05$). Thereafter, equivalence of the two PCB forms was tested with 224 nurses; comparable descriptive statistics for form A ($M = 101.95$, $SD = 8.12$, $\alpha = .92$) and form B ($M = 102.10$, $SD = 8.75$, $\alpha = .94$), and no significant difference between respondents' scores on the two forms, were found. Pearson's correlations between the item pairs (negative item, positive item) for each of the 14 themes were significantly correlated at $p < .001$. In 1991, Horner administered the PCB to 403 nurses and 394 laypersons to further evaluate the instrument.

Scores were subjected to principal axis component extraction and yielded a single factor with an eigenvalue of 9.36 that accounted for 33.4% of the variance. All 28 items loaded on factor 1, with factor loadings between .46 and .68.

Harrison (1995) further refined the PCB in a study with nurses and the family members of patients. Only one item, "The caring nurse respects the patient's spiritual beliefs," was significantly more important to nurses than to family members. This is consistent with other studies that have found differences between nurses' and others' rating of caring.

Roberts (1997) examined the associations between moral voice, PCB, and the feeling dimension on the Myers–Briggs Inventory with nursing students ($N = 61$) just entering their professional program of study. Pearson's correlations between the total scores on forms A and B of the PCB were $r = .73$ ($p = .01$). Roberts reported significant correlations between students' scores on altruism ($r = .33$), the value of caring ($r = .42$), and PCB total scores, and a nonsignificant inverse relationship between students' moral voice scores and PCB total scores ($r = -.16$).

The instruments are provided with this chapter. Dr. Horner requests that she be contacted when the instrument is used and provided with a summary report of findings.

TOOL 8.1

Professional Caring Behaviors—Form A

Directions: Read each statement, then indicate the degree to which you agree or disagree that the statement indicates professional caring.

Strongly Disagree = SD; Disagree = D; Agree = A; Strongly Agree = SA

1. The caring nurse explains things in a way that is over the patient's head.	SD	D	A	SA
2. The caring nurse uses a gentle tone of voice during procedures.	SD	D	A	SA
3. The caring nurse takes a few minutes just to talk.	SD	D	A	SA
4. The caring nurse understands and shares in the patient's experiences.	SD	D	A	SA
5. The caring nurse is poorly organized when providing care.	SD	D	A	SA
6. The caring nurse touches patients roughly when they are hurting.	SD	D	A	SA
7. The caring nurse seems to be "going through the motions" without any real feeling.	SD	D	A	SA
8. The caring nurse straightens up patient rooms to look nicer.	SD	D	A	SA
9. The caring nurse enters rooms without knocking.	SD	D	A	SA

(continued)

TOOL 8.1

Professional Caring Behaviors—Form A (*continued*)

10. The caring nurse listens carefully to complaints.	SD	D	A	SA
11. The caring nurse learns of patients' special needs.	SD	D	A	SA
12. The caring nurse gives shots in a manner that causes patients less pain and stress.	SD	D	A	SA
13. The caring nurse speaks in a harsh manner.	SD	D	A	SA
14. The caring nurse expresses concern for patients.	SD	D	A	SA
15. The caring nurse does not show real interest in patients' problems.				
16. The caring nurse takes time with patients' families.	SD	D	A	SA
17. The caring nurse does not attend to patients' spiritual beliefs.	SD	D	A	SA
18. The caring nurse remembers patients as real people.	SD	D	A	SA
19. The caring nurse is abrupt and hurried in completing work.	SD	D	A	SA
20. The caring nurses looks unfriendly at patients.	SD	D	A	SA
21. The caring nurse does not give information to patient's family.	SD	D	A	SA
22. The caring nurse is not concerned about patient problems.	SD	D	A	SA
23. The caring nurse leaves soiled linens and dressings in patients' rooms.	SD	D	A	SA
24. The caring nurse touches the patient appropriately.	SD	D	A	SA
25. The caring nurse gives carefully thought-out answers.	SD	D	A	SA
26. The caring nurse respects patients' spiritual needs.	SD	D	A	SA
27. The caring nurse does not listen when patients talk about problems and concerns.	SD	D	A	SA
28. The caring nurse gives warm smiles.	SD	D	A	SA

TOOL 8.2

Professional Caring Behaviors—Form B

Directions: Read each statement, then indicate the degree to which you agree or disagree that the statement indicates professional caring.

Strongly Disagree =SD; Disagree =D; Agree =A; Strongly Agree = SA

1. The caring nurse does a procedure without an explanation.	SD D A SA
2. The caring nurse leaves soiled equipment in the patient's room.	SD D A SA
3. The caring nurse's face reflects kindness and concern.	SD D A SA
4. The caring nurse answers the call light in a short period of time.	SD D A SA
5. The caring nurse is well organized.	SD D A SA
6. The caring nurse treats patients like objects.	SD D A SA
7. The caring nurse talks in a warm friendly manner.	SD D A SA
8. The caring nurse gives support to patients' families.	SD D A SA
9. The caring nurse gives opinions without regard for the patient's spiritual beliefs.	SD D A SA
10. The caring nurse is concerned with patients' problems.	SD D A SA
11. The caring nurse ignores patients when they are upset or crying.	SD D A SA
12. The caring nurse shows interest when patients describe problems.	SD D A SA
13. The caring nurse answers before patients have finished talking.	SD D A SA
14. The caring nurse takes a long time to bring pain medication.	SD D A SA
15. The caring nurse finds some way to make the patient's room more pleasant.	SD D A SA
16. The caring nurse moves patients roughly.	SD D A SA
17. The caring nurse seldom smiles.	SD D A SA
18. The caring nurse stays with patients who are experiencing discomfort.	SD D A SA
19. The caring nurse does not look at patients while doing routine procedures.	SD D A SA
20. The caring nurse listens to patients' problems when they need to talk.	SD D A SA
21. The caring nurse gives clear explanations about procedures, tests, and medicines.	SD D A SA
22. The caring nurse ignores the patient's family.	SD D A SA
23. The caring nurse touches patients in a supportive manner.	SD D A SA

(continued)

TOOL 8.2

Professional Caring Behaviors—Form B (*continued*)

24. The caring nurse respects patient's spiritual beliefs.	SD	D	A	SA
25. The caring nurse speaks in a loud sharp voice.	SD	D	A	SA
26. The caring nurse has trouble managing equipment.	SD	D	A	SA
27. The caring nurse calls patients by their proper name.	SD	D	A	SA
28. The caring nurse does not appear concerned by patients' complaints.	SD	D	A	SA

REFERENCES

Harrison, E. (1995). Nurse caring and the new health care paradigm. *Journal of Nursing Care Quality, 9*(4), 14–23. doi:10.1097/00001786-199507000-00004

Roberts, H. T. (1997). The measurement of caring relationships in associate degree nursing students (Doctoral dissertation, Iowa State University). *Dissertation Abstracts International, 58*(06), 2108A. (UMI No. PUZ 9737752)

REFERENCES

Nyberg Caring
Assessment Scale

Jan Nyberg

Nyberg's Caring Assessment (also referred to as the Caring Attributes Scale, or CAS) was developed based on caring attributes reported in the literature. Nyberg (1990) reports basing scale development on the work of Watson and "theoretically related caring theorists," including Mayeroff and Noddings. She was interested in the effects of caring and economics on nursing practice. It is interesting that her instrument is not focused on behavior but on attributes, which she uses in an attempt to philosophically and operationally capture the subjective aspect of caring. The caring attributes are such dimensions as deep respect for the needs of others, a belief that others have potential, and commitment to relationship. In developing the tool, she focused on the human care element of nursing. For example, items from the carative factors (Watson, 1979) are helping/trusting relationship, understanding spiritual aspects, solving problems creatively, and being sensitive to self and others sustaining hope.

The original instrument was formulated during Nyberg's doctoral studies at the University of Colorado. The original questions for the instrument were derived directly from the literature: the first seven items from Watson's (1979, 1985) carative factors, and the others from Gaut (1984), Noddings (1984), and Mayeroff (1971).

Since the instrument was an outcome of the author's doctoral studies, the literature review was vigorous and extensive. The conceptual definitions became the operational definitions as the questionnaire was developed. Thus construct and content validity were the outcome of the method of development of this measurement scale.

In the original study, Nyberg developed the Nyberg Caring Assessment Scale for the purpose of finding out if the caring attributes were important to the study subjects, how the nurses actually used the caring attributes, and how

© Springer Publishing Company DOI:10.1891/9780826195425.0009

their supervisors used them. The questionnaires were sent to nurses at multiple hospitals. That made it possible to study the data from unit to unit, from staff and supervisors, and from hospital to hospital. By also collecting information about economic factors at the hospitals (using hours per patient day), the researcher was able to use correlation coefficients to see if hospitals with higher caring scores have more hours of patient care.

Three hundred fifty questionnaires were sent to a random sample of nurses, and 135 were returned. The overall population from which this random sample was drawn consisted of 22,793 nurses from seven hospitals. During the developmental work on the questionnaire, a Cronbach's alpha of .80 to .97 was found. During the actual study, 135 returned questionnaires had an alpha of .85 to .97. Table 9.1 provides a matrix for Nyberg's CAS (Tool 9.1).

The Nyberg Caring Assessment Scale was first published in 1990. Since that time, the author has received dozens of requests to use the scale from scholars and practicing nurses around the world. In the majority of cases, the questionnaire has been used to measure the results of changing nursing practice, such as the implementation of primary nursing or relationship-centered nursing. While permission to use the scale was given in all instances, reports of the results of the studies were not provided.

Construct and content validity were achieved through the development of the questionnaire; however, there is very little information available on construct validity. This instrument has potential for further use and refinement, but to date, the use of the CAS has not been reported in additional research studies. The instrument is copyrighted, and the author requests that she be contacted for permission and advice regarding its use.

TABLE 9.1 Matrix of Nyberg Caring Assessment Scale

INSTRUMENT	PUBLICATION SOURCE	DEVELOPED TO MEASURE	INSTRUMENT DESCRIPTION	PARTICIPANTS	REPORTED VALIDITY/ RELIABILITY	CONCEPTUAL-THEORETICAL BASIS OF MEASUREMENT	LATEST CITATION IN NURSING LITERATURE
Nyberg Caring Assessment Scale (1989, 1990)	Nyberg (1990)	Caring attributes of nurses (more subjective human element than behaviors)	20 items on 5-point Likert Scale Four separate rating scales on items	N = 135 nurses from a random sample mailing of questionnaire	Cronbach's alpha reported at .87–.98 No discussion of construct or content validity, except use of theory factors, previously tested (Cronin & Harrison, 1988)	Draws directly from caring theory literature Specific items from Watson's carative factors and others from Noddings, Gaut, and Mayeroff	Nyberg (1990) McCartan and Hargie (2004)

TOOL 9.1

Nyberg Caring Assessment Scale

Are these caring attributes things you actually use in your day-to-day practice?

Always use in practice 5

Often use in practice 4

Sometimes use in practice 3

Occasionally use in practice 2

Cannot use in practice 1

Do you:

	1	2	3	4	5
1. Have deep respect for the needs of others.					
2. Not give up hope for others.					
3. Remain sensitive to the needs of others.					
4. Communicate a helping, trusting attitude toward others.					
5. Express positive and negative feelings.					
6. Solve problems creatively.					
7. Understand that spiritual forces contribute to human care.					
8. Consider relationships before rules.					
9. Base decisions on what is best for the people involved.					
10. Understand thoroughly what situations mean to people.					
11. Go beyond the superficial to know people well.					
12. Implement skills and techniques well.					
13. Choose tactics that will accomplish goals.					
14. Give full consideration to situational factors.					
15. Focus on helping others to grow.					
16. Take time for personal needs and growth.					
17. Allow time for caring opportunities.					
18. Remain committed to a continuing relationship.					
19. Listen carefully and be open to feedback.					
20. Believe that others have a potential that can be achieved.					

Source: Reprinted with permission of the author. ©Copyright Nyberg.

REFERENCES

Gaut, D. A. (1984). A theoretic description of caring as action. In M. M. Leininger (Ed.), *Care: The essence of nursing and health* (pp. 27–44). Thorofare, NJ: Charles B. Slack.

Mayeroff, M. (1971). *On caring.* New York, NY: Harper & Row.

McCartan, P. H., & Hargie, O. D. (2004). Assertiveness and caring: Are they compatible? *Journal of Clinical Nursing, 13*(6), 707–713. doi:10.1111/j.1365-2702.2004.00964.x

Noddings, N. (1984). *Caring: A feminine approach to ethics and moral development.* Berkeley, CA: University of California Press.

Nyberg, J. (1990). The effects of care and economics on nursing practice. *Journal of Nursing Administration, 20*(5), 13–18. doi:10.1097/00005110-199005000-00006

Watson, J. (1979). *Nursing: The philosophy and science of caring.* Boston, MA: Little, Brown.

Watson, J. (1985). *Nursing: Human science and human care.* Norwalk, CT: Appleton-Century-Crofts.

Caring Ability Inventory

Ngozi O. Nkongho

The Caring Ability Inventory (CAI) was developed by Nkongho (1990) to measure the ability to care when one is involved in a relationship with others. The conceptual basis for the instrument was derived from caring literature and the author's identification of four theoretical assumptions: (1) caring is multidimensional (with attitudinal and cognitive components); (2) the potential to care is present in all individuals; (3) caring can be learned; and (4) caring is quantifiable. Other aspects of caring are drawn upon as background for the instrument, but the direct conceptual influence was Mayeroff's (1971) view of caring: "helping another to grow and actualize himself . . . a way of relating to someone that involves development" (p. 23). Other indicators of caring from Mayeroff that informed the development of the instrument are knowing, alternating rhythm, patience, honesty, trust, humility, hope, and courage (Nkongho, 1990).

During the early developmental stages of the CAI, Mayeroff's framework was used to formulate the original items. Items were derived in two ways: through a review of caring literature, which yielded 61 items, and through the development of 10 open-ended questions that were asked of 15 consenting adults. Nineteen additional items were derived from these 15 interviews; thus, the first version consisted of a total of 80 items—34 positive statements and 46 negative statements. The 80 items were placed on a 7-point Likert scale.

The 80-item version was subjected to additional testing with the use of 543 participants and a factor analysis of the items. From this process, subscales emerged that capture aspects such as knowing, courage, and patience, which are congruent with Mayeroff's theory. The knowing subscale has 14 items, the courage subscale has 13 items, and the patience subscale has 10 items. The final version of the CAI consists of 37 items representing three of Mayeroff's theoretical elements of caring. Item responses are summed for each subscale, yielding a total score for each subscale. Higher scores indicate greater degree of caring if the item is positively phrased; scoring is reversed if the item is negatively worded.

Additional reliability and validity were assessed through Cronbach's alphas and test–retest administration (after a 2-week period). The alpha coefficient for each of the subscales ranged from .71 to .84 ($N = 537$); the test–retest r ranged from .64 to .80 ($N = 38$).

Two experts in content area established content validity. Revisions were made and resubmitted to content reviewers, which resulted in a content validity index using the method outlined by Waltz et al. (1984). The content validity index was reported as .80. Construct validity was established by correlation with the Tennessee Self-Concept Scale as well as discrimination between groups (female and male practicing nurses and college students). The t-tests on mean scores of groups were both statistically significant.

The various reliability and validity tests indicate the CAI is both reliable and valid for measuring caring elements of knowing, courage, and patience. As a self-report measure, the CAI is easy to administer and may be used for different professional groups (e.g., engineers, social workers, physicians, and nurses). Identifying individuals on the high or low dimensions of caring may serve as a guide for counseling, guidance, and self-growth. The CAI has potential for use in both academic and clinical settings.

The CAI has sophisticated psychometric properties that support its use and that help to ensure its measurement confidence (Table 10.1; Tool 10.1). The CAI has been used in academic and clinical settings by different national and international professional groups (Cossette, Cote, Pepin, Ricard, & D'Aoust, 2006; Fjortoft, 2003; Hegedus, 1999; Simmons & Cavanaugh, 2000).

TABLE 10.1 Matrix of Caring Ability Inventory

INSTRUMENT	AUTHOR CONTACT INFORMATION	PUBLICATION SOURCE	DEVELOPED TO MEASURE	INSTRUMENT DESCRIPTION	PARTICIPANTS	REPORTED VALIDITY/ RELIABILITY	CONCEPTUAL– THEORETICAL BASIS OF MEASUREMENT	LATEST CITATION IN NURSING LITERATURE
Caring Ability Inventory (1990)	Ngozi O. Nkongho, PhD, RN Associate Professor Lehman College, Department of Nursing The City University of New York Bronx, NY 10468 Phone: 718-960-8794	Nkongho (1990)	Ability to care when involved in relationship	Self-administered 7-point Likert with 37 items	*n* = 462 college students, varied majors	Cronbach's alpha for each factor (range: .71–.84)	General review of caring theory literature	Nkongho (1990)
				Three major factors: knowing, courage, patience	*n* = 75 nurses attending a professional conference	Factor analysis for collapsing items	Development informed by Mayeroff's eight critical elements of caring	
				Measured with subscales		Content validity established with experts	Simmons and Cavanaugh (2000)	
						Test-retest *r* = .64–.80		
						Construct validity between group discrimination and correlation established with Tennessee Self-Concept Scale		
						—	Cossette et al. (2006)	Fjortoft (2000)
				—				Barrera et al. (2006)

121

TOOL 10.1

Caring Ability Inventory

Please read each of the following statements and decide how well it reflects your thoughts and feelings about other people in general. There is no right or wrong answer. Using the response scale, from 1 to 7, circle the degree to which you agree or disagree with each statement directly on the booklet. Please answer all questions.

	1	2	3	4	5	6	7	
	strongly disagree					strongly agree		

	STRONGLY DISAGREE						STRONGLY AGREE
	1	2	3	4	5	6	7
1. I believe that learning takes time.	1	2	3	4	5	6	7
2. Today is filled with opportunities.	1	2	3	4	5	6	7
3. I usually say what I mean to others.	1	2	3	4	5	6	7
4. There is very little I can do for a person who is helpless.	1	2	3	4	5	6	7
5. I can see the need for change in myself.	1	2	3	4	5	6	7
6. I am able to like people even if they don't like me.	1	2	3	4	5	6	7
7. I understand people easily.	1	2	3	4	5	6	7
8. I have seen enough in this world for what I need to know.	1	2	3	4	5	6	7
9. I make the time to get to know other people.	1	2	3	4	5	6	7
10. Sometimes I like to be involved and sometimes I do not like being involved.	1	2	3	4	5	6	7
11. There is nothing I can do to make life better.	1	2	3	4	5	6	7
12. I feel uneasy knowing that another person depends on me.	1	2	3	4	5	6	7
13. I do not like to go out of my way to help other people.	1	2	3	4	5	6	7
14. In dealing with people, it is difficult to let my feelings show.	1	2	3	4	5	6	7
15. It does not matter what I say, as long as I do the correct thing.	1	2	3	4	5	6	7
16. I find it difficult to understand how the other person feels if I have not had similar experiences.	1	2	3	4	5	6	7

(continued)

TOOL 10.1

Caring Ability Inventory (*continued*)

17. I admire people who are calm, composed, and patient.	1	2	3	4	5	6	7
18. I believe it is important to accept and respect the attitudes and feelings of others.	1	2	3	4	5	6	7
19. People can count on me to do what I say I will.	1	2	3	4	5	6	7
20. I believe that there is room for improvement.	1	2	3	4	5	6	7
21. Good friends look after each other.	1	2	3	4	5	6	7
22. I find meaning in every situation.	1	2	3	4	5	6	7
23. I am afraid to "let go" of those I care for because I am afraid of what might happen to them.	1	2	3	4	5	6	7
24. I like to offer encouragement to people.	1	2	3	4	5	6	7
25. I do not like to make commitments beyond the present.	1	2	3	4	5	6	7
26. I really like myself.	1	2	3	4	5	6	7
27. I see strengths and weaknesses (limitations) in each individual.	1	2	3	4	5	6	7
28. New experiences are usually frightening to me.	1	2	3	4	5	6	7
29. I am afraid to be open and let others see who I am.	1	2	3	4	5	6	7
30. I accept people just the way they are.	1	2	3	4	5	6	7
31. When I care for someone else, I do not have to hide my feelings.	1	2	3	4	5	6	7
32. I do not like to be asked for help.	1	2	3	4	5	6	7
33. I can express my feelings to people in a warm and caring way.	1	2	3	4	5	6	7
34. I like talking with people.	1	2	3	4	5	6	7
35. I regard myself as sincere in my relationships with others.	1	2	3	4	5	6	7
36. People need space (room, privacy) to think and feel.	1	2	3	4	5	6	7
37. I can be approached by people at any time.	1	2	3	4	5	6	7

Source: Reprinted with permission of Springer Publishing. Copyright © 1988 Springer Publishing.

TOOL 10.2

Scoring Information

Items to be summed for each subscale:

Knowing: 2, 3, 6, 7, 9, 19, 22, 26, 30, 31, 33, 34, 35, 36
Courage: 4, 8, 11, 12, 13, 14, 15, 16, 23, 25, 28, 29, 32
Patience: 1, 5, 10, 17, 18, 20, 21, 24, 27, 37
Items to be reverse-scored: 4, 8, 11, 12, 13, 14, 15, 16, 23, 25, 28, 29, 32

The nurse group comprised 75 practicing nurses attending a national conference. Participants came from all areas of the country. To determine ranges for low, medium, and high norm scores, .5 standard deviation on either side of the mean was considered to be the middle range of scores. Scores above this were considered high, and scores below this were considered low. See the following table for low, medium, and high norms for the nurse group.

The college students group consisted of 424 females and 103 males attending a large university in metropolitan New York. The students represented a wide variety of ability, ethnic, and socioeconomic groups. Low, medium, and high groups were determined in the same way as previously. See the following table for low, medium, and high norms for female and male college students.

Low, Medium, and High Norms for CAI and Its Subscales for Nurses

SUBSCALE	LOW	MEDIUM	HIGH
Knowing	Below 76.4	76.4–84.0	Above 84.0
Courage	Below 62.5	62.5–74.0	Above 74.0
Patience	Below 61.0	61.0–65.2	Above 65.2
Total CAI	Below 203.1	203.1–220.3	Above 220.3

Low, Medium, and High Norms for CAI and Its Subscales for Female and Male College Students

SUBSCALE	FEMALES (N = 424)			MALES (N = 103)		
	LOW	MEDIUM	HIGH	LOW	MEDIUM	HIGH
Knowing	<68.8	68.8–79.5	>79.5	<64.6	64.6–75.1	>75.11
Courage	<62.14	62.14–73.06	>73.06	<54.41	54.41–66.56	>66.56
Patience	<58.05	58.05–64.35	>64.35	<53.4	53.4–62.4	>62.4
Total CAI	<190.29	190.29–211.12	>211.12	<178.00	178.00–199.36	>199.36

LATEST CITATION IN NURSING LITERATURE

Azócar, S., Rivera Fuentes, N., & Pérez Villalobos, C. (2016). Caring abilities in nursing students from a Chilean traditional university. *Ciencia y Enfermeria, 22,* 117–127. doi:10.4067/S0717-95532016000200009

Benson, G., Martin, L., Ploeg, J., & Wessel, J. (2012). Longitudinal study of emotional intelligence, leadership, and caring in undergraduate nursing students. *Journal of Nursing Education, 51*(2), 95–101. doi:10.3928/01484834-20120113-01

Cheng, L., Liu, Y., Ke, Y., & Wang, W. (2016). Comparison of caring ability between Chinese and American nursing students. *Western Journal of Nursing Research, 39*(2), 290–304. doi:10.1177/0193945916656613

Fjortoft, N. (2004). Caring pharmacists, caring teachers. *American Journal of Pharmaceutical Education, 68*(1), 1–2. doi:10.5688/aj680116

Gutshall, C. (2011). Measuring the ability to care in pre-service teachers. *Southeastern Regional Association of Teacher Educators (SRATE) Journal, 20*(1), 33–41. Retrieved from https://eric.ed.gov/?id=EJ948705

Khalaila, R. (2014). Simulation in nursing education: An evaluation of students' outcomes at their first clinical practice combined with simulations. *Nurse Education Today, 34,* 252–258. doi:10.1016/j.nedt.2013.08.015

Larin, H., Benson, G., Wessel, J., Martin, L., & Ploeg, J. (2014). Changes in emotional-social intelligence, caring, leadership and moral judgment during health science education programs. *Journal of the Scholarship of Teaching and Learning, 14*(1), 26–41. doi:10.14434/josotl.v14i1.3897

Mayeroff, M. (1971). *On caring.* New York, NY: Harper & Row.

Rosanelli, C., da Silva, L., & de Rivero Gutierrez, M. (2016). Cross-cultural adaptation of the Caring Ability Inventory to Portuguese. *Acta Paulista de Enfermagem, 29*(3). doi:10.1590/1982-0194201600048

Waltz, C. F., Strickland, O. L., & Lenz, E. R. (1984). *Measurement in nursing research.* Philadelphia, PA: F. A. Davis.

Zhang, J., Gao, M., Li, W., & Lei, H. (2012). The level of humanistic caring ability among nursing undergraduates. *Chinese Journal of Nursing Education, 2012*(07).

Zhang, Y., Zhang, P., Xu, C., & Kong, L. (2013). Correlation between caring ability of surgical nurses and patient satisfaction in tertiary hospitals. *Journal of Nursing Science, 2013*(14).

REFERENCES

Barrera, O., Galvis, L., Moreno, F., Pinto, A. N., Pinzón, R., Romero, G., & Sánchez, H. (2006). Caring ability of family caregivers of chronically diseased people. *Investigacióny Educación en Enfermería, 24*(1), 36–46.

Cossette, S., Cote, J. K., Pepin, J., Ricard, N., & D'Aoust, L.-X. (2006). A dimensional structure of nurse–patient interaction from a caring perspective: Refinement of the Caring Nurse–Patient Interaction Scale (CNPI Short Scale). *Journal of Advanced Nursing, 55*(2), 198–214. doi:10.1111/j.1365-2648.2006.03895.x

Fjortoft, N. (2000). Caring pharmacists, caring teachers. *American Journal of Pharmaceutical Education, 68*(1), 1–2.

Fjortoft, N., & Zgarrick, D. (2003). An assessment of pharmacists' caring ability. *Journal of the American Pharmacists Association, 43*(4), 483–487. doi:10.1331/154434503322226220

Hegedus, K. S. (1999). Providers' and consumers' perspective of nurses' caring behaviours. *Journal of Advanced Nursing, 30*(5), 1090–1096. doi:10.1046/j.1365-2648.1999.01198.x

Nkongho, N. (1990). The Caring Ability Inventory. In O. L. Strickland & C. R. Waltz (Eds.), *Measurement of nursing outcomes* (Vol. 4, pp. 3–16). New York, NY: Springer Publishing.

Simmons, P. R., & Cavanaugh, S. (2000). Relationships among student and graduate caring ability and professional school climate. *Journal of Professional Nursing, 16*(2), 76–83. doi:10.1016/S8755-7223(00)80019-8

Caring Behavior Checklist and Client Perception of Caring Scale

Anna M. McDaniel and Lisa A. Bagnall

The Caring Behavior Checklist (CBC) and the Client Perception of Caring Scale (CPC) were developed by McDaniel (1990) to measure caring behaviors of nurses as they care for clients. As conceptual background for the instrument development, McDaniel (1990) distinguished between the notions of caring for and caring about. The process of caring (which involves caring about) was conceptualized at four levels:

■ Acknowledgment of need for care (involves existential I–thou relationship)

■ Decision to care (involves commitment on behalf of well-being of other)

■ Actions (acts and behaviors intended to promote welfare of other—external manifestations of internal processes)

■ Actualization (ultimate result of caring process and perception of other as being cared for and about—satisfaction in both nurse and other)

For development of the instruments, caring behaviors were defined as those verbal and nonverbal actions denoting care performed by the nurse—this was operationalized based on the subjective and affective responses of clients to the nurse's caring behaviors (Table 11.1). The differences in what defines caring behaviors and how they are demonstrated are noted in the verbal and nonverbal acts a nurse uses to convey concern for client safety and well-being (Papastavrou et al., 2012). The CBC (Tool 11.1) was designed to measure the presence or absence of specific actions denoting care, not to quantify the degree or amount of care (McDaniel, 1990). The CPC (Tool 11.2) is a questionnaire designed to measure the client's response to the caring behaviors of the nurse. The items for the CPC were developed from studies that described clients' reactions to nurse–client interactions, in order to get at the more essential structure of the caring interaction as experienced by the client. The CPC is administered to the client after the observation period. This tool has 10 items, which respondents are asked to rate on a 6-point rating scale; items are summed to obtain the score. The potential range of scores is from 10 to 60; high scores indicate a high degree of caring as perceived by the client, and low scores indicate a low degree of caring as perceived by the client.

The CBC consists of 12 items that represent caring behaviors. It requires a trained observer to score a nurse–client interaction for a period of 30 minutes; each behavior is dichotomously scored as either present or absent. The range of scores is from 0 to 12; high scores indicate a high number of behaviors were observed; low scores indicate a low number of observed caring behaviors.

The two instruments were designed to be used together to capture the caring process. They were originally intended for hospital-setting use and administration. However, the CBC and CPC may be adapted for use in the simulation environment for measuring and facilitating the development of caring behaviors in nursing students. Dunnington and Farmer's (2015) study showed that incorporating caring scenarios within simulation increased caring behaviors in Bachelor of Science in Nursing (BSN) students. However, transpersonal caring behaviors and attention to the human spirit had the lowest scores (Dunnington & Farmer, 2015). The researchers indicated that interacting with a mannequin and not a human may be the reason for these low scores. Additional research is needed to better understand the relationship among teaching theoretical concepts of caring, simulation exercises, and the subsequent effects on caring behaviors in nursing students.

Both reliability and validity were established for both instruments. The content validity index described by Waltz and associates (1984) was used to determine content validity for Caring Behaviors Checklist. Content validity was calculated as .80. Reliability of CPC was established with internal consistency, with standardized item alpha calculated as .81. Item-to-total correlation averaged .41. Reliability of the CBC was determined through interrater agreements. Two trained raters simultaneously scored the items independently on each of the 21 interactions. Agreement on each of the 12 items ranged from .76 to 1.00; 8 of the 12 items had scores of .90 or above. Efforts to estimate construct validity by correlating the CPC against the Empathy Scale (LaMonica, 1981) were not conclusive, possibly due to the low number of subjects.

Studies from 2007 onward have shown that the CBC and CPC instruments remain valid and reliable instruments for identifying caring behaviors and the correlated patient perception of nursing caring. The two instruments used together continue to show promise for capturing external behaviors as well as client perceptions around a shared caring occasion. New studies using patient-reported outcomes for confirming construct validity are recommended. The instruments are copyrighted by the author. Anyone using these instruments should contact the author for permission. The matrix in Table 11.1 outlines key properties of both instruments.

TABLE 11.1 Matrix of Caring Behavior Checklist and Client Perception of Caring Scale

INSTRUMENT	AUTHOR CONTACT INFORMATION	PUBLICATION SOURCE	DEVELOPED TO MEASURE	INSTRUMENT DESCRIPTION	PARTICIPANTS	REPORTED VALIDITY/ RELIABILITY	CONCEPTUAL– THEORETICAL BASIS OF MEASUREMENT	LATEST CITATION IN NURSING LITERATURE
Caring Behavior Checklist	Anna McDaniel, PhD, RN, FAAN Dean and the Linda Harman Aiken Professor University of Florida College of Nursing, Gainesville, Florida Email: annammcdaniel@ufl.edu Phone: 352-273-6324	McDaniel (1990)	Caring processes (external observable)	12 items of observable behavior; dichotomous scoring of each item by trained observers	105 BSN students from two traditional BSN programs	Interrater reliability .92 overall of 12 items Content validity index .80	Informed by philosophical views in general caring literature Interest in *caring about* as well as *caring for* guided instrument development	Dunnington and Farmer (2015) Jasmine (2007) Owens (2006)
Client Perception of Caring Scale	Anna McDaniel, PhD, RN, FAAN Dean and Linda Harman Aiken Professor University of Florida College of Nursing, Gainesville, Florida Email: annammcdaniel@ufl.edu Phone: 352-273-6324	McDaniel (1990)	Client's perceptions of nursing caring (detect both caring and noncaring behavior as perceived by clients)	Designed to be used with CBC in hospital setting 10 items rated on 6-point scale (scores ranging from 10 to 60)	Junior-level nursing students in BS nursing program (*N* not given)	Content validity index = 1.00 Alpha .81 reliability Item-to-total correlation .41 Construct validity not significant after correlation with empathy scale	General caring theory literature Conceptual model of caring process developed to guide instrument	Jasmine (2007) Owens (2006)

TOOL 11.1

Caring Behavior Checklist

Directions: Observe the nurse–client interaction for 30 minutes. Check whether the following behaviors were present (check 1) or absent (check 0).

VERBAL CARING BEHAVIORS	ABSENT (0)	PRESENT (1)
Verbally responds to an expressed concern.		
Explains procedure prior to initiation.		
Verbally validates patient's physical status.		
Verbally validates patient's emotional status.		
Shares personal observations or feelings (self-disclosing) in response to patient's expression of concern.		
Verbally reassures patient during care.		
Discusses topics of patient's concern other than current health problems.		
NONVERBAL CARING BEHAVIORS		
Sits down at bedside.		
Touches patient exclusive of procedure.		
Sustains eye contact during patient interaction.		
Enters patient room without solicitation.		
Provides physical comfort measures.		

TOOL 11.2

Client Perception of Caring Scale

Directions: Please rate your interpretation of the following items. The scale ranges from (1) not at all to (6) very much.

1. I felt that this nurse really listened to what I was saying.

1	2	3	4	5	6
☐	☐	☐	☐	☐	☐
Not at all					Very much

2. I felt reassured when this nurse cared for me.

1	2	3	4	5	6
☐	☐	☐	☐	☐	☐
Not at all					Very much

3. I felt that this nurse really valued me as an individual.

1	2	3	4	5	6
☐	☐	☐	☐	☐	☐
Not at all					Very much

4. I felt free to talk to this nurse about what concerned me.

1	2	3	4	5	6
☐	☐	☐	☐	☐	☐
Not at all					Very much

5. I felt the nurse could tell when something was bothering me.

1	2	3	4	5	6
☐	☐	☐	☐	☐	☐
Not at all					Very much

6. I felt this nurse was more interested in his/her "job" than my needs.

1	2	3	4	5	6
☐	☐	☐	☐	☐	☐
Not at all					Very much

(continued)

TOOL 11.2

Caring Behaviors Inventory (*continued*)

7. I felt secure with this nurse taking care of me.

1	2	3	4	5	6
☐	☐	☐	☐	☐	☐
Not at all					Very much

8. I felt frustrated by this nurse's attitude.

1	2	3	4	5	6
☐	☐	☐	☐	☐	☐
Not at all					Very much

9. I could tell this nurse really cared about me.

1	2	3	4	5	6
☐	☐	☐	☐	☐	☐
Not at all					Very much

10. I could tell that this nurse wanted to make me feel comfortable.

1	2	3	4	5	6
☐	☐	☐	☐	☐	☐
Not at all					Very much

REFERENCES

Dunnington, R. M., & Farmer, S. R. (2015). Caring behaviors among student nurses interacting in scenario-based high fidelity human patient simulation. *International Journal for Human Caring, 19*(4), 44–49. doi:10.20467/1091-5710-19.4.44

Jasmine, T. (2007). *The elderly client's perception of caring behaviors.* Retrieved from https://search.proquest.com/docview/304721621?pq-origsite=gscholar

LaMonica, E. (1981). Construct validity of an empathy instrument. *Research in Nursing and Health, 4,* 389–400. doi:10.1002/nur.4770040406

McDaniel, A. M. (1990). The caring process in nursing: Two instruments for measuring caring behaviors. In O. Strickland & C. Waltz (Eds.), *Measurement of nursing outcomes* (pp. 17–27). New York, NY: Springer Publishing.

Owens, R. S. (2006). The caring behaviors of the home health nurse and influence of medication adherence. *Home Healthcare Nurse, 24*(8), 517–526. doi:10.1097/00004045-200609000-00010

Papastavrou, E., Efstathiou, G., Tsangari, H., Suhonen, R., Leino-Kilpi, H., Patiraki, E., . . . Merkouris, A. (2012). A cross-cultural study of the concept of caring through behaviours: Patients' and nurses' perspectives in six different EU countries. *Journal of Advanced Nursing, 68,* 1026–1037. doi:10.1111/j.1365-2648.2011.05807.x

Waltz, C. F., Strickland, O. L., & Lenz, E. R. (1984). *Measurement in nursing research.* Philadelphia, PA: F. A. Davis.

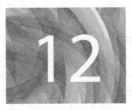

Caring Assessment Tools: CAT-V, CAT-Admin, and CAT-Edu

Joanne R. Duffy

Background

The Caring Assessment Tools (Caring Assessment Tool [CAT], Caring Assessment Tool-administrative version [CAT-admin], and the Caring Assessment Tool–educational version [CAT-edu]) were originally developed by Duffy in 1990 and 1992 and were based on Watson's (1985) Theory of Human Caring. Each item corresponded to a carative factor; several items taken together were intended to reflect an entire carative factor. Items were written in simple, easy-to-understand English at the eighth-grade level of reading comprehension. In the absence of other measures of nurse caring, the CAT was initially developed for use with hospitalized acute care patients to assess the degree of nurse caring and link it to important nursing-sensitive outcomes.

Development

After choosing a conceptual foundation, an item pool of 130 items was developed from the patients' points of view. Content and face validity were supported by an eight-member panel of experts. Panelists were instructed to comment on three areas: (1) appropriateness of each item as a nurse-caring behavior, (2) the representativeness of each item to the carative factors (Watson, 1979), and (3) general clarity of each item. Panelists used a scale of 1 (very low caring) to 5 (very high caring) to rate their responses to each item. Nineteen items were worded negatively

© Springer Publishing Company DOI:10.1891/9780826195425.0012

and/or overlapped with other items; they were intentionally designed to minimize the chance of error. Cut points of means greater than 3.5 and less than 1.5 for recoded items were established. Means were calculated for each item; those items meeting the criteria were retained. One hundred items met the retention criteria. Three recommendations were made (all within one domain of caring) for wording changes. These recommendations were used to revise the tool (CAT II), which was then resubmitted to the panel for a second review. All panelists responded in support of content validity.

Eighty-six randomly selected hospitalized medical–surgical patients were then recruited to measure internal consistency reliability. Cronbach's coefficient alpha was .97 (Duffy, 1990). The wording of eight items was slightly revised in 2000 (CAT III) to capture the realities of outpatient healthcare; internal consistency reliability remained high.

A shorter instrument that decreased subject burden while accurately and reliably measuring caring was needed to meet the increasing demands of relationship-centered professional practice in the United States. In 2006, five U.S. hospitals participated in a study of the tool. A convenience sample of hospitalized adults was recruited from hospitals in urban/suburban areas in Virginia, Maryland, Illinois, New Jersey, and the District of Columbia. The targeted subjects were adults who were hospitalized for at least 2 days to ensure that some interaction with professional nurses had occurred. Although the intended subjects were hospitalized medical–surgical patients, none was critical or unstable. Since the number of variables in this study was large (100 items), data from the five hospitals were merged to form the largest data set possible for analysis. The total sample size was 557. Included were adults from all diagnostic, socioeconomic, sex, and ethnic groups.

With the use of exploratory factor analysis, eight independent factors emerged, internal consistency remained high for the total tool (.96) and for each of the eight factors (.797–.963), and items were reduced. The scale mean was 141.20 with a standard deviation of 28.41. A revised factor labeling scheme was created by an expert panel and compared to existing nursing theory and research to provide a clear representation of what it means to be caring, as perceived by the patients in this sample (Duffy, Hoskins, & Seifert, 2007). The generalizability of this study was limited, however, because of the nonrandom sample, lack of adjustment for demographic and/or institution-specific characteristics that could have confounded results, and data accuracy problems.

Yet, the reduction of items to 36 (while maintaining high overall internal consistency) provided a more efficient method for assessing caring. The final tool (CAT-IV) determined the degree of nurse caring as perceived by patients. Questions were directed at how often nurses performed specific activities in the healthcare situation, were designed to be completed by the subject, and were printed in 14-point font. Responses indicated how frequently an activity occurred. The revised tool was designed to be administered after the patient had experienced some interaction with nurses (i.e., in the acute care setting, at least 24 hours after the patient's admission). The overall score, a summation of the scores from individual items, ranged from 36 to 180. In general, higher total scores indicated a greater degree of caring.

Over time, the CAT-IV has commonly been used by students, researchers, and administrators to assess the quality of patient–RN relationships, the relationship between nurse caring and important patient outcomes, as the basis for nursing interventions, for performance improvement initiatives, to determine effectiveness of caring-based professional practice models, and to provide support for RN professional advancement (Duffy, 2018). The CAT-IV is frequently used in acute care; however, it has also been employed in outpatient settings, is available in Spanish and Japanese, and was used by nursing students to assess relationship competency.

Because of the emerging clinical evidence between relationship quality and positive patient outcomes, the increasing emphasis on patient-centered care, the significance of the RN's role in provision of services to hospitalized individuals, and the limitations of the prior study, further evaluation of the CAT was warranted. In 2014, Duffy, Brewer, and Weaver collected data from 1,111 patients in 12 U.S. hospitals in four geographically distinct regions to (a) confirm the factor structure of the construct, caring relationships, and (b) to perform item reduction for ease of administration in the hospital setting (Duffy et al., 2014). In this study, the factor structure of the CAT was examined with a confirmatory factor analysis based on an orthogonal eight-factor structure described previously (Duffy, Hoskins, et al., 2007). The null hypothesis of fit of that model to observed data was rejected and an alternative exploratory analysis was performed to identify a more appropriate structure. A single factor provided acceptable fit to the 36-item CAT measure (70% of variance reproduced; confirmatory fit index [CFI] = .98) and high internal consistency (coefficient alpha = .977). Retained items that had factor loadings of at least .70 and item–total correlations of at least .70 produced a 27-item revised CAT, with a single-factor solution, explaining 73% of the variance. Coefficient alpha for that 27-item measure was also high (.967).

The resulting CAT-V is a revised and shortened version of the CAT-IV included in the second edition of this book. The CAT-V is a theoretically based instrument, low in burden and high in reliability, designed to meet the need of researchers, nurse leaders, nurses, and others for data on caring relationships. Evidence supported a single dimension of the concept, caring, while reduced items and high internal consistency resulted in a tool with little burden for use in clinical settings and multiple patient populations. Since the development of the CAT-V, the instrument has been used by researchers to describe, compare, or evaluate patient-centered environments and patient–nurse relationships, by nurse leaders and students, and even has been evaluated for electronic use in a hospitalized older adult population (Duffy, Kooken, Wolverton, & Weaver, 2012).

CARING ASSESSMENT TOOL–ADMINISTRATION VERSION

Background
In addition to the CAT-V, the CAT-admin was developed in the early 1990s and has evolved over time. The CAT-admin was designed to reflect staff nurses' perceptions of their managers' caring behaviors for administrative nursing research.

Development of the CAT-Admin
The CAT-admin was developed in 1997 as an adaptation of the original CAT (Duffy, 1992). It comprised 94 items that were tailored to capture staff nurses' perceptions of their managers. The interpretation of each item and the meaning related to a specific carative factor was left in its original form, and content validity was established by an expert panel. A Likert-type scale with scores ranging from 1 (never) to 5 (always) was used to rate each item, and the total score (possible range 94–470) was interpreted as low to high caring, with lower scores indicating the nurse perceives less caring from the nurse manager. Some of the items were reverse-coded and recoded prior to analysis. The CAT-admin was tested in a study of both undergraduate and master's-level nursing students. Alpha internal consistency reliability was measured at .9849. A qualitative question was added to the original tool to expand and enrich data collection.

A sample of 56 full-time and part-time nurses was used in the tool revision. A Cronbach's alpha of .98 was reported for internal consistency. Stepwise multiple regression was used to clarify the interrelationships between variables' unit type, number of employees, and nursing turnover. Duffy's 1992 and 1993 citations of the tool's use have reported a correlation between caring and patient satisfaction for the CAT, and a correlation between nurse manager caring and staff nurse satisfaction for the CAT-admin.

In 2008, an exploratory factor analysis was carried out to further the development of this instrument (CAT-admin-II). Data for this study were collected from four U.S. hospitals in different geographic locations (the Mid-Atlantic, South, Southwest, and Midwest). The data were merged into one large set with 1,850 respondents. The majority of the sample were female subjects, the mean years subjects had worked as RNs was 7.0, and mean years subjects had worked at their current jobs was 5.98. The majority of the sample had a bachelor's degree (59%); the remainder was evenly divided between associate degree and diploma-prepared nurses. A principal component analysis revealed six factors with eigen values greater than 1, which explained 67.75% of the variance, but the first three factors accounted for 63.44% of the variance. These results and the scree plot and varimax rotation techniques were used to force a three-factor solution. Factor labels chosen for the three factors are shared decision making, human respect, and noncaring. When Cronbach's alpha was used to measure internal consistency reliability, the total instrument measured .942; factor 1 independently measured .971, factor 2 measured .958, and factor 3 measured .972.

The CAT-admin-II represented a shortened version of the original tool (39 items) designed to capture staff nurses' perceptions of their managers.

While the identified and newly labeled factors are consistent with prior work, several theorized factors did not load independently on this version. To validate whether staff nurses' perceptions of their managers' caring behaviors were different from patients' perceptions of nurse caring, 17 RNs who were attending a graduate course were asked the question: Think of a nurse manager/administrator you perceived as caring. What behaviors or attitudes did he or she use that conveyed caring to you? Of these, all participants reported human respect, and 15 participants reported valuing or collaborating in decision making as caring. In all, staff nurses' perceptions of caring did not include all those factors associated with caring in a patient sample. Rather, staff nurses in the sample perceived their managers' respect and attitudes/behaviors conveying mutual understanding and collaborative decision making as caring. This study suffered limitations in terms of the size and generalizability of the sample.

In 2016, a full psychometric testing of the CAT was undertaken for the purposes of evaluating the validity and reliability of the CAT-admin. Three specific aims were to (1) evaluate and construct validity of the CAT-admin, (2) estimate the internal consistency, and to (3) conduct item reduction analysis to reduce administrative and participant burden. A convenience sample of 1,143 acute care hospital staff nurses (RNs) were recruited from seven hospitals located in three states in the Midwestern, Mid-Atlantic, and Southern Regions of the United States (both Magnet® and non-Magnet–designated hospitals). Inclusion criteria were permanent staff RNs employed for a minimum of 6 months, allowing for time to establish and reflect upon relationships that had developed with the nurse manager.

Using the original 94-item CAT-admin, the survey was administered through electronic data collection over a period of several months. Confirmatory analysis was used to determine the dimensionality of the construct, nurse manager caring behaviors. The null hypothesis was that an eight-factor solution fit the theoretical model. The null hypothesis was rejected because none of the measures examined for goodness of fit measures supported the null hypothesis. A new exploratory factor analysis was completed that supported a one-factor solution that was conceptually labeled "caring behaviors." To decrease subject burden, the 94-item survey was reduced to 25 items using item reduction analysis including assessing minimum factor loadings of $\geq.60$ and evaluating survey item–total correlation and alpha. The Cronbach's alpha was reported to be .98. This revised 25-item CAT-Admin survey provides hospital administrators, nurse managers, and researchers with a sound, less burdensome instrument to collect valuable information about nurse manager–caring behaviors. Scores can be used to assess nurses' perceptions of manager caring, or nurse manager "caring competence," or to monitor improvements in nursing administrative practice (Wolverton et al., 2018).

CARING ASSESSMENT TOOL–EDUCATIONAL VERSION

Another version of the CAT, the CAT-educational version, or CAT-edu, designed for nursing educational use remains unchanged. This educational version of the instrument was tested on a convenience sample of 71 baccalaureate and master's nursing students. Internal consistency reliability data resulted in a Cronbach's alpha of .98 (Watson, 2008, p. 126). The CAT-edu consists of a 5-point Likert-type scale, similar to that used by the other versions, and has 94 items constructed for educational use. Several items in the CAT-edu are worded negatively and must be reverse-scored during analysis. This instrument was developed to measure students' perceptions of faculty caring behaviors. The CAT-edu instrument is included here.

SCORING GUIDELINES

For the three instruments, closed-response 5-point Likert-type scale items are used. Each item measures the frequency with which the behavior occurs in the work/learning environment. Scores range from 1 (never) to 5 (always). With the exception of the CAT-edu, individual item scores are summed for a total score interpreted as low or poor caring to high or superior caring. The CAT-edu requires reverse scoring prior to summation. Each tool has a different range of total scores based on the total number of items. This total score characterizes interval-level data, which allow for inferential correlational and comparative analyses. Based on a sample's measures of central tendency and dispersion, a more precise interpretation of total scores might be apparent. Similarly, each item could be interpreted as higher or lower caring in the same manner.

Ongoing development of the caring behavior tools, such as caring capacity and caring intention tools, is being considered. Most importantly, as assessments of a unique domain of nursing, the tools provide researchers, students, and others with opportunities to advance the evidence base for nursing practice and improve the quality of patient care.

AVAILABILITY AND ACCESSIBILITY OF THE CAT TOOLS

These three versions of the CAT are copyrighted by the author. They can be administered via paper and pencil or electronically. Permission for use and accessing the tools can be done by visiting www.quality-caring.com directly for additional information and licensing details. Table 12.1 presents a matrix of key data for each of the instruments; item examples can be found in Tools 12.1 to 12.3.

TABLE 12.1 Description of Most Recent Versions of the Caring Assessment Tools

INSTRUMENT	AUTHOR CONTACT INFORMATION	HOW TO ACCESS	DEVELOPED TO MEASURE	INSTRUMENT DESCRIPTION	REPORTED VALIDITY AND RELIABILITY	THEORETICAL BASIS
CAT-V	Joanne R. Duffy, PhD, RN, FAAN Indiana University Indianapolis, IN	Visit: www.quality -caring.com	Patients' perceptions of nurse-caring behaviors or patients' perceptions of "feeling cared for" by nurses	27 items administered to patients, either self-reported or reported with assistance	Content validity established (Duffy, 1990); excellent internal consistency reliability (alpha = .967); factor analysis revealed a single factor provided acceptable fit (Duffy et al., 2014)	Initially developed based on Watson's Caring Theory (1985). Latest version supports one dimension of caring—interpreted as a combination of behaviors, skills, and attitudes may be intertwined to meet the needs of patients at a given moment in time

(continued)

TABLE 12.1 Description of Most Recent Versions of the Caring Assessment Tools (*continued*)

INSTRUMENT	AUTHOR CONTACT INFORMATION	HOW TO ACCESS	DEVELOPED TO MEASURE	INSTRUMENT DESCRIPTION	REPORTED VALIDITY AND RELIABILITY	THEORETICAL BASIS
CAT-Admin	Cheryl L. Wolverton, PhD, RN Franciscan Health Indianapolis, IN	Visit: www.quality -caring.com	Staff nurses' perceptions of nurse–manager caring behaviors: Addresses RNs' perceptions of the RN–nurse manager relationship	25 items administered to staff nurses (RNs) and self-reported via paper and pencil or electronically	Content validity established (Duffy, 1990); excellent internal consistency reliability (alpha = .98); factor analysis revealed a single factor, labeled "caring behaviors," provided acceptable fit (Wolverton et al., 2018)	Duffy (2018) Quality-Caring Model
CAT-edu	Joanne R. Duffy, PhD, RN, FAAN Indiana University Indianapolis, IN	Visit: www.quality -caring.com	Students' perceptions of faculty-caring behaviors; addresses students' perceptions of the student–teacher relationship	95 self-administered items	Content validity established (Duffy, 1990); internal consistency reliability excellent (alpha = .98) (J. Duffy, personal communication, 2001)	Watson's Caring Theory (1985)

TOOL 12.1

Caring Assessment Tool Version V©

Directions: All of the statements in this survey refer to nursing activities that occur in a healthcare situation. There are five possible responses to each item. For each statement, please check how often you think each activity is occurring during your healthcare.

Since I have been a patient here, the nurse/s:

ITEM	NEVER 1	RARELY 2	OCCASIONALLY 3	FREQUENTLY 4	ALWAYS 5
1. Help me to believe in myself					
2. Make me feel as comfortable as possible					
3. Support me with my beliefs					
4. Pay attention to me when I am talking					
5. Help me see some good aspects of my situation					
6. Help me feel less worried					
7. Anticipate my needs					
8. Allow me to choose the best time to talk about my concerns					
9. Are concerned about how I view things					
10. Seem interested in me					
11. Respect me					
12. Are responsive to my family					
13. Acknowledge my inner feelings					
14. Help me understand how I am thinking about my illness					

(continued)

TOOL 12.1

	NEVER 1	RARELY 2	OCCASIONALLY 3	FREQUENTLY 4	ALWAYS 5
Caring Assessment Tool Version V© (*continued*)					
ITEM					
15. Help me explore alternative ways of dealing with my health problems					
16. Ask me what I know about my illness					
17. Help me to figure out questions to ask other healthcare professionals					
18. Support my sense of hope					
19. Respect my need for privacy					
20. Ask me how I think my healthcare treatment is going					
21. Treat my body carefully					
22. Help me with my special routine needs for sleep					
23. Encourage my ability to go on with life					
24. Help me deal with my bad feelings					
25. Know what is important to me					
26. Talk openly to my family					
27. Show respect for those things that have meaning to me					

THIS IS THE END OF THE SURVEY. THANK YOU FOR YOUR VALUABLE TIME. If there is anything else you think the nurse ought to do differently, please write your answer below.

Source: © Joanne R. Duffy, PhD, RN, FAAN 2010.

TOOL 12.2

Caring Assessment Tool—Adm©

Directions: All of the statements in this survey refer to activities that occur in healthcare work environments. There are five possible responses to each item. For each statement, please check how often you think each activity occurs during your workday/night.

Since I have been a staff nurse here, my nurse leader (manager):

ITEM	NEVER 1	RARELY 2	OCCASIONALLY 3	FREQUENTLY 4	ALWAYS 5
1. Keeps me informed					
2. Allows me to choose the best time to talk about my concerns					
3. Openly shows concern for me					
4. Asks me about how I like to do my work					
5. Helps me deal with my bad feelings					
6. Expresses human emotions when he/she is with me					
7. Is patient with me even when I am difficult					
8. Is interested in information I have to offer about the work					
9. Accepts what I say, even if it is negative					
10. Is aware of my feelings					
11. Helps me find solutions regarding my work problems					
12. Asks me how I think my work is going					
13. Asks me what I think about nursing/healthcare					

(*continued*)

TOOL 12.2

Caring Assessment Tool—Adm© (*continued*)					
ITEM	NEVER 1	RARELY 2	OCCASIONALLY 3	FREQUENTLY 4	ALWAYS 5
14. Provides me with literature about my work					
15. Checks with me to make sure I understand what is going on in the workplace					
16. Makes sure my coworkers know what I need					
17. Makes me feel safe					
18. Helps me feel special					
19. Keeps me challenged					
20. Allows me time off to be with my family/friends					
21. Helps me achieve my work goals					
22. Understands my unique situation					
23. Is concerned about how I view things					
24. Knows what is important to me					
25. Acknowledges my inner feelings					

THIS IS THE END OF THE SURVEY. THANK YOU FOR YOUR VALUABLE TIME. If you were asked to advise nurse leaders on what they need to do differently, what would you advise?

Source: Wolverton, C. L., Lasiter, S., Duffy, J. R., Weaver, M. T., & McDaniel, A. M. (2018). Psychometric testing of the caring assessment tool: Administration (CAT-Adm©). *SAGE Open Medicine, 6*. doi:10.1177/2050312118760739.

TOOL 12.3

Caring Assessment Tool—Educational Version©

Directions: All of the statements in this survey refer to activities that occur among people in a nursing school. There are five possible responses to each item. For each statement, please circle how often you think each activity is occurring during your education.

Since I have been a student nurse here, my instructors:

ITEM	NEVER 1	RARELY 2	OCCASIONALLY 3	FREQUENTLY 4	ALWAYS 5
1. Listen to me					
2. Accept me as I am					
3. Treat me kindly					
4. Ignore me					
5. Answer my questions					
6. Include me in their discussions					
7. Respect me					
8. Are more interested in their own problems					
9. Pay attention to me					
10. Enjoy working with me					
11. Use my name when they talk to me					
12. Are available to me					
13. Have no time for me					
14. Seem interested in me					
15. Support me with my beliefs					
16. Help me to believe in myself					
17. Keep me informed					
18. Fail to keep their promises to me					
19. Encourage me to think for myself					
20. Encourage me to ask questions					

(continued)

TOOL 12.3

	Caring Assessment Tool—Educational Version© (continued)				

ITEM	NEVER 1	RARELY 2	OCCASIONALLY 3	FREQUENTLY 4	ALWAYS 5
21. Help me see some good aspects of my situation					
22. Encourage me to continue studying here					
23. Anticipate my needs					
24. Encourage me to talk about my concerns					
25. Openly show concern for me					
26. Ask me about my family					
27. Never show any emotion					
28. Ask me how I would do things					
29. Help me deal with any negative feelings					
30. When appropriate, share personal information with me					
31. Express human emotions when they are with me					
32. Respond honestly to my questions					
33. Initiate conversations with me					
34. Check on me frequently					
35. Look me in the eye when they talk to me					
36. Refuse to tell me aspects about my performance when I ask					
37. Pay attention to me when I am talking					

(continued)

TOOL 12.3

Caring Assessment Tool—Educational Version© (continued)					
ITEM	NEVER 1	RARELY 2	OCCASIONALLY 3	FREQUENTLY 4	ALWAYS 5
38. Act as if they disapprove of me					
39. Encourage me to talk about whatever is on my mind					
40. Are patient with me even when I am difficult					
41. Are interested in information I have to offer					
42. Talk about me openly in front of other faculty members					
43. Accept what I say, even when it is negative					
44. Seem annoyed if I speak my true feelings					
45. Are aware of my feelings					
46. Don't want to talk to me					
47. Allow me to talk about my true feelings without any risk to my grades					
48. Question me about my past experiences in nursing					
49. Help me set career goals that I am able to accomplish					
50. Help me find solutions to my problems					
51. Deal with my school problems in ways that are impractical for me					
52. Help me with all of my academic problems, not just parts of them					

(continued)

TOOL 12.3

ITEM	NEVER 1	RARELY 2	OCCASIONALLY 3	FREQUENTLY 4	ALWAYS 5
Caring Assessment Tool—Educational Version© (continued)					
53. Help me deal with difficult situations					
54. Help me understand my feelings					
55. Ask me how I think my school work is going					
56. Help me explore alternative ways of dealing with my academic problems					
57. Know when to go to a higher authority					
58. Provide me with literature regarding my work and areas of interest					
59. Use terms I don't understand					
60. Know what they are doing					
61. Help me to learn about nursing and/or healthcare					
62. Discourage me from asking questions					
63. Check in with me to make sure I understand					
64. Tell me what to expect					
65. Make me feel as comfortable as possible					
66. Respect my need for confidentiality					
67. Make sure that clinical instructors know my strengths and weaknesses					

(continued)

TOOL 12.3

Caring Assessment Tool—Educational Version© (*continued*)					
ITEM	NEVER 1	RARELY 2	OCCASIONALLY 3	FREQUENTLY 4	ALWAYS 5
68. Know what to do in an emergency					
69. Never ask what I need					
70. Protect me from situations where I could get harmed					
71. Know a lot about my work habits					
72. Spend time with me					
73. Make me feel secure regarding my performance in school					
74. Appreciate my family demands					
75. Limit or interfere with my basic routines					
76. Make sure I have time out for my own needs					
77. Keep me challenged					
78. Monitor my skill level					
79. Make sure my grades are accurate					
80. Make me wait a long time for an appointment when I need help					
81. Help me feel less worried					
82. Allow me the time to be with my spouse and special family/friends					
83. Discourage me from interacting with others					
84. Help me achieve my career goals					
85. Don't care whether I get a break					

(continued)

TOOL 12.3

Caring Assessment Tool—Educational Version© *(continued)*

ITEM	NEVER 1	RARELY 2	OCCASIONALLY 3	FREQUENTLY 4	ALWAYS 5
86. Respect my needs when scheduling class and/or clinicals					
87. Understand my unique situation					
88. Have no idea how school is affecting me					
89. Are concerned about how I view things					
90. Know what is important to me					
91. Acknowledge my inner feelings					
92. Help me cope with the stress of my work					
93. Show respect for those things that have meaning for me					
94. Are out of touch with my daily world					

THIS IS THE END OF THE SURVEY. THANK YOU FOR YOUR VALUABLE TIME. If you were asked to advise nurse faculty members on what they need to do differently, what would you advise?

Source: © Duffy (1992).

REFERENCES

Duffy, J. (1990). *An analysis of relationships among nurse caring behaviors and selected outcomes of care in hospitalized medical and/or surgical patients.* Retrieved from Dissertations and Theses database. (AAT 9027657)

Duffy, J. (1992). The impact of nurse caring on patient outcomes. In D. A. Gaut (Ed.), *The presence of caring in nursing* (pp. 113–136). New York, NY: National League for Nursing.

Duffy, J. (1993). Caring behaviors of nurse managers: Relationship to staff nurse satisfaction and retention. In D. A. Gaut (Ed.), *A global agenda for caring* (pp. 365–378). New York, NY: National League for Nursing.

Duffy, J. (2018). *Quality caring in nursing and health care.* New York, NY: Springer Publishing.

Duffy, J., Brewer, B. B., & Weaver, M. T. (2014). Revision and psychometric properties of the caring assessment tool. *Clinical Nursing Research, 23*(1), 80–93. doi:10.1177/1054773810369827

Duffy, J., Hoskins, L. M., & Seifert, R. F. (2007). Dimensions of caring: Psychometric properties of the Caring Assessment Tool. *Advances in Nursing Science, 30*(3), 1–12. doi:10.1097/01.ANS.0000286622.84763.a9

Duffy, J., Kooken, W., Wolverton, C., & Weaver, M. (2012). Evaluating patient-centered care: Feasibility of electronic data collection in hospitalized older adults. *Journal of Nursing Care Quality, 27*(4), 307–315. doi:10.1097/ncq.0b013e31825ba9d4

Watson, J. (1979). *Nursing: The philosophy and science of caring*. Boston, MA: Little, Brown.

Watson, J. (1985). *Nursing: Human science and human care, a theory of nursing*. Norwalk, CT: Appleton-Century-Crofts.

Watson, J. (2008). *Assessing and measuring caring in nursing and health science* (2nd ed.). New York, NY: Springer Publishing.

Wolverton, C. L., Lasiter, S., Duffy, J. R., Weaver, M. T., & McDaniel, A. M. (2018). Psychometric testing of the caring assessment tool: Administration (CAT-Adm©). *SAGE Open Medicine, 6*. doi:10.1177/2050312118760739

Peer Group Caring Interaction Scale and Organizational Climate for Caring Questionnaire

Linda Hughes[‡]

No significant change to or use of this instrument has been reported since the first edition of this book. However, W. Gabbert (personal communication, June 4, 2007) reports using the organizational climate version in her dissertation research with an online nursing student population.

The original Peer Group Rating Scale (PGRS) was designed by Hughes (1993) to measure the climate for caring as experienced by a student peer group. The PGRS is one of two investigator-developed instruments that focus on the climate for caring among students in nursing education. The second tool developed by Hughes is the Organizational Climate for Caring Questionnaire (OCCQ). The original Peer Group Caring Interaction Scale (PGCIS) instrument was empirically derived from items that were generated in a qualitative study conducted with 10 junior nursing students. There was no identified conceptual–theoretical basis for the instrument, except for a general interest in identifying behavioral and interactional aspects of caring as experienced by students. Indirectly, theories of caring and educational theory are represented in the direction, nature, and application of the instrument. Caring curricular ideas and educational theories of caring presented by Bevis and Watson (2000), along with Noddings (1994), are built into the assumptions upon which the original study was built, although they are not explicitly identified as the theoretical–conceptual basis of the instrument development.

[‡]Deceased

The PGCIS consists of two subscales: giving assistance and modeling. The PGCIS was pretested with a convenience sample of one junior student enrolled in the school of nursing. Content validity was determined by two nurse educators with expertise in the concept of caring.

The refined PGCIS was then used in a pilot study of 873 nursing students at 87 schools of nursing drawn from a population that was randomly selected from the 1992 listing of state-approved schools of nursing. The sample represents a response rate of 73% for school systems at the organizational level, and 54% for individual students.

After additional item analysis to detect internal consistency, a 16-item scale emerged as the final version, with a Cronbach's alpha for both subscales reported at .91. The mean interitem correlation for the two subscales was .60, suggesting minimum redundancy among the items.

The final 16-item version of the PGCIS was subjected to additional exploratory factor analysis. Hughes (1993) reported there were no residuals that exceeded the established criterion of .10. Thus, empirical support has been established for the two-subscale structure of the PGCIS. Scores from a second investigator-developed instrument, the Organizational Climate Description Questionnaire (Hughes, unpublished research, 2000), were used to construct an additional intercorrelation matrix. A statistically significant and moderately positive correlation ranging from .59 ($p < .001$) to .69 ($p < .001$) was found between relevant subscales for the PGCIS scores and scores on the Organizational Climate Description Questionnaire.

Hughes concludes that the preliminary support for the PGCIS demonstrates that the tool is a reliable and valid approach to measuring peer group caring in baccalaureate schools of nursing. She further suggests that the PGCIS has potential applicability in the evaluation of the "hidden" curriculum, as described by Bevis and Watson (2000); thus, it can be used to examine educative strategies designed to enhance students' caring interactions. The PGCIS is one of the few measurements of caring that are designed for use in nursing education, and the only one found to focus on peer group climate. This instrument is copyrighted, and the author requests that she be contacted for permission and additional information. The original work for the development of this instrument was supported by the National Center for Nursing Research at the National Institutes of Health (NIH). The matrix framework in Table 13.1 provides key summary data for the PGCIS (Tool 13.1).

The OCCQ (Tool 13.2) is a sister measurement tool to the PGCIS. It is a newly reported instrument and has not yet been published. This instrument was developed as part of the author's doctoral dissertation (Hughes, 1993, 2001).

The OCCQ was constructed and refined over a series of three pilot studies designed to capture dimensions of a caring climate experienced by nursing students. The investigator's interest was related to normative educational processes and the environmental contexts within which caring can be learned. The student-perceived organizational climate for caring within the context of faculty–student interactions was the focus for study and instrument construction. OCCQ

TABLE 13.1 Matrix of Peer Group Caring Interaction Scale and Organizational Climate for Caring Questionnaire

INSTRUMENT	PUBLICATION SOURCE	DEVELOPED TO MEASURE	INSTRUMENT DESCRIPTION	PARTICIPANTS	REPORTED VALIDITY/ RELIABILITY	CONCEPTUAL–THEORETICAL BASIS OF MEASUREMENT	LATEST CITATION IN NURSING LITERATURE
Peer Group Caring Interaction Scale and Organizational Climate for Caring Questionnaire (1993, 1998)							Organizational Climate for Caring Questionnaire used by W. Gabbert in dissertation research with online nursing students (hybrid version) Email: Wrennah. gabbert @angelo .edu

items were based upon data obtained during individual interviews with 10 junior students enrolled at five baccalaureate schools of nursing who were asked to describe a climate of caring within the context of their interactions with faculty.

The conceptual–theoretical basis of the instrument is Noddings's (1994) conceptualizations of the components of a moral education for a caring curriculum. The OCCQ consists of four subscales, which correspond directly with Noddings's framework for caring in education: modeling, dialogue, practice, and confirmation. The modeling subscale has 14 items that describe caring behaviors that can be modeled by teachers during their interactions with students. The dialogue subscale has nine items that describe the open exchange of thoughts, ideas, or opinions between teachers and students. The practice subscale has nine items that focus on students' clinical practice experiences. The confirmation subscale has seven items that address the role of teachers in building students' self-esteem by expressing confidence in their abilities and potential as students and future nurses.

Two content experts helped to establish the content validity of the OCCQ (Hughes, 1993, 2001). Three pilot studies to develop the psychometric properties of the OCCQ were conducted with junior students enrolled at the National League for Nursing–accredited baccalaureate schools of nursing, which were randomly selected from a list of state-approved schools of nursing. The samples consisted of 180 students from 20 schools for the first pilot study, 363 students from 27 schools for the second pilot study, and 853 students from 87 schools for the third pilot study.

Hughes used data from the third pilot study to establish psychometric properties. Coefficient alphas for the OCCQ subscales ranged from .88 to .92 (Hughes, 2001). Scores on the OCCQ and subscales on two other scales were correlated to assess convergent validity. Correlations ranged from .50 to .86. Separate factor analyses using maximum likelihood estimation were completed in the second and third pilots, in which four factors resulted: modeling/dialogue, practice, confirmation, and uncaring behaviors.

Hughes (2001) reports that the combined findings of the studies on the OCCQ suggest that this instrument offers a reliable and valid approach to the measurement of the organizational climate for caring in schools of nursing. This concept is conceptualized as a variable that mediates the relationship between student outcomes and the educational process. Assessment of the organizational climate for caring within the context of faculty–student relationships can be useful in the evaluation of nursing educational programs. The OCCQ is the only tool on caring identified for this project that specifically addresses organizational climate for caring in nursing education. While no published reports exist yet for the OCCQ, this tool has promise for future refinement, testing, and use in nursing educational research, both at the individual student perceptional level and at the organizational climate level.

This instrument is copyrighted by Hughes. The author requests that anyone wishing to use the OCCQ contact her for more information. Any published research using the instrument should indicate Hughes as the author of the instrument. Table 13.1 presents a matrix of key properties for the OCCQ.

TOOL 13.1

Peer Group Caring Interaction Scale

Developed by

Linda C. Hughes, PhD, RN

Associate Professor, School of Nursing

University of Texas Medical Branch

301 University Blvd.

Galveston, TX 77555-1029

(409) 772-8247

Directions: Please respond to each of the following statements by circling the number that best describes the climate or atmosphere at YOUR school of nursing. Make your responses according to how things are at your school; NOT how you would like them to be or how you think they should be.

	STRONGLY DISAGREE	MODERATELY DISAGREE	SLIGHTLY DISAGREE	SLIGHTLY AGREE	MODERATELY AGREE	STRONGLY AGREE
1. Students at this school anticipate the needs of their classmates.	1	2	3	4	5	6
2. Students at this school talk with each other about their problems and concerns.	1	2	3	4	5	6
3. Students at this school share ideas with each other about how best to take care of patients.	1	2	3	4	5	6
4. Students at this school talk to their classmates about things they wish they had done better while in a patient care setting.	1	2	3	4	5	6
5. Students at this school will help a classmate ONLY WHEN it is in their best interest to do so.	1	2	3	4	5	6
6. Students at this school think it should be left up to the teachers to work with students who need extra help.	1	2	3	4	5	6

(continued)

157

TOOL 13.1

Peer Group Caring Interaction Scale (*continued*)

	STRONGLY DISAGREE	MODERATELY DISAGREE	SLIGHTLY DISAGREE	SLIGHTLY AGREE	MODERATELY AGREE	STRONGLY AGREE
7. There is a lot of camaraderie among the students at this school.	1	2	3	4	5	6
8. Students at this school notice when a classmate is having problems.	1	2	3	4	5	6
9. Students at this school get advice and suggestions from their classmates when completing homework assignments.	1	2	3	4	5	6
10. Students at this school can count on their classmates for help.	1	2	3	4	5	6
11. Students at this school are TOO BUSY to help their classmates.	1	2	3	4	5	6
12. Students at this school are a source of encouragement to each other.	1	2	3	4	5	6
13. Students at this school help each other by sharing class notes, books, or articles.	1	2	3	4	5	6
14. Students at this school get opinions from their classmates about things that happen to them while in a patient care setting.	1	2	3	4	5	6
15. Students at this school talk with their classmates about how it feels to care for patients with whom they are uncomfortable .	1	2	3	4	5	6
16. There is TOO MUCH competition among the students at this school.	1	2	3	4	5	6

TOOL 13.2

Organizational Climate for Caring Questionnaire

Developed by Linda Hughes, PhD, RN

Associate Professor, School of Nursing

University of Texas Medical Branch

301 University Blvd.

Galveston, TX 77555-1029

(409) 772-8247

Directions: Please respond to each of the following statements by circling the number that best describes the climate or atmosphere at YOUR school of nursing. Make your responses according to how things are at your school; NOT how you would like things to be.

	STRONGLY DISAGREE	MODERATELY DISAGREE	SLIGHTLY DISAGREE	SLIGHTLY AGREE	MODERATELY AGREE	STRONGLY AGREE
1. The teachers at this school are always cheering the students on.	1	2	3	4	5	6
2. Students at this school are given the reason for decisions that affect them.	1	2	3	4	5	6
3. There is an open exchange of ideas among teachers and students at this school.	1	2	3	4	5	6
4. Students at this school get a lot of uplifting encouragement from the teachers.	1	2	3	4	5	6
5. The teachers at this school sincerely want to see students succeed.	1	2	3	4	5	6
6. The teachers at this school are easy to talk to.	1	2	3	4	5	6
7. The teachers at this school tell students up front what is expected of them.	1	2	3	4	5	6

(continued)

TOOL 13.2

Organizational Climate for Caring Questionnaire (continued)

	STRONGLY DISAGREE	MODERATELY DISAGREE	SLIGHTLY DISAGREE	SLIGHTLY AGREE	MODERATELY AGREE	STRONGLY AGREE
8. The teachers at this school DO NOT make students feel stupid for asking questions.	1	2	3	4	5	6
9. The teachers at this school help students have confidence in themselves.	1	2	3	4	5	6
10. The teachers at this school take a personal interest in students.	1	2	3	4	5	6
11. Students at this school can depend on the clinical teachers to help them do a good job of taking care of patients.	1	2	3	4	5	6
12. Students at this school can count on a pat on the back from their teachers when they perform well.	1	2	3	4	5	6
13. Students at this school can NEVER be sure how the teachers will treat them from one day to the next.	1	2	3	4	5	6
14. The clinical teachers at this school sometimes put students down in front of other people.	1	2	3	4	5	6
15. The teachers at this school understand how it feels to be a student.	1	2	3	4	5	6
16. The teachers at this school take the time to make sure that students understand what they are learning.	1	2	3	4	5	6
17. The teachers at this school make it a point to tell students that they have confidence in their ability to become good nurses.	1	2	3	4	5	6

#	Statement	1	2	3	4	5	6
18.	Conflicts between teachers and students at this school can be resolved through one-to-one meetings.	1	2	3	4	5	6
19.	The teachers at this school tell students what they are doing wrong RATHER THAN what they are doing right.	1	2	3	4	5	6
20.	At this school, it is very much "I'm the instructor and you're the student and this is how we do it."	1	2	3	4	5	6
21.	The teachers at this school recognize when students are having problems.	1	2	3	4	5	6
22.	The clinical teachers at this school make it possible for students to do their best when taking care of patients.	1	2	3	4	5	6
23.	The teachers at this school enjoy being around students.	1	2	3	4	5	6
24.	The teachers at this school are usually TOO BUSY to take time to really listen to students' problems or concerns.	1	2	3	4	5	6
25.	The teachers at this school deal with students fairly.	1	2	3	4	5	6
26.	Students and teachers at this school share personal experiences with each other.	1	2	3	4	5	6
27.	Students at this school think it is a WASTE OF TIME to talk with teachers about their problems.	1	2	3	4	5	6
28.	The teachers at this school take students' opinions into account when deciding about school policies and procedures.	1	2	3	4	5	6
29.	The clinical teachers at this school ADD to the anxiety that students feel in the clinical setting.	1	2	3	4	5	6
30.	The clinical teachers at this school give more attention to evaluating students than to helping students meet patients' needs.	1	2	3	4	5	6

(continued)

TOOL 13.2

Organizational Climate for Caring Questionnaire (*continued*)

	STRONGLY DISAGREE	MODERATELY DISAGREE	SLIGHTLY DISAGREE	SLIGHTLY AGREE	MODERATELY AGREE	STRONGLY AGREE
31. Students at this school feel free to state their ideas or opinions around the teachers.	1	2	3	4	5	6
32. The clinical teachers at this school help students problem-solve difficult patient simulations.	1	2	3	4	5	6
33. It is safe for students at this school to openly disagree with the teachers.	1	2	3	4	5	6
34. The teachers at this school treat each student as an individual.	1	2	3	4	5	6
35. The clinical teachers at this school set a good example for students in their behaviors with patients and families.	1	2	3	4	5	6
36. The clinical teachers at this school are genuinely concerned about the patients to whom the students are assigned.	1	2	3	4	5	6
37. As nurses, the teachers at this school know what they are doing.	1	2	3	4	5	6
38. The teachers at this school are readily available to students.	1	2	3	4	5	6
39. The clinical teachers at this school make it easy for students to perform well in the clinical setting.	1	2	3	4	5	6

REFERENCES

Bevis, E. O., & Watson, J. (2000). *Toward a caring curriculum.* Sudbury, MA: Jones and Bartlett.

Hughes, L. (1993). Peer group interactions and the students-perceived climate for caring. *Journal of Nursing Education, 32*(2), 78–83.

Noddings, N. (1984). *Caring: A feminine approach to ethics and moral development.* Berkeley, CA: University of California Press.

REFERENCES

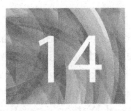

Caring Efficacy Scale

Carolie Coates

The Caring Efficacy Scale (CES) was developed by Dr. Carolie Coates, currently a consultant in the area of measurement and program evaluation. It was designed to assess an individual's confidence in (or sense of efficacy about) his or her ability to express a caring orientation and establish a caring relationship with patients. The conceptual theoretical basis for the scale is Bandura's self-efficacy theory (1977) from the discipline of social psychology and Watson's theory of transpersonal human caring from nursing. The most current version of the instrument is intended to be used to evaluate outcomes of nursing education in a new advanced program with a formal caring philosophy and caring curriculum (Watson & Phillips, 1992). The original CES self-report was developed so it could be administered to nursing students, clinical preceptors, supervisors, alumni, and alumni employers to assess caring efficacy as an outcome of nursing curriculum at the University of Colorado School of Nursing.

The original version, drafted in the late 1980s and refined for application in 1992, had 46 items that attempted to measure caring attitudes, skills, and behaviors on a 6-point Likert scale with a self-report format. Since then the CES has undergone a series of additional testing and revision, resulting in the current 30-item self-report scale and a parallel 30-item form designed for use by nurse preceptors/supervisors to rate individual nurses. The current CES form is balanced for positive and negative items. For accreditation assessment, the two original forms for self-report and supervisors were reduced to 12-item short versions consisting of the top 12 loading items in a factor analysis (Coates, 1997).

The initial version was tested on a sample of 47 novice nurses; this study produced promising reliability and validity information and provided guidance for reduction of items based on interitem correlation. Later samples consisted of 110 graduating nurses (BS, ND, and MS), 119 alumni (BS, ND, and MS), 117 employers of alumni, and 67 clinical preceptors supervising BS, ND, and MS nursing students. Nursing education evaluation studies using both the long and short forms of the CES produced good scale reliability data. Form A, with 30 items (consisting of more positive than negative items), yielded an alpha of .85, and form B, with 30 items (balanced for positively and negatively worded items), yielded an alpha of .88. The alpha for the short form of the supervisor scale was .84.

Faculty members who are very familiar with Watson's theory rated each of the 30 items in form B in terms of Watson's carative factors in order to establish content validity (Coates, 1997). A factor analysis conducted on the short form produced a three-factor solution accounting for 69% of the variance (Coates, 1996). Items loading on factor 1 (accounting for 41% of the variance) referred to sense of efficacy in establishing caring relationships with clients.

Assessment of the degree of relationship between the CES as a measure of caring and the clinical evaluation tool (CET) used by the university in accreditation studies as a measure of clinical competence provided additional concurrent validity evidence. The CET achieved alphas of .85 for student self-ratings and .95 for supervisor ratings of students. Positive correlations were found between graduates' ratings of care (CES) and their clinical competence ratings (form A: $r = .34$, $p = .05$; form B: $r = .37$, $p = .01$). Similar results occurred with alumni responses ($r = .63$, $p = .01$). More importantly, alumni self-ratings on the CET correlated positively with employers' independent ratings on the CET ($r = .46$, $p = .01$).

In a more recent unpublished application to assess the effects of a 3-day training based on empowerment and Watson's caring theory, the CES achieved alphas of .91 on the pretest utilization of the scale and .84 on the posttest (Coates, 1999). The sample consisted of 118 healthcare workers in a rehabilitation hospital. Significant short-term change (posttest within 4–6 weeks) was established through use of the CES ($p = .000$). The CES correlated in predictable ways with other outcome measures; it correlated positively with personal accomplishment (from the Maslach Burnout Inventory), and negatively with reliance on powerful others, reliance on chance, depersonalization, and the job stress inventory. This additional research adds further credibility to the use of the tool in both clinical settings and educational program evaluation.

This tool is guided by theories from both social psychology and nursing caring theory. It has been tested in nursing education and clinical care settings. It has psychometric sophistication in its development, use, and refinement. The Likert form makes it relatively easy to use. It is one of the few caring measurement tools that offer content validity with reference to the carative factors in Watson's theory. Coates reports that many schools of nursing in the United States have requested permission to use the CES as a student outcome measure. It is a copyrighted instrument, and the author requests that those interested in using it contact her for permission. Table 14.1 provides a matrix of the CES (Tool 14.1) with overall summary information.

TABLE 14.1 Matrix of Caring Efficacy Scale

INSTRUMENT	AUTHOR CONTACT INFORMATION	PUBLICATION SOURCE	DEVELOPED TO MEASURE	INSTRUMENT DESCRIPTION	PARTICIPANTS	REPORTED VALIDITY/ RELIABILITY	CONCEPTUAL-THEORETICAL BASIS OF MEASUREMENT	LATEST CITATION IN NURSING LITERATURE
Caring Efficacy Scale (1992, 1995)	Carolie Coates, PhD Research and Measurement Consultant 1441 Snowmass Ct. Boulder, CO 80305 Phone: 303-499-5756 Email: coatescj@ home.com	Coates (1997)	Assess conviction or belief in one's ability to express a caring orientation, develop caring relationship with patients	Original instrument had 46 items Current instrument has 12 items 6-point Likert-type scale Current instrument has 30 items (both self-report and supervisor format)	$n = 110$ nursing students $n = 119$ alumni $n = 117$ alumni employers $n = 67$ clinical supervisors	Cronbach's alpha Form A = .85 Form B = .88 Form B (short version) = .84 Content validity against theory and Watson's carative factors Significant positive correlation between clinical evaluation tool (alpha .85 and .95) and CES	Bandura's social psychology Self-Efficacy Scale and Watson's caring theory and 10 carative factors	Coates (1997) Sadler (2003)

TOOL 14.1

Caring Efficacy Scale

Instructions: When you are completing these items, think of your recent work with patients/clients in clinical settings. Circle the number that best expresses your opinion.

Rating Scale:

−3 strongly disagree

−2 moderately disagree

−1 slightly moderate

+1 slightly agree

+2 moderately agree

+3 strongly agree

	STRONGLY DISAGREE					STRONGLY AGREE
1. I do not feel confident in my ability to express a sense of caring to my clients/patients.	−3	−2	−1	+1	+2	+3
2. If I am not relating well to a client/patient, I try to analyze what I can do to reach him/her.	−3	−2	−1	+1	+2	+3
3. I feel comfortable in touching my clients/patients in the course of caregiving.	−3	−2	−1	+1	+2	+3
4. I convey a sense of personal strength to my clients/patients.	−3	−2	−1	+1	+2	+3
5. Clients/patients can tell me almost anything and I won't be shocked.	−3	−2	−1	+1	+2	+3
6. I have an ability to introduce a sense of normalcy in stressful conditions.	−3	−2	−1	+1	+2	+3
7. It is easy for me to consider the multifacets of a client's/patient's care, at the same time as I am listening to them.	−3	−2	−1	+1	+2	+3
8. I have difficulty in suspending my personal beliefs and biases in order to hear and accept a client/patient as a person.	−3	−2	−1	+1	+2	+3

(continued)

TOOL 14.1

Caring Efficacy Scale (*continued*)

	STRONGLY DISAGREE					STRONGLY AGREE
9. I can walk into a room with presence of serenity and energy that makes clients/patients feel better.	−3	−2	−1	+1	+2	+3
10. I am able to tune into a particular client/patient and forget my personal concerns.	−3	−2	−1	+1	+2	+3
11. I can usually create some way to relate to almost any client/patient.	−3	−2	−1	+1	+2	+3
12. I lack confidence in my ability to talk to clients/patients from backgrounds different from my own.	−3	−2	−1	+1	+2	+3
13. I feel if I talk to clients/patients on an individual, personal basis, things might get out of control.	−3	−2	−1	+1	+2	+3
14. I use what I learn in conversations with clients/patients to provide more individualized care.	−3	−2	−1	+1	+2	+3
15. I don't feel strong enough to listen to the fears and concerns of my clients/patients.	−3	−2	−1	+1	+2	+3
16. Even when I'm feeling self-confident about most things, I still seem to be unable to relate to clients/patients.	−3	−2	−1	+1	+2	+3
17. I seem to have trouble relating to clients/patients.	−3	−2	−1	+1	+2	+3
18. I can usually establish a close relationship with my clients/patients.	−3	−2	−1	+1	+2	+3
19. I can usually get patients/clients to like me.	−3	−2	−1	+1	+2	+3

(continued)

TOOL 14.1

Caring Efficacy Scale (*continued*)

	STRONGLY DISAGREE					STRONGLY AGREE
20. I often find it hard to get my point of view across to patients/clients when I need to.	−3	−2	−1	+1	+2	+3
21. When trying to resolve a conflict with a client/patient, I usually make it worse.	−3	−2	−1	+1	+2	+3
22. If I think a client/patient is uneasy or may need some help, I approach that person.	−3	−2	−1	+1	+2	+3
23. If I find it hard to relate to a client/patient, I'll stop trying to work with that person.	−3	−2	−1	+1	+2	+3
24. I often find it hard to relate to clients/patients from a different culture than mine.	−3	−2	−1	+1	+2	+3
25. I have helped many clients/patients through my ability to develop close, meaningful relationships.	−3	−2	−1	+1	+2	+3
26. I often find it difficult to express empathy with clients/patients.	−3	−2	−1	+1	+2	+3
27. I often become overwhelmed by the nature of the problems clients/patients are experiencing.	−3	−2	−1	+1	+2	+3
28. When a client/patient is having difficulty communicating with me, I am able to adjust to his/her level.	−3	−2	−1	+1	+2	+3
29. Even when I really try, I can't get through to difficult clients/patients.	−3	−2	−1	+1	+2	+3
30. I don't use creative or unusual ways to express caring to my clients patients.	−3	−2	−1	+1	+2	+3

Source: Coates, C. (1997). The Caring Efficacy Scale: Nurses' self-reports of caring in practice settings. *Advanced Practice Nursing Quarterly, 3*(1), 53–59. © Reprinted by permission of author.

The CES is copyrighted. This is the 30-item self-report form. Please contact Carolie J. Coates, PhD, Research and Measurement Consultant, 1441 Snowmass Court, Boulder, Colorado 80305, USA, to formally request to use the CES. (An administrator/supervisor version [30 items] is also available, as well as short forms [12 items] of the self-report and administrator/supervisor version.) Telephone and Fax +(303) 499-5756; email: coatescj@home.com (1/9/2001).

REFERENCES

Bandura, A. (1977). Self-efficacy: Toward a unified theory of behavioral change. *Psychological Review, 84*(2), 191–215.

Coates, C. J. (1996). *Development of the Caring Efficacy Scale: Self-report and supervisor versions.* Unpublished manuscript. Denver, CO: University of Colorado Health Sciences Center.

Coates, C.J. (1997). The Caring Efficacy Scale: Nurses' self-reports of caring in practice settings. *Advanced Practice Nursing Quarterly, 3*(1), 53–59.

Coates, C. J. (1999). *Outcome evaluation of Center for Healing and Renewal staff professional development training.* Unpublished manuscript. Boulder, CO: Boulder Community Hospital.

Sadler, J. (2003). A pilot study to measure the caring efficacy of baccalaureate nursing students. *Nursing Education Perspectives, 24*(6), 295–299.

Watson, J., & Phillips, S. (1992). A call for educational reform: Colorado nursing doctorate model as exemplar. *Nursing Outlook, 40*(1), 20–26.

Holistic Caring Inventory

Christine L. Latham

Caring is increasingly becoming relevant to healthcare that is often fraught with misconstrued communication (Latham, Ringl, & Hogan, 2011); weak, misguided, and sometimes demeaning coworker relationships (Latham, Ringl, & Hogan, 2013); and challenging management circumstances for frontline nurse managers, who are the center of many clinical and administrative decisions that impact patient care and workplace culture (Brousseau, Cara, & Blais, 2017). Even within complex health-care environments, nurses strive to be caring in their interactions with patients. However, since most healthcare facilities use general patient care surveys, this important characteristic of nursing is not captured. In an analysis of caring theories (L'etourneau, Cara, & Goudreau, 2017) the authors proposed that the therapeutic and dignity-preserving aspects of caring in nursing practice were fundamental to the profession and have a positive impact on patient care services and outcomes.

OVERVIEW OF THE HOLISTIC CARING INVENTORY

To meet the need to capture this important component of nursing practice, the Holistic Caring Inventory (HCI) was created to measure patient perspectives of caring by nurses. The instrument item blueprint for item development was based on caring research and Howard's Humanistic Caring Model (Howard, 1975). The conceptual framework for item construction is depicted in Figure 15.1.

An overview of the development of this measure included multiple levels of psychometric evaluation. The first use with hospitalized patients determined their perspectives of caring interactions with nurses, level of social desirability, and convergent and discriminant validity (Latham, 1996). The tool was subsequently used with two additional groups of hospitalized patients and another outpatient setting participant group to determine relationships between patient anxiety and satisfaction (Williams, 1998). One of the three studies by Williams (1998) used a simplified reading-level version of the HCI with oncology

© Springer Publishing Company DOI:10.1891/9780826195425.0015

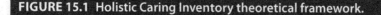

FIGURE 15.1 Holistic Caring Inventory theoretical framework.

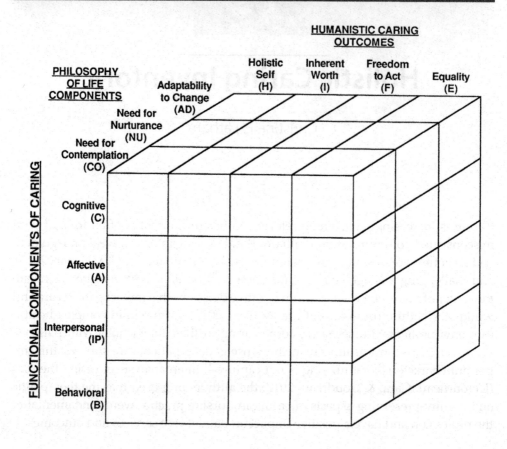

outpatients. While reliability estimates were positive, further validation work was recently completed to verify the relevance of this tool in today's healthcare environment. There have been other requests to use the HCI, but there are no subsequent publications to date regarding the findings.

BACKGROUND OF HCI DEVELOPMENT

Research Basis of the HCI

Both research and theory were used to construct the original items of the HCI. The original HCI item construction was influenced by research conducted on caring by Larson (1981, 1984), Mayer (1986), and Hall, Roter, and Katz (1988). Nurses and oncology patients had differences of opinion as to what was most favored by individuals receiving nursing care. Nurses favored psychosocially oriented behaviors, while patients preferred task-oriented behaviors (Larson, 1984). Mayer's (1986) subsequent study of a similar group of patients and nurses had similar results. However, the physical care modalities may hold greater symbolic significance for oncology patients, as was determined by analyses of patient ratings of instrumental (task-oriented) and expressive (psychosocial) behaviors of healthcare professionals (Hall et al., 1988). Hall and associates completed an analysis of 41 audio- and videotaped qualitative studies, and they found that patient satisfaction was most significantly related to the interpersonal competency of the caregiver, with provider information-giving rated as the second most important caregiver behavior. The researchers hypothesized that caregivers' task behaviors (e.g., information giving, technical competence, and the use of pertinent questions to ascertain the patient's perceptions) symbolize a caring attitude in that the provider shows concern for the patient in performing the required tasks. On the other hand, providers' socioemotional behavior (e.g., social conversation, positive talk, and interpersonal competence) was also found to influence patient satisfaction. Patients' perceptions of adequate caregiver task behavior seemed to influence their ratings of the providers' socioemotional competence, but the opposite effect of caregiver socioemotional skills on task delivery perceptions was not evident. This was confirmed by early studies by Auerbach, Martelli, and Mercuri (1983), who found that when information was delivered to patients in an unconcerned manner, the staff was rated as being dominant, hostile, and unfriendly. However, positive ratings were given when staff relayed information in a personal manner (i.e., with indicators of both verbal and nonverbal concern). The HCI was developed from studies of healthcare provider behaviors and patient reactions to various types of caring behaviors rather than ranking the importance of behaviors.

Theoretical Basis of HCI Development
Theory on holistic caring was also used to delineate the concepts for item construction. The theoretical framework for the HCI to capture caring provided by nurses was based on Howard's Humanistic Caring philosophy, as depicted in Figure 15.1. The philosophy underlying Howard's Humanistic Caring Model includes people's innate need for adaptability (AD), nurturance (NU), and contemplation (CO; Howard, 1975). The outcomes for interaction with caring from others include treatment as an equal and a whole person, and feelings of inherent worth and freedom to act. These model concepts were combined with patient expectations of nursing behaviors that include information giving (C, cognitive), assisting with feelings (A, affective), effective verbal communication (IP, interpersonal), caring nonverbal communication/behavior (B, behavioral), and intuition and empathy about the patient's current situation (PERC, perceptive ability). Care that addresses the whole person includes physical, psychological, sociocultural, and spiritual care realms. Figure 15.1, the "Holistic Caring Framework," integrates these different domains of humanistic, holistic caring and served as a blueprint for item development. Finally, the Fry (1968) readability formula was used to estimate the HCI reading level, which was determined to be at the sixth to seventh grade level. Subsequent work by Williams (1998) also reestablished an even lower reading level for outpatient oncology patients.

PSYCHOMETRIC EVALUATION OF THE HCI

Validity Estimates

Five methods were used to estimate validity of the tool. Initial content validity was established by a small qualitative study with nursing doctoral students to verify that the items reflected the theoretical framework. Following this, two doctorally prepared nurse scientists established a content validity index (CVI) of 1.00, using a minimal item mean of 3.0 (quite relevant ratings). A third test of validity focused on a pilot study of 30 patients to confirm item clarity. In a larger study of 120 hospitalized patients, discriminant validity was established with Kiesler's (1987) Impact Message Inventory (Latham, 1988). The Impact Message Inventory measures the interpersonal impact of others. Low correlations of .20 ($p < .01$) were found with the Impact Message Inventory's hostile subscale, and .16 ($p < .05$) with its submissive subscale. The total HCI and Impact Message Inventory score correlation was .15 ($p < .05$), which lent further evidence of discriminant validity between the two instruments. Finally, further support of concurrent validity was established in a subsequent study with 218 patients by Latham (1996), who found a moderate correlation of .39 ($p < .001$) between the Interpretive Caring Subscale and the Supportive Behavior Checklist (Gardner & Wheeler, 1987).

Additional psychometric estimates were established by a rotated varimax factor analysis to confirm four subscales. The factor analysis determined that four HCI factors explained 56.6% of the variance of the total scores. Factor analysis included mean interitem correlations (.34) and item-total correlations (ranging from .41 to .71). The four factors were physical, interpretive, spiritual, and sensitive caring (Latham, 1988). Table 15.1 lists items that loaded into four subscales labeled as physical, interpretive, spiritual, and sensitive caring. "Physical caring" refers to caring about the patient's physical status, "interpretive caring" refers to the nurse's ability to interpret the potential impact of patients' conditions and feelings, "spiritual caring" reflects caring about patients' spiritual needs, and "sensitive caring" relates to the nurse's sensitivity to patients' feelings and individuality.

In the original factor analyses, simple structure was present in the final factor analysis for all but two items, and all but one item (item 11) had high factor loadings. In the first derivation of the tool, item 11 was deleted from further analysis due to lack of factor loading (not higher than .19), and poor item-total correlation. On closer inspection, it was determined that item 11 can be interpreted in several different ways, depending on the individual's need or preference to be alone or with others, in this case, healthcare providers and nurses. Further examination of the four subscales revealed that there were low to moderate interscale correlations ranging from .11 to .58. Finally, total score correlations with the 10-item version of the Marlowe–Crowne Desirability Scale ($-.14$, $p < .05$) indicate that respondents did not answer in a socially desirable manner (Crowne & Marlowe, 1964), but rather chose to be truthful concerning their experience with care from nurses.

TABLE 15.1 Item Content Reflecting Holistic Caring Framework and Final Subscales

REALM OF CARE[a]	ITEM #	ITEM CONTENT[b]	SUBSCALES[c]
Physical Concerns	#1	IP-NU	Physical Caring
	#2	C-NU	Physical Caring
	#3	C-AD	Physical Caring
	#4	A/C-NU	Physical Caring
	#5	B-AD	Physical Caring
	#6	B-CO	Physical Caring
	#7	PERC-AD	Physical Caring
	#8	A-NU	Physical Caring
	#9	C-NU	Physical Caring
	#10	C-NU	Physical Caring
Psychological Concerns	#11	B-NU	Sensitive Caring
	#12	B-CO	Sensitive Caring
	#13	PERC/IP-AD	Interpretive Caring
	#14	PERC/CO-NU	Sensitive Caring
	#15	IP/NU-AD	Interpretive Caring
	#16	A-CO	Sensitive Caring
	#17	B-NU	Sensitive Caring
	#18	IP-AD	Sensitive Caring
	#19	C/PERC-AD	Interpretive Caring
	#20	B-AD	Sensitive Caring
Sociocultural Concerns	#21	C-AD	Interpretive Caring
	#22	B-CO	Interpretive Caring
	#23	A-NU/AD	Interpretive Caring
	#24	IP-AD	Sensitive Caring
	#25	A-NU/AD	Interpretive Caring
	#26	IP-NU	Interpretive Caring
	#27	B-AD	Interpretive Caring

(continued)

TABLE 15.1 Item Content Reflecting Holistic Caring Framework and Final Subscales (*continued*)

REALM OF CARE[a]	ITEM #	ITEM CONTENT[b]	SUBSCALES[c]
Sociocultural Concerns	#28	IP/PERC-AD	Interpretive Caring
	#29	IP/PERC-CO	Interpretive Caring
	#30	PERC-NU	Sensitive Caring
Spiritual Concerns	#31	B-NU	Spiritual Belief Systems
	#32	C-NU	Sensitive Caring
	#33	B-CO	Spiritual Belief Systems
	#34	C/PERC-AD	Spiritual Belief Systems
	#35	IP-AD	Spiritual Belief Systems
	#36	B/AD	Spiritual Belief Systems
	#37	A-AD	Spiritual Belief Systems
	#38	PERC-NU/CO	Spiritual Belief Systems
	#39	B-AD	Spiritual Belief Systems
	#40	A-NU	Spiritual Belief Systems

[a]Realm of nursing care is included in the first column.
[b]Item content in third column: Includes holistic care by healthcare provider (abbreviations referring to interpersonal [IP], cognitive [C], behavioral [B], and affective [A] realms of care) and personal outlook on life (second abbreviations referring to need for Nurturance [NU], Adaptability to Change [AD], and Contemplation [CO]).
[c]Final subscale for each item from factor analysis.

Reliability Estimates

Initial reliability was strong for the four caring subscales. Cronbach's alphas were .89 for interpretative caring, .91 for spiritual caring, and .90 for the other two subscales (physical and sensitive caring). Two subsequent studies using this tool indicated Cronbach's alphas ranged from .87 to .94 (Williams, 1998). In a fourth study, following rewording of the items to attain a lower reading level, one outpatient group was found to have internal consistency ratings ranging from .83 to .87, with a Cronbach's alpha of .53 for the physical caring subscale. In this last study, the rewording of the items may have contributed to the lower reliability levels.

Reaffirmation of Validity

This instrument has been refined and retested for validity since its initial development in 1988. In 2018 several items were reworded for clarity, and a study was conducted to reestablish content validity. Two negatively stated items that originally were deleted from the HCI were reworded to be positively stated (items 11 and 40), and items 4, 21, 30, 31, and 34 were reworded for simplicity and current language use. Two nurse scientists representing expertise in mental health and pediatrics/family care, and a medical anthropologist with expertise in medical sociology and cultural competence, ranked the items on a 4-point scale of not relevant (1) to very relevant (4). The CVI from the three raters was found to be .925 for scores over 3 on a 1 to 4 CVI scale with 1 = not relevant to 4 = very relevant, confirming the updated language, appropriate reflection of original theoretical underpinnings, and relevancy of the tool.

HCI SCORING AND INTERPRETATION OF FINDINGS

The HCI is a 40-item, 4-point Likert scale with 10 items, each representing four subscales that include physical, interpretive, spiritual, and sensitive caring. See Table 15.1 for items that correspond to each subscale.

Each item is scored as "strongly disagree" (1) to "strongly agree" (4). A mean score of 1 indicates that caring was not perceived, 2 means that some caring was evident, and scores of 3 and 4 reflect moderate to high levels of caring (Latham, 1998, 2009). A score between 1 and 2 indicates that an individual does not feel cared for in a holistic sense; a score of 2 to 3 indicates that caring is somewhat evident, and a score greater than 3 indicates that caring is very evident to the patient. Both subscale scores and the total score can be used for results. An individual's total score is a summated mean of all four subscales.

The interpretation of the four subscales indicates how the patients perceive nurses view them in a holistic manner that includes social, physical, psychological, and spiritual components. "Physical caring" is not evaluated from a technical perspective, but rather from the psychosocial view of obtaining information about physiological needs, interrelationships of physical and emotional components of their condition, and the ability of the nurse to assist patients to meet their needs. "Sensitirve caring" involves listening to patients' feelings, and anticipating and showing concern for their needs. "Interpretive caring" is assistance provided by nurses to make sense of their condition and the trajectory of their illness, the meaning of their feelings, and how their illness will affect other areas of their lives. "Spiritual caring" involves showing respect for patients' belief systems and spiritual needs.

A copy of the HCI is included (Tool 15.1). It is hoped, in this age of patient-centered care, that nurses focus on the individual who is receiving care and their support system. Nursing care is often measured by patient satisfaction with general aspects of the care received, answering patient or family questions, and completing tasks. The general surveys used to determine patient satisfaction do not capture the essence of the nurse–patient connection that involves humanistic caring. Caring about patients is a focus that needs more emphasis so that it can be taken into consideration when evaluating healthcare economics and patient outcomes (Turkel, 2001).

In summary, humanistic caring is a process where nurses meet patients at their level of understanding and life experience with the goal of intersubjective transactions that nurture and promote well-being and existential growth. These philosophical perspectives and concepts are the foundation of providing holistic care that goes beyond task-oriented physical care and measures nurses' ability to convey information, assist with feelings, employ empathy to be perceptive to patients' needs, and use appropriate verbal and nonverbal communication. Holistic care incorporates psychosocial and spiritual components to better connect with patients. The HCI is an instrument that can be used to estimate the extent that nurses care about an individual from the patient's perspective, and while nurses provide physical care, they also relate information, assist with feelings, and make connections that nurture respect and dignity with positive concern and empathy.

TOOL 15.1

Holistic Caring Inventory (Latham, 1988, 2018)

General Directions: For the remaining statements, think of one particular registered nurse who had the greatest effect on you during your healthcare experience.

	1	2	3	4
EXAMPLE: The following statement is an example of how to answer this survey.	**STRONGLY DISAGREE**	**DISAGREE**	**AGREE**	**STRONGLY AGREE**
I am able to get information from nurses to help me deal with my condition.		X		

This answer indicates that the person did not always get information from the registered nurse about his or her condition.

Instructions: Place a checkmark in the appropriate box to the right of each statement. Keep a specific registered nurse in mind, who has taken care of you during your current illness.

	1	2	3	4
The following 10 statements refer to getting physical help from a nurse.	**STRONGLY DISAGREE**	**DISAGREE**	**AGREE**	**STRONGLY AGREE**
1. I am able to discuss my physical problems with the nurse.				
2. The nurse is sensitive to the possible effect that information may have on my recovery.				
3. The information given by the nurse about my physical problems helps me to adjust to my condition.				

(continued)

TOOL 15.1

Holistic Caring Inventory (Latham, 1988, 2018) *(continued)*

	STRONGLY DISAGREE	DISAGREE	AGREE	STRONGLY AGREE
4. The nurse considers my feelings when giving me information about my physical condition.				
5. The nurse shows concern about how my physical condition will affect other areas of my life.				
6. The nurse allows time for me to think over my physical problems.				
7. The nurse shares his/her view of my physical condition with me.				
8. The nurse helps me with my feelings about changes happening to my body.				
9. The nurse understands my condition, and this helps me to deal with physical problems.				
10. The nurse knows when I need help in dealing with physical problems.				

The following 10 statements refer to the way the nurse deals with your feelings.	1 STRONGLY DISAGREE	2 DISAGREE	3 AGREE	4 STRONGLY AGREE
11. The nurse is attentive to my needs when I am depressed or feeling down.				
12. The nurse listens to my feelings when taking care of me.				
13. The nurse helps me to interpret the meaning of my feelings.				
14. The nurse shares her/his feelings about my situation to help me understand my condition.				
15. The nurse helps me to discuss my feelings when I need to make changes.				
16. The nurse is sensitive to my feelings when I am trying to understand my condition.				

(continued)

TOOL 15.1

Holistic Caring Inventory (Latham, 1988, 2018) (continued)

17. The nurse shows concern for my feelings.				
18. The nurse openly discusses my feelings to help me to adjust to being ill.				
19. The nurse shares how he/she sees my feelings affecting others who are close to me.				
20. The nurse reacts to my feelings in a way that helps me to adjust to a new situation.				

	1	2	3	4
The following 10 statements refer to how nurses handle other important areas of your life.	**STRONGLY DISAGREE**	**DISAGREE**	**AGREE**	**STRONGLY AGREE**
21. The nurse gives information about how my condition will affect other areas of my life.				
22. The nurse allows me time to reflect on how my condition will affect my family, friends, etc.				
23. With my permission, the nurse talks about my condition to family, friends, or other people to whom I go for help.				
24. When I have a new condition, I find that the nurse is easy to talk to.				
25. The nurse helps my feelings about my relationships with others.				
26. The nurse discusses how my condition will affect my sexuality.				
27. The nurse shows concern about how my condition will affect the work or job with which I am normally involved.				
28. The nurse shares her/his view of how my family or friends are reacting to my situation.				

(continued)

TOOL 15.1

Holistic Caring Inventory (Latham, 1988, 2018) (*continued*)

	1 STRONGLY DISAGREE	2 DISAGREE	3 AGREE	4 STRONGLY AGREE
29. I find the nurse is interested in knowing what I have done or would like to do during my lifetime.				
30. The nurse is aware of my idiosyncrasies and other things important to my care.				
The next 10 statements refer to how the nurse handles your need for hope and spiritual needs.				
31. While ill, I feel the nurse shows concern for my beliefs.				
32. The nurse considers my need for some hope when telling me about my condition.				
33. I find that the nurse encourages me to reflect on hope for my future.				
34. The nurse recognizes that my beliefs may help me to adjust to new situations in my life.				
35. The nurse openly discusses how this situation fits into the rest of my life.				
36. The nurse helps me obtain guidance when I can't deal with difficult feelings.				
37. The nurse accepts my need to sometimes feel like the situation is out of my hands.				
38. The nurse is able to sense times when I need help from a higher power.				
39. When requested, the nurse assists me in obtaining religious or spiritual advice to help me deal with health-related situations.				
40. The nurse respects my thoughts, practices, and belief systems.				

REFERENCES

Auerbach, S. M., Martelli, M. F., & Mercuri, L. G. (1983). Anxiety, information, interpersonal impacts, and adjustment to a stressful health care situation. *Journal of Personality and Social Psychology, 44*(6), 1284–1296. doi:10.1037/0022-3514.44.6.1284

Brousseau, S., Cara, C. M., & Blais, R. (2017). A humanistic caring quality of work life model in nursing administration based on Watson's philosophy. *International Journal of Human Caring, 21*(1), 2–8. doi:10.20467/1091-5710-21.1.2

Crowne, D. P., & Marlowe, D. (1964). *The approval motive: Studies in evaluative dependence.* New York, NY: Wiley.

Fry, E. (1968). A readability formula that saves time. *Journal of Reading, 11*(7), 575–578. Retrieved from https://www.jstor.org/stable/40013635

Gardner, K. G., & Wheeler, E. C. (1987). Patients' perceptions of support. *Western Journal of Nursing Research, 9*(1), 115–131. doi:10.1177/019394598700900110

Hall, J. A., Roter, D. L., & Katz, N. R. (1988). Meta-analysis of correlates of provider behavior in medical encounters. *Medical Care, 28*(7), 657–675. doi:10.1097/00005650-198807000-00002

Howard, J. (1975). Humanization and dehumanization of health care: A conceptual view. In J. Howard & A. Straus (Eds.), *Humanizing health care.* New York, NY: John Wiley.

Kiesler, D. J. (1987). *Manual for the impact message inventory: Research edition.* Palo Alto, CA: Consulting Psychologists Press.

Larson, P. (1981). Oncology patients' and professional nurses' perceptions of important nurse caring behaviors. *Dissertation Abstracts International, 42*(3), 0528B. (UMI No. 8116511)

Larson, P. (1984). Important nurse caring behaviors perceived by patients with cancer. *Oncology Nursing Forum, 11*, 46–50.

Latham, C. L. (1988, March). *Measurement of caring in recipient-provider interactions.* Paper presented at the Second Measurement of Clinical and Educational Nursing Outcomes Conference, San Diego, CA.

Latham, C. L. (1996). Predictors of patient outcomes following interactions with nurses. *Western Journal of Nursing Research, 18*(5), 548–564. doi:10.1177/019394599601800506

Latham, C. L. (2009). Holistic caring inventory. In J. Watson (Ed.), *Assessing and measuring caring in nursing and health science* (2nd ed., pp.171–178). New York, NY: Springer Publishing.

Latham, C. L., Ringl, K., & Hogan, M. (2011). Professionalization and retention outcomes of a university-service mentoring program partnership. *Journal of Professional Nursing, 27*(6), 344–353. doi:10.1016/j.profnurs.2011.04.015

Latham, C. L, Ringl, K., & Hogan, M. (2013). Combating workplace violence with peers. *Nursing Management, 44* (9), 30–39. doi:10.1097/01.NUMA.0000429005.47269.f9

L'etourneau, D., Cara, C., & Goudreau, J. (2017). Humanizing nursing care: An analysis of caring theories through the lens of humanism. *International Journal for Human Caring, 21*(1), 32–40. doi:10.20467/1091-5710.21.1.32

Mayer, D. (1986). Cancer patients' and families perceptions of nurse caring behaviors. *Topics in Clinical Nursing, 8*(2), 63–69.

Turkel, M. C. (2001). Struggling to find a balance: The paradox between caring and economics. *Nursing Administration, 26*(1), 67–82. doi:10.1097/00006216-200110000-00016

Williams, S. (1998). Quality of patient care: Patient perspectives. *Journal of Care Quality, 12*(6), 18–25. doi:10.1097/00001786-199808000-00006

Caring Dimensions Inventory

Roger Watson and Amandah Hoogbruin

The Caring Dimensions Inventory (CDI) is a quantitative tool to measure caring that was developed at the University of Edinburgh, Scotland. The conceptual–theoretical basis for the tool was guided by an empirical rather than theoretical approach to caring that acknowledges some of the general caring theory literature. The theoretical approaches used were those that supported the operationalization of caring through specific taxonomies and measurements. Several studies using this instrument have been reported in the literature, although the authors indicate that they have not systematically gathered information on the extent of its use.

Some of Leininger's (1981) major caring taxonomic constructs, along with Grobe and Hughes's (1993) nursing intervention lexicon and taxonomy, were identified as helpful notions. In addition to a review of academic literature, a grounded critique of popular articles in UK nursing journals and newspapers was conducted to detect how the concept of caring was presented to the readerships of such publications. Any articles that used the key words "care" or "caring" between 1983 and 1993 in the *British Journal of Nursing* and the *Nursing Times*, the *Nursing Standard*, and *Professional Nursing* were gleaned for meaning of the concept. From 63 articles reviewed and retrieved through a computerized system, 14 themes emerged. The most common were the nurse–patient relationship (36 articles), nursing interventions (17 articles), nursing attitudes (16 articles), nursing skills (15 articles), and communication (16 articles; Watson & Lea, 1997). In the development of the CDI, general categories of care were developed from the literature review. The four most popular themes were used to classify the CDI questions, as they were believed to describe general categories of care. A total of 25 core items was included on the CDI.

© Springer Publishing Company DOI:10.1891/9780826195425.0016

The CDI questionnaire was administered to nurses and student nurses in a local health trust and to a student sample in a neighboring health trust between August 1994 and January 1995. From a distribution of 3,024 questionnaires, 1,452 were returned, representing a 47% rate of return. Cronbach's alpha was used to establish reliability and internal consistency of the 25 core items at .91. Additional construct analysis was conducted to determine if there was a significant relationship between age and sex and CDI. The Mokken scale and SPSS PC+ along with a Spearman's correlation of age were used to conduct sophisticated analysis. Kruskal–Wallis one-way ANOVA of CDI Mokken scale scores for male and female subjects was carried out, yielding statistically significant results ($p < .05$) suggesting a relationship between age and CDI Mokken scale score, and differences between males and females. An interesting finding was that older nurses perceive more technical aspects of nursing work, in addition to psychosocial aspects, as being caring. Males tend to perceive nursing (caring) in more psychosocial terms than females (Watson & Lea, 1997). Content validity was demonstrated through the content findings of previous quantitative research on caring, as well as presentation of caring in popular nursing journals. The instrument is copyrighted by the authors, and they request that anyone using the tool contact them for permission. The matrix in Table 16.1 outlines the key elements of the CDI (Tool 16.1) along with latest citations of the work, referred to as the "Edinburgh CDI."

TABLE 16.1 Matrix of Caring Dimensions Inventory

INSTRUMENT	AUTHOR CONTACT INFORMATION	PUBLICATION SOURCE	DEVELOPED TO MEASURE	INSTRUMENT DESCRIPTION	PARTICIPANTS	REPORTED VALIDITY/ RELIABILITY	CONCEPTUAL– THEORETICAL BASIS OF MEASUREMENT	LATEST CITATION IN NURSING LITERATURE
Caring Dimensions Inventory (1997)	Roger Watson, PhD, RN, FI Biol FHEA, FRSA Editor, *Journal of Clinical Nursing* Professor of Nursing School of Nursing and Midwifery The University of Sheffield, Sheffield S10 2TN Phone: + 44-114-222-9848 Fax: + 44-114-222-9712 Email: roger.watson@ sheffield.ac.uk Amandah (Lea) Hoogbruin, PHD, RN Nursing Faculty Kwantlen University College 12666–72nd Avenue Surrey, BC V3W 2 MB Email: amandah .hoogbruin@ kwantlen.ca	Watson and Lea (1997)	Perceptions of caring from large sample of nurses	5-point Likert scale with 41 questions (25 core questions regarding perceptions of caring)	$N = 1,452$ nurses and nursing students	Cronbach's alpha = .91 Mokken scaling and Spearman's correlation of age Kruskal–Wallis one-way ANOVA for males vs. females ($p < .05$) for age and sex differences in perceptions of caring	Empirical approach vs. theoretical basis, although caring theory that supported operationalizing of caring was influential	Lea, Watson, and Deary (1998) Watson, Deary, and Hoogbruin (2001) Watson (2003) Watson et al. (2003)

TOOL 16.1

Caring Dimensions Inventory

Stem Question: Do you consider the following aspects of nursing practice to be caring?

Response on 5-point Likert scale: 1 (strongly disagree) to 5 (strongly agree)

	1	2	3	4	5
1. Assisting a patient with an activity of daily living (washing, dressing, etc.)	1	2	3	4	5
2. Making a nursing record about the patient	1	2	3	4	5
3. Feeling sorry for a patient	1	2	3	4	5
4. Getting to know the patient as a person	1	2	3	4	5
5. Explaining a clinical procedure to a patient	1	2	3	4	5
6. Being neatly dressed when working with a patient	1	2	3	4	5
7. Sitting with a patient	1	2	3	4	5
8. Exploring a patient's lifestyle	1	2	3	4	5
9. Reporting a patient's condition to a senior nurse	1	2	3	4	5
10. Being with a patient during a clinical procedure	1	2	3	4	5
11. Being honest with a patient	1	2	3	4	5
12. Organizing the work of others for a patient	1	2	3	4	5
13. Listening to a patient	1	2	3	4	5
14. Consulting with the doctor about a patient	1	2	3	4	5
15. Instructing a patient about an aspect of self-care (washing, dressing, etc.)	1	2	3	4	5
16. Sharing your personal problems with a patient	1	2	3	4	5
17. Keeping relatives informed about a patient	1	2	3	4	5
18. Measuring the vital signs of a patient (e.g., pulse and blood pressure)	1	2	3	4	5
19. Putting the needs of a patient before your own	1	2	3	4	5
20. Being technically competent with a clinical procedure	1	2	3	4	5
21. Involving a patient with his or her care	1	2	3	4	5
22. Giving reassurance about a clinical procedure	1	2	3	4	5
23. Providing privacy for a patient	1	2	3	4	5
24. Being cheerful with a patient	1	2	3	4	5
25. Observing the effects of a medication on a patient	1	2	3	4	5

Source: From Watson, R., & Lea, A. (1997). The Caring Dimensions Inventory (CDI): Content validity, reliability and scaling. *Journal of Advanced Nursing, 25*, 87–94. doi:10.1046/j.1365-2648.1997.1997025087.x. Reprinted by permission of the authors.

REFERENCES

Hughes, L. (1993). Peer group interactions and the students-perceived climate for caring. *Journal of Nursing Education, 32*(2), 78–83.

Lea, A., Watson, R., & Deary, I. J. (1998). Caring in nursing: A multivariate analysis. *Journal of Advanced Nursing, 28*(3), 662–671. doi:10.1046/j.1365-2648.1998.00799.x

Leininger, M. M. (1981). The phenomenon of caring: Importance, research questions and theoretical considerations. In M. M. Leininger (Ed.), *Caring: An essential human need* (pp. 2–15). Thorofare, NJ: Charles B. Slack.

Watson, R. (2003). Intrarater reliability of the Caring Dimensions Inventory and Nursing Dimensions Inventory. *Journal of Clinical Nursing, 12*(5), 786–787. doi:10.1046/j.1365-2702.2003.00712.x

Watson, R., Deary, I. J., & Hoogbruin, A. L. (2001). A 35-item version of the caring dimensions inventory (CD-35) multivariate analysis and application to a longitudinal study involving nursing students. *International Journal of Nursing Studies, 38*(5), 511–521. doi:10.1016/S0020-7489(00)00107-3

Watson, R., Hoogbruin, A. L., Rumeu, C., Beunza, M., Barbarin, B., MacDonald, J., & McCready, T. (2003). Differences and similarities in the perception of caring between Spanish and UK nurses. *Journal of Clinical Nursing, 12*(1), 85–92. doi:10.1046/j.1365-2702.2003.00671.x

Watson, R., & Lea, A. (1997). The Caring Dimensions Inventory (CDI): Content validity, reliability and scaling. *Journal of Advanced Nursing, 25,* 87–94. doi:10.1046/j.1365-2648.1997.1997025087.x

Caring Attributes, Professional Self-Concept, and Technological Influences Scale

David G. Arthur

Arthur and colleagues in Hong Kong (1999) developed a complex caring instrument and tested it with 1,957 registered nurses in 11 different countries. The purpose was to develop an understanding of caring and to compare the responses to caring items with responses to items related to professional self-concept and technological influences across different countries and cultures. The conceptual–theoretical basis of the study was informed by the empirical work of Lea and Watson (1996; Watson & Lea, 1997) and the conceptual and multidimensional construct development of Wolf and associates (1994). In addition, theoretical, practical, and pedagogical perspectives were generated from such works from the general nursing-caring literature as Leininger (1981), and Watson (1988). Of all the instruments in this book, this instrument has the most global focus and scope; its testing, use, and continued development have taken place across several different countries (Table 17.1).

The Caring Attributes, Professional Self-Concept, and Technological Influences (CAPSTI) scale was developed through a pilot study using a convenience sample of nurses from Hong Kong, Beijing, and Macau (Tools 17.1 and 17.2). The themes and language that emerged from this sample were reviewed for content validity by a sample of experts. Specific items emerged from a combination of sources: the literature, the sample, and the experts. The instrument was administered to an additional sample of 100 nurses in Hong Kong in order to establish — reliability and validity. A Cronbach's alpha of greater than .7 was found for each of the three parts of the instrument (Arthur et al., 1999). Apart from 7 demographic items, the instrument consists of 44 items in Part 1, in which items 1 to 30 measure the Professional Self Concept (PSCNI), and items 31 to 34 are technological influences questions (TIQ). Part 2 is the Technological Influences Scale (TIS) which determines the technological influence of different hospital units, while Part 3 consists of 60 items related to caring attributes (CAQ).

Each of the three parts of the instrument uses a Likert scale, on which a high ranking indicates a positive attitude or belief. Individual scores and group scores were obtained for the components of the PSCNI (professional practice, satisfaction, and communication), technological influences (Technological Influences Questionnaire [TIQ] and Technological Influences Survey [TIS]), and caring attributes (including theoretical, practical, and pedagogical perspectives).

The international sample was gathered by an international team of collaborators who were invited to participate in the project via a letter. Colleagues in six countries agreed to participate, and later other interested colleagues agreed to participate. Each site was asked to translate the instrument into the local language, to administer the instrument to a randomly selected sample of 250 registered nurses working in a clinical hospital setting, and to send the completed questionnaires to the Hong Kong research team. Eventually 11 countries participated, which meant that the instruments needed to be translated into Chinese and Korean, and the results were entered into a comprehensive database for descriptive and inferential analysis.

A total of 1,957 questionnaires from 11 different countries were analyzed. Cronbach's alphas were reported as follows: PSCNI = .89; TIQ = .75; TISQ = .94; and CAQ = .88. Face and construct validity of the CAPSTI were established from the literature and the original pilot study. Significant correlations were found between and among the different parts of the CAPSTI. Pearson's correlation coefficients were reported at $p < .0001$, between the PSCNI and caring attributes ($r = .51$), between the PSCNI and TIQ = .13, and between the caring attributes and the TIQ = .16. Mean scores on the different parts of the instrument differed between and among the various countries. For example, on the caring attributes dimension, the Chinese (Beijing) sample had the lowest mean score, while the Filipino sample was significantly different from all the samples except those from South Africa and Sweden. The Canadian sample was significantly different from the Korean sample. The items that solicited the highest mean for the total sample were "Creating a sense of trust," "A confident relationship between a nurse and a patient is one based on trust, truth, and respect," "Allowing the patient to express feelings," "Paying attention to the patient when he/she is talking," and "Listening to the patient." Only the Canadian and South African samples reported the highest scores on "Treating patients' information confidentially." All respondents gave the caring attributes scores greater than 3, the arbitrary midpoint of the caring continuum.

The Filipino sample had the highest mean score for caring attributes. A caring, trusting relationship between the nurse and the patient was one of the aspects of caring commonly reported by most of the international samples. Additional detailed differences between and among the different countries are reported by Arthur and associates (1999).

This research is the first to develop and empirically test and measure caring across different countries. Moreover, it is an ambitious study that has attempted to compare and contrast caring attributes in relation to professional self-concept and technological influences in an international sample. The CAPSTI has been reported to be reliable and valid, helping to create a composite picture of caring among nurses in various countries and cultures. The CAPSTI was administered in a study of 560 Korean RNs, and the relationship between caring attributes and technological influences was examined (Choon, Arthur, & Sohng, 2002). A factor analysis supported the factor structure, with some variation accounted for by cultural differences.

Building on this research, Arthur, Pang, and Wong (2001) conducted a psychometric analysis based on the original international sample and refined the instrument, resulting in the CAPSTI-2. Factor analysis revealed a four-factor structure with a reduced number of items (31) clustered in four dimensions: caring communication, caring involvement, caring advocacy, and learning to care. O'Brien, Arthur, Woods, and Watson (2004) used the CAPSTI-2 with a sample of 380 New Zealand nurses. This supported the validity (with some modification due to local culture) and reliability of the modified instrument.

Most recently the CAPSTI-2 has been used to compare the caring attributes of Hong Kong and Thai psychiatric nurses (Arthur, Chong, Rujorakarn, Wong, & Wongpanarak, 2004) and to explore caring attributes and perceptions of workplace change among gerontological nurses in England, Scotland, and Hong Kong (Schofield, Tolson, Arthur, Davies, & Nolan, 2005). While the majority of the items composing the CAPSTI-2 were used in these studies, minor modifications were made to suit the culture and/or branch of nursing being examined.

Arthur and Randle (2007) report that a longitudinal study using the CAPSTI-2 with other psychological outcome variables to correlate students' entry behaviors and performances in a nursing program with selected outcome variables is being conducted in Singapore.

The refined CAPSTI-2 is emerging as a reliable and valid measure for nursing studies on caring attributes, and normative databases are being developed in various branches of nursing and in various cultures. This offers useful direction for both descriptive and experimental studies in the future, and the instrument may prove to be a useful predictor of nursing performance both clinically and educationally. It continues to be refined and used and tested extensively in various parts of the world. For example, since the last edition of this text, an application of the caring instrument (Caring Attributes Questionnaire [CAQ]) was demonstrated in an Iranian study where the authors (Bagherian, Sabzevari, Mirzaei, & Ravari, 2017) refined the instrument through factor analysis and examined the relationship between caring attributes and technology in a sample of 200 critical care nurses. In a Portuguese study (Almeida, Almeida, Escola, & Rodrigues, 2016) using a rigorous translation method and testing, the CAQ again showed its versatility and application for further research. The psychometric properties of the scale were assessed and strongly supported based on its application to a sample of 341 individuals (nurses, physicians, final-year nursing and medical students). Since 2013 five studies using the PSCNI alone have been conducted in samples in Korea, China, and Turkey, again showing the versatility of the tool for use in

TABLE 17.1 Matrix of Caring Attributes, Professional Self-Concept, and Technological Influences (CAPSTI and CAPSTI-2) Scale

INSTRUMENT	AUTHOR CONTACT INFORMATION	PUBLICATION SOURCE	DEVELOPED TO MEASURE	INSTRUMENT DESCRIPTION	PARTICIPANTS	REPORTED VALIDITY/ RELIABILITY	CONCEPTUAL–THEORETICAL BASIS OF MEASUREMENT	LATEST CITATION IN NURSING LITERATURE
Caring attributes, professional self-concept, and technological influences scale (2001)	David Arthur, PhD, RN Professor and Dean School of Nursing and Midwifery The Aga Khan University Karachi Pakistan Email: david.arthur@aku.edu	Arthur et al. (1999)	Multidimensional construct of caring internationally	Uses three subscales of caring attributes and three subscales of 13 theoretical, 41 practical items, and 7 pedagogical items	$N = 1,957$ RNs from 11 countries (Hong Kong, Australia, Canada, China, Korea, New Zealand, the Philippines, Scotland, Singapore, South Africa, Sweden)	Cronbach's alpha = .75 overall PSCNI = .89, TIQ = .75,TISQ = .94, CAQ = .88	Items designed to reflect theoretical, practical, and pedagogical perspectives of caring Items in three categories generated by caring theory literature (e.g., Leininger, Benner, Watson, Morse)	Arthur et al. (1999)

CAPSTI-2 (2001)	David Arthur, PhD, RN Professor and Dean School of Nursing and Midwifery The Aga Khan University Karachi Pakistan Email: david.arthur@aku.edu	Arthur et al. (2001)	Multidimensional construct of caring across cultures and in different branches of nursing	31 items measure caring attributes in four dimensions: caring communication, caring involvement, caring advocacy, and learning to care	N = 1,957 RNs from 11 countries (Hong Kong, Australia, Canada, China, Korea, New Zealand, the Philippines, Scotland, Singapore, South Africa, Sweden)	Caring communication: 10 items, α = .84, factor analysis % of variance = 15.96 Caring involvement: 8 items, α = .79, factor analysis % of variance = 11.67 Caring advocacy: 7 items, α = .78, factor analysis % of variance = 9.83 Learning to care: 5 items, α = .62, factor analysis % of variance = 7.02	Items designed to reflect theoretical, practical, and pedagogical perspectives of caring Items in three categories generated by caring theory literature (e.g., Leininger, Benner, Watson, Morse) Refined by psychometric analysis and factor analysis	Arthur and Randle (2007)

different samples and across cultures (A-ri & In Sook, 2013; Dong & Choi, 2016; Eun Jin, Se Young, & Kyung Mi, 2013; Guo, Liu, & Yu, 2016; Kantek & Simsek, 2017). Both instruments have also contributed to the discourse and debate on nursing characteristics and behaviors, and are widely cited in articles that address the important constructs of caring and self-concept in nurses. This instrument is copyrighted by Arthur, whose contact information is provided in Table 17.1.

TOOL 17.1

Caring Attributes, Professional Self-Concept, and Technological Influences Scale: Nursing Studies Section Opinion Survey

This questionnaire was developed by nurses from the Department of Health Sciences at the Hong Kong Polytechnic University.

This is an international study involving nurses from different countries including: Australia, Canada, China, Hong Kong, Japan, Macau, the Philippines, Scotland, South Africa, South Korea, and Sweden.

By filling in the questionnaire you will be helping us develop a profile of how nurses in different cultures approach caring and professional issues in nursing.

This questionnaire consists of four parts that explore nurses' perceptions of caring, professional self-concept, and technological influences in their caring practice. In all four parts please express your opinion on the item statements.

All data will be kept confidential and only group results will be reported. It is not necessary to write your name.

Thank you for taking the time to complete the questionnaire.

Yours sincerely,

David Arthur, Thomas Wong, Samantha Pang

This study is funded by the University Grants Committee of Hong Kong. © *Arthur, Pang, Wong, 1997.*

Source: Reprinted by permission of the author. Copyright © David Arthur.

TOOL 17.2

Caring Attributes, Professional Self-Concept, and Technological Influences Scale

PART I

Answer each item by ranking your agreement on the 4-point scale: 1 = disagree, 2 = tend to disagree, 3 = tend to agree, 4 = agree. *By circling one symbol ("1" or "4") you are indicating your disagreement or agreement.*

Rank your degree of agreement with the following items. *How well does each item describe you and your work as a nurse?*

ITEM	1=DISAGREE	2=TEND TO DISAGREE	3=TEND TO AGREE	4=AGREE
1. When I am at work and the situation calls, I am able to think of alternatives.	1	2	3	4
2. I am a skillful nurse.	1	2	3	4

(continued)

TOOL 17.2

Caring Attributes, Professional Self-Concept, and Technological Influences Scale (*continued*)

ITEM	1=DISAGREE	2=TEND TO DISAGREE	3=TEND TO AGREE	4=AGREE
3. I am a competent leader.	1	2	3	4
4. I believe that flexibility is one of my attributes.	1	2	3	4
5. Competency is one of my characteristics.	1	2	3	4
6. When I am in charge, people work efficiently.	1	2	3	4
7. I generally look forward to going to work.	1	2	3	4
8. When confronted with nursing problems, my creativity helps me to solve them.	1	2	3	4
9. I do not believe I am particularly empathetic.	1	2	3	4
10. Nursing is a rewarding career.	1	2	3	4
11. Flexibility helps solve nursing problems.	1	2	3	4
12. I prefer a barrier between me and my patients.	1	2	3	4
13. I would rather not have the responsibility of leadership.	1	2	3	4
14. Work as a nurse is generally as I expected before I started.	1	2	3	4
15. I am quick to grasp the essentials of nursing problems, to see alternative solutions, and to select the most appropriate solution.	1	2	3	4
16. I think it is important to share emotions with patients.	1	2	3	4
17. Most of my colleagues seem willing to work with me as a leader.	1	2	3	4
18. I regret ever starting nursing.	1	2	3	4

(continued)

TOOL 17.2

Caring Attributes, Professional Self-Concept, and Technological Influences Scale (*continued*)

ITEM	1=DISAGREE	2=TEND TO DISAGREE	3=TEND TO AGREE	4=AGREE
19. On the whole I am satisfied with my creative approach to my work as a nurse.	1	2	3	4
20. Competency is the demonstrated ability to successfully apply knowledge and skills in the performance of complex tasks. I am a competent nurse.	1	2	3	4
21. I feel more comfortable not getting too emotionally close to the people with whom I work.	1	2	3	4
22. Decision making is one of my attributes.	1	2	3	4
23. Nursing is less satisfying than I thought it would be.	1	2	3	4
24. I usually perform skills as well as my other colleagues.	1	2	3	4
25. I feel trapped as a nurse.	1	2	3	4
26. My flexible approach brings out the best in my patients.	1	2	3	4
27. I think I will continue in nursing for most of my working life.	1	2	3	4
28. In nursing, it is important to have professional interaction with colleagues.	1	2	3	4
29. Most people would say nursing is a valuable profession.	1	2	3	4
30. I think I am respected as a nurse by other professionals.	1	2	3	4
31. I don't think there is any more spare time in nursing even though we have an increase in technology.	1	2	3	4
32. High technology requires high-tech skills.	1	2	3	4

(continued)

TOOL 17.2

Caring Attributes, Professional Self-Concept, and Technological Influences Scale (*continued*)

ITEM	1=DISAGREE	2=TEND TO DISAGREE	3=TEND TO AGREE	4=AGREE
33. The increase in technology in nursing has increased the workload of nurses.	1	2	3	4
34. The increase of technical tasks has downgraded the nursing profession.	1	2	3	4
35. The influx of technology has raised the profession of nurses.	1	2	3	4
36. Due to the application of technology, nurses often become frustrated when the inevitable death of a patient occurs.	1	2	3	4
37. Technology and the use of machines often interfere with providing adequate nursing care.	1	2	3	4
38. Nurses often neglect patients because of the influx of machines.	1	2	3	4
39. I'm not sure about the benefits of technology to my practice.	1	2	3	4
40. In general, technology enhances patient care and well-being.	1	2	3	4
41. Technology has resulted in nurses becoming increasingly professionally uncertain.	1	2	3	4
42. Mastery of technology has helped nurses control their work environment.	1	2	3	4
43. Technology is an activity that adds meaning to the work of nurses.	1	2	3	4
44. Mastery of technology is a useful tool in developing the professional status of nurses.	1	2	3	4

(continued)

TOOL 17.2

Caring Attributes, Professional Self-Concept, and Technological Influences Scale (*continued*)

PART II

These questions aim to explore your impression of the technological influences in a hospital.

Please give your response as quickly as you can.

1. *What is your present working unit?* _____

2. *In your experience as a nurse, how would you rate the technological influence in the following different units of a hospital? Please rate degree of technological influence in the following units.*

UNIT	1=VERY LOW	2=LOW	3= MODERATE	4=HIGH	5=VERY HIGH
Intensive Care Unit (ICU)	1	2	3	4	5
Cardiac Care Unit	1	2	3	4	5
Orthopedic and Traumatology Unit	1	2	3	4	5
Renal Unit	1	2	3	4	5
Geriatric Unit	1	2	3	4	5
Radiotherapy and Oncology Unit	1	2	3	4	5
Medical Unit	1	2	3	4	5
Surgical Unit	1	2	3	4	5
Neurosurgical Unit	1	2	3	4	5
Obstetrics Unit	1	2	3	4	5
Labor Room	1	2	3	4	5
Neonatal and Infant Care Unit	1	2	3	4	5
Neonatal ICU	1	2	3	4	5
Pediatric Unit	1	2	3	4	5
Burn Unit	1	2	3	4	5
Infection Control Unit	1	2	3	4	5
Operating Theater	1	2	3	4	5
Accident and Emergency Department	1	2	3	4	5
General Outpatient Department	1	2	3	4	5
Specialty Outpatient Department	1	2	3	4	5

(continued)

TOOL 17.2

Caring Attributes, Professional Self-Concept, and Technological Influences Scale (*continued*)

UNIT	1=VERY LOW	2=LOW	3= MODERATE	4=HIGH	5=VERY HIGH
Hematology Unit	1	2	3	4	5
Organ Transplantation Unit	1	2	3	4	5
Psychiatric Unit	1	2	3	4	5
Gynecology Unit	1	2	3	4	5
Ear, Nose, and Throat Unit	1	2	3	4	5
Neurological Unit	1	2	3	4	5
Sport Medicine Unit	1	2	3	4	5
Cardiothoracic Surgery Unit	1	2	3	4	5
Dental Unit	1	2	3	4	5
Ophthalmology Unit	1	2	3	4	5

PART III

The following items relate to *what caring means to you* as a nurse. Rank your degree of agreement. Try to write what you believe, not what others say, or what others might expect you to say.

ITEM	1= DISAGREE	2=TEND TO DISAGREE	3=TEND TO AGREE	4=AGREE
1. Caring is a natural human response and does not require any planning.	1	2	3	4
2. Caring is the central feature of nursing.	1	2	3	4
3. Caring nurses are motivated by a feeling or emotion to provide care for patients.	1	2	3	4
4. In plain language, caring is a "joint effort" between the nurse and the patient.	1	2	3	4
5. Caring is a planned nurse activity designed to meet patients' needs.	1	2	3	4
6. Caring is acting; it is not just a feeling.	1	2	3	4
7. Caring is a central virtue in nursing and focuses on the nurse as the moral agent.	1	2	3	4

(continued)

TOOL 17.2

Caring Attributes, Professional Self-Concept, and Technological Influences Scale (*continued*)

ITEM	1=DISAGREE	2=TEND TO DISAGREE	3=TEND TO AGREE	4=AGREE
8. Caring is aimed at preserving the dignity of the patient.	1	2	3	4
9. Caring is unique in nursing.	1	2	3	4
10. A nurse cannot care too much.	1	2	3	4
11. Caring makes no difference to the patients' health condition.	1	2	3	4
12. If a nurse ceases to care, he/she ceases to be a nurse.	1	2	3	4
13. Caring is a tool for technology.	1	2	3	4

Rank your degree of agreement with the following items. *When I am working with my patient, I am being caring when I am:*

ITEM	1=DISAGREE	2=TEND TO DISAGREE	3=TEND TO AGREE	4=AGREE
14. Treating everyone as an individual	1	2	3	4
15. Being empathic.	1	2	3	4
16. Avoiding the patient.	1	2	3	4
17. Listening to the patient.	1	2	3	4
18. Touching the patient when comfort is needed.	1	2	3	4
19. Allowing the patient to express feelings.	1	2	3	4
20. Talking to the patient.	1	2	3	4
21. Helping to make experiences more pleasant.	1	2	3	4
22. Demonstrating professional skills.	1	2	3	4
23. Putting the need of the hospital before the patient.	1	2	3	4
24. Communicating with the patient.	1	2	3	4
25. Providing the patient with encouragement.	1	2	3	4

(continued)

TOOL 17.2

Caring Attributes, Professional Self-Concept, and Technological Influences Scale (*continued*)

ITEM	1= DISAGREE	2=TEND TO DISAGREE	3=TEND TO AGREE	4=AGREE
26. Helping the patient clarify thinking.	1	2	3	4
27. Expecting the patient to do what I tell him/her.	1	2	3	4
28. Treating patients' information confidentially.	1	2	3	4
29. Helping the patient with his/her activities of daily living.	1	2	3	4
30. Giving the patient explanations concerning his/her care.	1	2	3	4
31. Not giving the patient all the information he/she needs.	1	2	3	4
32. Educating the patient about some aspects of self-care.	1	2	3	4
33. Keeping the relatives informed about the patient as negotiated with the patient.	1	2	3	4
34. Preventing any anticipated problems/dangers from occurring.	1	2	3	4
35. Knowing what to do in an emergency.	1	2	3	4
36. Creating a sense of trust.	1	2	3	4
37. Speaking up for the patient when it is perceived that something harmful will be done to the patient.	1	2	3	4
38. Speaking on behalf of the patient, in relation to his/her care.	1	2	3	4
39. Paying attention to the patient when he/she is talking.	1	2	3	4
40. Documenting care given to the patient.	1	2	3	4
41. Working collaboratively with colleagues to ensure continuity of care.	1	2	3	4
42. Not involving the patient in the planning of his/her care.	1	2	3	4

(continued)

TOOL 17.2

Caring Attributes, Professional Self-Concept, and Technological Influences Scale (*continued*)

Rank your degree of agreement with the following items. *How well does each item describe a caring nurse?*

ITEM	1= DISAGREE	2=TEND TO DISAGREE	3=TEND TO AGREE	3=AGREE
43. To be a caring nurse is to just ask someone how he/she is, and to look after and provide for that person.	1	2	3	4
44. To be a caring nurse is to care for another person and to help him/her.	1	2	3	4
45. To be a caring nurse is to do your best to make someone comfortable in his/her surroundings.	1	2	3	4
46. Caring nurses do not feel concern for the well-being of others.	1	2	3	4
47. To be a caring nurse is to help someone who is suffering from a disability and is unable to do things you can do.	1	2	3	4
48. A committed nurse is one who is prepared to work extra time with no pay.	1	2	3	4
49. The human expression of compassion is a necessary component of caring in an environment that is technologically cold and impersonal.	1	2	3	4
50. A competent nurse is someone who has respect for oneself, the profession, and patients.	1	2	3	4
51. A confident relationship between a nurse and a patient is one based on trust, truth, and respect.	1	2	3	4
52. A caring nurse is displaying conscience when he/she is morally aware of the relationship and the status of his/her actions on others.	1	2	3	4
53. A committed nurse is one who balances personal desires and professional obligations to provide care to patients.	1	2	3	4

(continued)

TOOL 17.2

Caring Attributes, Professional Self-Concept, and Technological Influences Scale (*continued*)

Rank your degree of agreement with how each item describes *how caring is learned and taught:*

ITEM	1= DISAGREE	2=TEND TO DISAGREE	3=TEND TO AGREE	4=AGREE
54. Caring is learned through instruction in counseling techniques.	1	2	3	4
55. Caring is learned by modeling in the clinical setting.	1	2	3	4
56. Caring cannot be learned or taught.	1	2	3	4
57. To care for a patient is an obligation according to a patient's needs, regardless of the nurse's experience or ability.	1	2	3	4
58. Nurses learn about caring in the nursing school.	1	2	3	4
59. Nurses learn about caring by observing other nurses work.	1	2	3	4
60. Nurses learn about caring from personal experience.	1	2	3	4

END

Thank you for your cooperation.

Source: Reprinted by permission of the author.

REFERENCES

Almeida, C., Almeida, F., Escola, J., & Rodrigues, V. (2016). The technological influence on health professionals' care: Translation and adaptation of scales. *Revista Latino-Americana de Enfermagem, 24*, e2681. doi:10.1590/1518-8345.0990.2681

A-ri, M., & In Sook, K. (2013). Relationship of perception of clinical ladder system with professional self-concept and empowerment based on nurses' clinical career stage. *Journal of Korean Academy of Nursing Administration, 19*(2), 254–264. doi:10.11111/jkana.2013.19.2.254

Arthur, D., Chong, C., Rujkorakarn, D., Wong, D., & Wongpanarak, N. (2004). A profile of the Caring Attributes of Hong Kong and Thailand Psychiatric Nurses. *International Journal of Mental Health Nursing, 13*(2):100-106. doi:10.1111/j.1440-0979.2004.00313.x

Arthur, D., Pang, S., & Wong, T. (2001). The effect of technology on the caring attributes of an international sample of nurses. *International Journal of Nursing Studies, 38*, 37–43. doi:10.1016/S0020-7489(00)00049-3

Arthur, D., Pang, S., Wong, T., Alexander, M. F., Drury, J., Eastwood, H., . . . Xiao, S. (1999). Caring attributes, professional self-concept and technological influences in a sample of registered nurses in eleven countries. *International Journal of Nursing Studies, 36*, 387–396. doi:10.1016/S0020-7489(99)00035-8

Arthur, D., & Randle, J. (2007). The professional self-concept of nurses: A review of the literature from 1992–2006. *Australian Journal of Advanced Nursing, 24*(3), 60–64.

Bagherian, B., Sabzevari, S., Mirzaei, T., & Ravari, A. (2017). Effects of technology on nursing care and caring attributes of a sample of Iranian critical care nurses. *Intensive and Critical Care Nursing, 39*, 18–27. doi:10.1016/j.iccn.2016.08.011

Choon, H. N., Arthur, D., & Sohng, K. Y. (2002). Relationship between technological influences and caring attitudes of Korean nurses. *International Journal of Nursing Practice, 8*, 247–256. doi:10.1046/j.1440-172X.2002.00374.x

Dong, H. J., & Choi, M. S. (2016). 간호대학생의 전문직 자아개념과 셀프리더십이 임상수행능력에 미치는 영향 [Influence of professional self-concept and self-leadership on clinical competence in nursing students]. *Journal of Korean Academy of Fundamentals of Nursing, 23*(4), 373–382. doi:10.7739/jkafn.2016.23.4.373

Eun Jin, O., Se Young, L., & Kyung Mi, S. (2013). Interpersonal relations, hope, professional self-concept and turnover intention according to adult attachment styles in early stage nurses. *Journal of Korean Academy of Nursing Administration, 19*(4), 491–500. doi:10.11111/jkana.2013.19.4.491

Guo, X., Liu, Y., & Yu, J. (2016). Status quo of professional self concept and subjective wellbeing of nurses in department of neurology and their correlation research. *Chinese Nursing Research, 30*(1B), 157–160. doi:10.3969/j.issn.1009-6493.2016.02.010

Kantek, F., & Şimşek, B. (2017). Factors relating to professional self-concept among nurse managers. *Journal of Clinical Nursing, 26*(23/24), 4293–4299. doi:10.1111/jocn.13755

Lea, A., & Watson, R. (1996). Caring research and concepts: A selected review of the literature. *Journal of Clinical Nursing, 5*, 71–77. doi:10.1111/j.1365-2702.1996.tb00230.x

Leininger, M. M. (1981). The phenomenon of caring: Importance, research questions and theoretical considerations. In M. M. Leininger (Ed.), *Caring: An essential human need* (pp. 2–15). Thorofare, NJ: Charles B. Slack.

O'Brien, A., Arthur, D., Woods, M., & Watson, P. (2004). A national survey of New Zealand registered nurses caring attributes, professional self-concept and technological influences. *Asian Journal of Nursing Studies, 7*(3), 43–55.

Schofield, I., Tolson, D., Arthur, D., Davies, S., & Nolan, M. (2005). An exploration of the caring attributes and perceptions of workplace change among gerontological nursing staff in England, Scotland and China (Hong Kong). *International Journal of Nursing Studies, 42*, 197–209. doi:10.1016/j.ijnurstu.2004.06.002

Watson, J. (1988). *Nursing. Human science and human care. A theory of nursing.* New York, NY: National League for Nursing.

Watson, R., & Lea, A. (1997). The Caring Dimensions Inventory (CDI): Content validity, reliability, and scaling. *Journal of Advanced Nursing, 25*, 87–94. doi:10.1046/j.1365-2648.1997.1997025087.x

Wolf, Z. R., Giardino, E. R., Osborne, P. A., & Ambrose, M. S. (1994). Dimensions of nurse caring. Image: *Journal of Nursing Scholarship, 26*(2), 107–111. doi:10.1111/j.1547-5069.1994.tb00927.x

Methodist Health Care System Nurse Caring Instrument

Gwen Sherwood

The Methodist Health Care System Nurse Caring Instrument was developed by the Nursing Quality Indicator Caring Subcommittee at Methodist Health Care System in Houston, Texas. Members of the subcommittee are Mary Shepherd, MS, RN, CNAA; Gwen Sherwood, PhD, RN; Mari Rude, MS, RN, CS, AOCN; and Lillian Eriksen, DSN, RN. This tool emerged from the nursing leadership team and a system-wide nursing quality indicator committee, which was concerned with quality indicators for which nursing would hold itself accountable. Nurses' caring was identified as a key indicator by the committee. The tool development was incorporated into an academic and clinical partnership between Methodist Hospital and the University of Texas School of Nursing, Houston. Thus, an outcome-based research study of nurses' caring became part of the initiative that generated the Nurse Caring Instrument.

There have been no substantive changes to the tool since the first edition of this book. However, the authors are responsive to any new inquiries.

The tool was designed to measure patient satisfaction with caring. The conceptual–theoretical basis of the instrument reflects a range of contemporary caring concepts from different caring theories. Items and dimensions were identified from a qualitative approach to content analysis from 42 publications. The result generated 12 dominant and 14 supportive dimensions of caring that became the core of the project. Content validity was achieved through focus groups consisting of 200 Methodist Hospital nurses, who identified 51 dimensions of caring. These were cross-referenced with the literature. Two focus groups of 21 patients further validated the final 12 dominant dimensions of caring that had been identified. The 12 dominant dimensions were care coordination, competence, teaching/learning, emotional support, respect for individuality, physical comfort, availability, helping/trusting relationship, patient/family involvement, physical environment, spiritual environment, and outcomes. The items are reflective of concepts from the caring literature and caring theory of Watson and others, as well as items that are familiar areas of assessment on other instruments.

The purpose of the process of instrument development was to develop a valid and reliable instrument, to test its psychometric properties for measuring patient satisfaction with nurses' caring, and to establish a baseline for measuring future changes. The instrument was tested with a sample of 369 medical-surgical patients who were mailed and responded to a 33-item instrument. From that sample the scale was refined to 20 items. An intraclass correlation (ICC) yielded an ICC of .98 with no interaction effect. Construct validity was established through a principal axis factoring with a varimax rotation. One factor that accounted for 75% of the variance emerged. Additional validity was apparent in mean scores for patient care units. For example, units that were expected to score higher on the scale did indeed report the highest mean scores.

Additional repeat measurements and refinements of the tool are underway. A repeat measure is planned to reevaluate caring-based outcomes. This repeat measure is to follow a year-long system-wide educational intervention for creating a caring community, including practice guidelines, and performance indicators for standards of care for the nursing staff at Methodist Health Care System.

The Nurse Caring Instrument is a first-generation caring assessment tool but has been tested with over 300 patients. It consists of 20 items on a Likert-type scale that are informed by content analysis of caring literature. Because this instrument is still in its infancy, there are no publication sources at this time. However, presentations on the development and testing of the instrument and findings to date have been delivered at international conferences (Shepherd, Rude, & Sherwood, 2000). Further analysis, testing, and validation of the instrument are underway. Methodist Hospital holds the copyright for the instrument and offers support for its ongoing refinement and use. The authors encourage anyone interested to contact them directly. Table 18.1 provides key information regarding the evolution and development of the Methodist Health Care System Nurse Caring Instrument to date (Tool 18.1).

TABLE 18.1 Matrix Of Methodist Health Care System Nurse Caring Instrument

INSTRUMENT	AUTHOR CONTACT INFORMATION	PUBLICATION SOURCE	DEVELOPED TO MEASURE	INSTRUMENT DESCRIPTION	PARTICIPANTS	REPORTED VALIDITY/ RELIABILITY	CONCEPTUAL– THEORETICAL BASIS OF MEASUREMENT	LATEST CITATION IN NURSING LITERATURE
Methodist Health Care System Nurse Caring Instrument (2000)	Mary Shepherd, MSN, RN, CNAA Nursing Project & Magnet Program Director Methodist Health Care System 6565 Fannin Street Houston, TX 77030-2707 Phone: 713-441-2531 Fax: 713-441-4427 Email: MLShepherd@tmhs.org	Unpublished	Valid and reliable instrument of nurses' caring; to operationalize caring as a core concept in patient satisfaction and outcome-based research on nurses' caring	20-item Likert-type scale Measures dominant components of caring	$N = 200$ nurses and 21 patients Revised version $N = 369$ medical-surgical patients	Intraclass correlation .98 Construct validity with principal axis factoring with varimax rotation Content validity with staff nurses	Empirically derived from range of caring literature Qualitative content analysis	None to date. Two formal research presentations: Sherwood, Ericksen, Shepherd, and Rude (2001)
	Gwen Sherwood, PhD, RN, FAAN Associate Dean for Academic Affairs The University of North Carolina Chapel Hill School of Nursing Carrington Hall Campus Box 7460 Chapel Hill, NC 27599-7400 Phone: 919-966-3734 Email: Gwen.sherwood@ unc.edu							Shepherd et al. (2000)

TOOL 18.1

Methodist Health Care System Nurse Caring Instrument

Directions: Please assist us in evaluating our nursing services by reading the following descriptions. For each description, CIRCLE the ONE NUMBER that BEST shows your opinion about the nursing care you received during your most recent hospital admission.

THE NURSING STAFF	SELDOM OR RARELY		OFTEN OR FREQUENT		ALWAYS OR ALMOST ALWAYS		DOES NOT APPLY
1. Communicated a helping and trusting attitude (Helping/Trusting)	1	2	3	4	5	6	7
2. Considered my needs when scheduling procedures or medications (Individual Respect)	1	2	3	4	5	6	7
3. Offered me a choice regarding my treatment plan (Individual Respect)	1	2	3	4	5	6	7
4. Helped me understand the changes in my life from my illness (Helping/Trusting)	1	2	3	4	5	6	7
5. Involved me in my care (Patient Involvement)	1	2	3	4	5	6	7
6. Involved my family and significant others in my care (Family Involvement)	1	2	3	4	5	6	7
7. Made me feel that if I needed nursing care again, I would come back to this hospital (Outcome)	1	2	3	4	5	6	7
8. Made me feel secure when giving me care (Emotional Support)	1	2	3	4	5	6	7
9. Made spiritual care and resources available to me (Spiritual)	1	2	3	4	5	6	7
10. Made sure other staff knew how to care for me (Care Coordination)	1	2	3	4	5	6	7

(continued)

TOOL 18.1

Methodist Health Care System Nurse Caring Instrument (*continued*)

THE NURSING STAFF	SELDOM OR RARELY		OFTEN OR FREQUENT		ALWAYS OR ALMOST ALWAYS		DOES NOT APPLY
11. Provided basic comfort measures (Physical Environment)	1	2	3	4	5	6	7
12. Demonstrated professional knowledge skills (Competence)	1	2	3	4	5	6	7
13. Provided good physical care (Physical Comfort)	1	2	3	4	5	6	7
14. Recognized that I may have special needs (Care Coordination)	1	2	3	4	5	6	7
15. Returned to check on me, not just when I called (Availability)	1	2	3	4	5	6	7
16. Showed concern for me (Emotional Support)	1	2	3	4	5	6	7
17. Taught me to care for myself whenever appropriate (Teaching/Learning)	1	2	3	4	5	6	7
18. Took care of my requests in a reasonable time (Availability)	1	2	3	4	5	6	7
19. Were honest with me (Helping/Trusting)	1	2	3	4	5	6	7
20. Were pleasant and friendly to me (Helping/Trusting)	1	2	3	4	5	6	7

Comments:

Source: ©The Methodist Hospital, Houston, Texas. Instrument developed by the Nursing Quality Indicator Subcommittee under the direction of Mary Shepherd, RN, MSN, CNAA. Reprinted with permission.

REFERENCES

Shepherd, M., Rude, M., & Sherwood, G. (2000, July 2). *Patient satisfaction with nurses caring instrument development for a nursing quality indicator.* 22nd International Association for Human Caring Conference, Boca Raton, FL.

Sherwood, G., Ericksen, L., Shepherd, M., & Rude, M. (2001, June 6). *Changing a community: A blueprint for operationalizing nurse caring behaviors.* Creating Communities of Caring. 23rd International Association of Human Caring Conference, Stirling, Scotland.

Relational Caring Questionnaires

Marilyn A. Ray and Marian C. Turkel

The Relational Caring Questionnaires (professional and patient) were initially developed by Turkel and Ray (2001) from grounded theory methodology. The questionnaires were refined through additional qualitative research and psychometric testing (Turkel & Ray, 2000, 2001).

Ray and Turkel view caring in healthcare organizations as a relational caring process within the economic context of quality, cost, and patient outcomes. The focus of their research trajectory was to understand the value of caring among nurses, patients, and administrators within hospital cultural and economic systems (Ray & Turkel, 1995, 1996, 2000).

From 1995 to 2001, Ray and Turkel used grounded theory to study the nurse–patient relationship within an economic context of military, for-profit, and not-for-profit healthcare organizations by interviewing over 250 registered nurses (RNs), patients, and hospital administrators from seven geographically and financially diverse hospitals. A formal theory of relational caring complexity was generated (Turkel & Ray, 2000).

Relational caring complexity theory demonstrates that the caring relationship among the nurse, patient, and administrator is complex and creative, is both a process and an outcome, and is a function of sets of economic variables and nurse–patient relational caring variables. Economic variables were identified as time, technical, and organizational resources. Nurse–patient relational caring variables were identified as caring, relationship, and education. The formal theory consisted of two parts: (1) relationship as a function of the intentionality and caring actions of nurses, patients, and administrators and (2) the monetary and moral values of those interactions within the economic content of organizations.

The research and theory show that nurses in the United States are practicing caring and valuing the nurse–patient relationship in a managed-care environment regulated by costs. Nurses, patients, and administrators are affected by external economic forces and the subsequent impact on the nurse–patient relationship. As demonstrated, one central tenet of the relational caring complexity theory is the concept of relational interconnectedness. The interactors (the nurse and the patient) are interconnected by means of the relationship itself and the relational process. Administrators are interconnected by means of the organizational system, which manages the economics. Often nursing practice is driven by the questions Who will pay? and How much will be paid? One nurse shared the following:

> Can you put a dollar value on how many minutes I spend with a patient? No, you can't. It takes 2 minutes to engage in a caring moment with one patient, 10 minutes for another, and one patient may need you for 2 hours. It's not comparable; each patient is a unique individual and you're the nurse. This caring moment is beyond the attachment of a dollar amount.

For patients, the concept of reimbursement is ambiguous and a maze of confusion. It is also difficult for patients to comprehend the economic value of caring, for fear that they may have to pay more for a caring relationship with a nurse. The perceived intangible nature of caring makes it difficult to quantify in monetary terms. One patient shared this feeling: "It should not add anything to the cost, not a nickel. When you're in the hospital, you want the care you need. And part of that is the nurse being caring."

Administrators make choices concerning how to allocate scarce economic resources because current external and internal economic forces also have an impact on them. Administrators are interconnected to the interactions between the nurse and the patient by virtue of their position within the organizational system. As such, administrators are interwoven into the process of caring between the nurse and the patient and are aware of their moral responsibility. This ethical awareness facilitates the choices administrators must make when allocating economic resources within the organization. An administrator embraced this ethical awareness with the following statement:

> The cuts from Medicare, Medicaid, and managed care are putting a tremendous responsibility on all of us. How do we do the things we have to do with less money? What is it that I can do that will make it easier for nurses to have time for the patients? How do I provide for that with the dollars I have to spend? How do you make those judgments? How do I ensure I'm making the right choices for the patients? These are questions we are faced with everyday.

In continuing research conducted by Ray, Turkel, and Marino (2002), qualitative interviews revealed that losing trust was a dominant theme and the result of organizations being driven by economic survival. Administrators recognized that trust must be rebuilt to create a better practice environment. RNs viewed the rebuilding of trust as integral to the recruitment and retention of professional nurses. Strategies identified to rebuild trust included respecting the nursing staff, communicating with the nursing staff, maintaining visibility, and engaging in participative decision making.

The Relational Caring Questionnaires were developed from a synthesis of all qualitative data. The professional form consists of 26 items based on three subscales of caring: administrative culture, professional ethics, and trust. Questions 1, 2, 4, 5, 6, and 19 to 26 relate to administrative culture. Questions 3, 7, and 9 relate to trust and questions 8, and 10 to 18 relate to professional ethics. The patient form consists of 15 items based on the subscales of professional ethics, trust, and caring. Questions 7, 8, and 11 relate to professional ethics, questions 1 to 4 and 6 relate to trust, and questions 5, 9, 10, and 12 to 15 relate to caring.

Psychometric evaluation was a lengthy process and involved reliability and validity testing from 1996 to 2002. Numerous revisions were made during the process. Specific details are provided in Table 19.1. Reliability testing involved test–retest and was measured by Cronbach's alpha. The final version of the professional questionnaire has an overall reliability of .86, and the patient version has an overall reliability of .89.

Content reliability was assessed by six experts using the content validity index. The majority (75%) agreed that all items were quite or very relevant to the construct of both questionnaires.

The Valentine (1991) Caring Questionnaires were used to compute convergent (concurrent) validity coefficients. The coefficient for the professional form (.14) was low, suggesting they measured somewhat different concepts. In contrast, the coefficient for the patient form was .54, moderate in size.

Factor analysis was used to verify construct validity. Exploratory factor analysis (principal axis factor extraction with varimax rotation) on the professional form yielded four factors, which explained 47% of the variance. Fourteen items loaded on the first factor with a minimum loading coefficient of .490. Six items loaded on the second factor with a minimum loading coefficient of .515. Three items loaded on the third factor with a minimum loading coefficient of .569. Four items loaded on the fourth factor with a minimum loading coefficient of .481. The reliability for the factors/subscales was .73 (caring), .83 (administrative culture), .78 (professional ethics), and .72 (trust).

Exploratory factor analysis (principal axis factor extraction with oblique rotation) on the patient form yielded four factors, which explained 64% of the variance. Nine items loaded on the first factor with a minimum loading coefficient of .483. Three items loaded on the second factor with a minimum loading coefficient of −.565. Two items loaded on the third factor with a minimum loading coefficient of .492. Three items loaded on the fourth factor with a minimum loading coefficient of −.596. One item did not load on any factors. Reliabilities of the three retained factors/subscales in order were .94 (professional ethics), .85 (trust), and .81 (caring). Based on factor analysis and reliability analysis results, the two reverse-coded items on the patient form were dropped from further consideration.

TABLE 19.1 Matrix of Relational Caring Questionnaires

INSTRUMENT	AUTHOR CONTACT INFORMATION	PUBLICATION SOURCE	DEVELOPED TO MEASURE	INSTRUMENT DESCRIPTION	PARTICIPANTS	REPORTED VALIDITY/ RELIABILITY	CONCEPTUAL-THEORETICAL BASIS OF MEASUREMENT	LATEST CITATION IN NURSING LITERATURE
Relational Caring Questionnaire—Professional Form (2001)	Marilyn Ray, PhD, RN, CTN, FAAN Professor Emerita Florida Atlantic University Christine E. Lynn College of Nursing 8487 Via D'Oro Boca Raton, FL 33433 Phone: 561-470-8109 Email: mray@health.fau.edu	Turkel and Ray (2001)	Organizational caring (professional form) and nurse-caring behavior (patient form)	Professional form: 26 items, 5-point Likert scale	Qualitative research from 1995 to 2001 with over 250 RNs, patients, and administrators from seven diverse hospitals	Professional form reliability .86 Content validity established by panel of six experts ≥75% items very relevant	Qualitative research finding from interviews with over 250 RNs, patients, and administrators	Turkel and Ray (2001)
Relational Caring Questionnaire—Patient Form (2001)	Marian Turkel, PhD, RN, NEA-BC, FAAN Associate Professor Florida Atlantic University Christine E. Lynn College of Nursing 8487 Via D'Oro Boca Raton, FL 33433 Office 561-297-3264 Cell 312-203-3944 Email: mturkel@ health.fau.edu	Ray and Turkel (2005)		Patient form: 15 items, 5-point Likert scale	Psychometric testing from 1996 to 2003 with 447 RNs and administrators and 234 patients from seven diverse hospitals	Convergent or concurrent validity determined with Valentine Caring Questionnaire .14 Construct validity, exploratory factor analysis	Turkel and Ray (2000)	Ray and Turkel (2005)

Four factors explained 47% of the variance.	Ray et al. (2002)	Final report. National Technical Information Service. U.S. Government Repository, 2007
First factor loading coefficient .490; reliability .73		
Second factor loading coefficient .515; reliability .83		
Third factor loading coefficient .569; reliability .78		
Fourth factor loading coefficient .481; reliability .72		
Patient form reliability .86		
Content validity established by panel of six experts		
$\geq$75% items very relevant		

(continued)

TABLE 19.1 Matrix of Relational Caring Questionnaires (*continued*)

INSTRUMENT	AUTHOR CONTACT INFORMATION	PUBLICATION SOURCE	DEVELOPED TO MEASURE	INSTRUMENT DESCRIPTION	PARTICIPANTS	REPORTED VALIDITY/ RELIABILITY	CONCEPTUAL-THEORETICAL BASIS OF MEASUREMENT	LATEST CITATION IN NURSING LITERATURE
Relational Caring Questionnaire—Patient Form (2001)						Convergent or concurrent validity determined with Valentine Caring Questionnaire .54 Construct validity Exploratory factor analysis Four factors explained 64% of the variance Based on analysis, three factors retained First factor loading coefficient .483; reliability .94 Second factor loading coefficient −.565; reliability .85		
Relational Caring Questionnaire—Professional Form (2001, 2005, 2007)	Marilyn Ray Professor Emerita Florida Atlantic University Christine E. Lynn College of Nursing	Turkel and Ray (2001)	Organizational caring (professional form) and nurse-caring	Professional form: 26 items, 5-point Likert scale	Qualitative research from 1995 to 2001 with over 250	Third factor loading coefficient −.596; reliability .81 Professional form reliability .86	Qualitative research finding from interviews with over 250 RNs, patients, and administrators	Turkel and Ray (2001)

						Turkel and Ray (2000)	Ray and Turkel (2005)
	8487 Via D'Oro Boca Raton, FL 33433 Phone: 561-470-8109 Email: mray@health.fau.edu	behavior (patient form)		RNs, patients, and administrators from seven diverse hospitals			
Relational Caring Questionnaire— Patient Form (2001, 2005, 2007)	Marian Turkel PhD, RN, NEA-BC, FAAN Associate Professor Florida Atlantic University Christine E. Lynn College of Nursing 8487 Via D'Oro Boca Raton, FL 33433 Work: 561-297-3264 Cell: 312-203-3944 Email: mturkel@health.fau.edu	Ray and Turkel (2005)	Patient form: 15 items, 5-point Likert scale	Psychometric Testing from 1996 to 2003 with 447 RNs and administrators and 234 patients from seven diverse hospitals	Content validity established by panel of six experts ≥75% items very relevant. Convergent or concurrent validity determined with Valentine Caring Questionnaire .14. Construct validity, exploratory factor analysis		

(continued)

TABLE 19.1 Matrix of Relational Caring Questionnaires (*continued*)

INSTRUMENT	AUTHOR CONTACT INFORMATION	PUBLICATION SOURCE	DEVELOPED TO MEASURE	INSTRUMENT DESCRIPTION	PARTICIPANTS	REPORTED VALIDITY/ RELIABILITY	CONCEPTUAL- THEORETICAL BASIS OF MEASUREMENT	LATEST CITATION IN NURSING LITERATURE
Relational Caring Questionnaire— Patient Form (2001, 2005, 2007)						Four factors explained 47% of the variance First factor loading coefficient .490; reliability .73 Second factor loading coefficient .515; reliability .83 Third factor loading coefficient .569; reliability .78 Fourth factor loading coefficient .481; reliability .72 Patient form reliability .86 Content validity established by panel of six experts ≥75% items very relevant	Ray et al. (2002)	Final report. National Technical Information Service. U.S. Government Repository, 2007

Convergent or concurrent validity determined with Valentine Caring Questionnaire .54

Construct validity, exploratory factor analysis

Four factors explained 64% of the variance

Based on analysis, three factors retained

First factor loading coefficient .483; reliability .94

Second factor loading coefficient −.565; reliability .85

Third factor loading coefficient −.596; reliability .81

Between 2002 and 2004, the two final questionnaires were distributed to RNs, patients, and administrators at five hospitals (Ray & Turkel, 2005). Overall mean scores on the questionnaires were then compared to economic and patient outcomes data. It is interesting to note that the hospital with the highest mean score (3.30) for the professional questionnaire had the lowest ratio (3.36) of full-time equivalents per adjusted occupied bed and the lowest number of patient falls. The hospital with the highest patient mean score (4.50) had the lowest cost ($1,265) per adjusted patient day. These findings validate what RNs verbalized in the qualitative research: "Living the caring values in everyday practice makes a difference in nursing practice and patient outcomes."

One limitation is that these findings reflect data collected from only five hospitals. However, the Relational Caring Questionnaires are reliable and valid instruments for measuring caring in healthcare organizations. The researchers are confident that others will be able to use these questionnaires to assess organizational caring in terms of economic and patient outcomes.

CONTEMPORARY APPLICATION OF RELATIONAL CARING QUESTIONNAIRES

The Relational Caring Questionnaires remain relevant in the current healthcare economic culture with a focus on economic value–based outcomes and the patient experience. The subscales of trust, caring, and professional ethics make explicit the link between caring and economic outcomes. The questionnaires have international applicability and are being used by doctoral students in France, Indonesia, and Iran; by undergraduate students in France; and by hospital-based RNs in Portugal.

Lane-Mathern, Casterline, and Templin (2014) conducted a research study, Nurse-Perception of Organizational Culture of Caring. The purpose of this study was to measure the perception of organizational caring by the nursing staff as a baseline for implementing strategies to improve the caring culture. Ray's Theory of Bureaucratic Caring (Ray, 1989, 2013) was the guiding framework for the study. The research question was: What is the organizational culture of caring as perceived by direct care and indirect care nursing staff? All RNs employed at the medical center ($N = 3,000$) were invited to participate in this descriptive study. Organizational culture of caring was measured via an online Survey Monkey using theRelational Caring Questionnaire Professional Form (Ray & Turkel, 2007). Several demographic questions were included: age, years in nursing, and years employed by this organization. Respondents were asked to identify themselves as a direct bedside care nurse (at the bedside >50%) and nondirect care nurse (at the bedside <50%).

Nearly 900 nurses responded to the online survey; 85% identified themselves as direct bedside care nurses. There was a statistically significant difference in overall mean scores between direct care (88.25) and indirect care (97.0) nursing staff ($t = 5.6$, df 851, $p < .0001$). The caring subscale had more "agree" and "strongly agree" responses from both groups of nurses, but statistical differences in overall aggregate mean scores were observed in all subscales ($p < .0001$). There was a significantly positive correlation between overall score and age ($p < .025$) and overall score and years of nursing experience ($p < .007$). Overall score and years employed by the organization correlated at $p = .054$. In this sample, younger nurses and nurses with less experience perceived the organization as less caring.

The results of this study support Ray's theory that organizational caring is impacted by economic elements that include time, technology, and resources. Study findings suggest a need for increased collaboration and trust between nursing leadership and direct bedside staff, to create a culture of caring that improves support, communication, and opportunities for shared decision making.

Relational Caring Questionnaire©
(Professional Form)
Ray and Turkel, 2005, 2007, 2017

INTRODUCTION

Nursing is important to healthcare in the United States. This questionnaire is designed to assist nursing and healthcare organizations/hospitals to understand the important components of organizational caring. Your completion of this questionnaire implies consent to participate in this study. Assisting in this research will *not* in any way affect your status as a professional in this hospital or any healthcare facility.

This is strictly voluntary. Do not write your name on this questionnaire.

DEMOGRAPHIC INFORMATION

Directions
Mark an "**X**" in the box or add the information requested that applies to you.

1. Gender: ☐ Female ☐ Male

2. Highest Completed Education

☐ Associate Degree   ☐ BS (Non-Nursing) ☐ BSN

☐ MS (Non-Nursing)   ☐ MS (Nursing)   ☐ Doctoral Degree

3. Age:

☐ 21–25 ☐ 26–35 ☐ 36–45 ☐ 46–55

☐ 56–65 ☐ 66–70 ☐ Over 70

4. Cultural Background: Black or African American ☐

(Check *all* that apply)   Hispanic or Latino American ☐

White or Caucasian American ☐

Asian American ☐

North American Indian ☐

Other (Specify)   (_____)

5. Job Status: Administrator (Non-Nurse) ☐

Administrator (Nurse) ☐

RN ☐

6. Years of Nursing and/or Administrative Experience:

Under 2 ☐   2–5 ☐   6–10 ☐   11–15 ☐

16–20 ☐   21–25 ☐   26–30 ☐   Over 30 ☐

Questionnaire Directions and Example

BACKGROUND

Caring is important within healthcare organizations. Your responses to the statements on the following questionnaire will help identify and give researchers the opportunity to analyze your answers regarding factors important to the concept of organizational caring.

DIRECTIONS

Please answer the 26 numbered statements. Using a pen or pencil, mark an **X** in the circle that represents your response. Mark only one circle for each question. If your answer is that you "Agree" with the statement, then you would mark an **X** in the (4) for the statement as shown in the following example.

EXAMPLE

2. Nurses are treated with respect by other professionals in the organization. This frequently happens within the organization where I work.

Strongly Disagree	Disagree	Neither Agree Nor Disagree	Agree	Strongly Agree
(1)	(2)	(3)	**(X)**	(5)

1. Nurses are valued as individuals. This frequently happens within the organization where I work.

Strongly Disagree	Disagree	Neither Agree Nor Disagree	Agree	Strongly Agree
(1)	(2)	(3)	(4)	(5)

2. Nurses are treated with respect by other professionals. This frequently happens within the organization where I work.

Strongly Disagree	Disagree	Neither Agree Nor Disagree	Agree	Strongly Agree
(1)	(2)	(3)	(4)	(5)

3. Nurses are able to live their values in practice. This frequently happens within the organization where I work.

Strongly Disagree	Disagree	Neither Agree Nor Disagree	Agree	Strongly Agree
(1)	(2)	(3)	(4)	(5)

(continued)

4. Nurses are involved in policy decisions that affect patient care. This frequently happens within the organization where I work.

Strongly Disagree	Disagree	Neither Agree Nor Disagree	Agree	Strongly Agree
(1)	(2)	(3)	(4)	(5)

5. We see administrators making rounds and helping out when needed. This frequently happens within the organization where I work.

Strongly Disagree	Disagree	Neither Agree Nor Disagree	Agree	Strongly Agree
(1)	(2)	(3)	(4)	(5)

6. The focus of administrators is working on the budget and attending meetings. This frequently happens within the organization where I work.

Strongly Disagree	Disagree	Neither Agree Nor Disagree	Agree	Strongly Agree
(1)	(2)	(3)	(4)	(5)

7. Nurses receive effective communication from administrators, which means we know exactly what is going on and why decisions are made. This frequently happens within the organization where I work.

Strongly Disagree	Disagree	Neither Agree Nor Disagree	Agree	Strongly Agree
(1)	(2)	(3)	(4)	(5)

8. Nurses are counted only as numbers. This frequently happens within the organization where I work.

Strongly Disagree	Disagree	Neither Agree Nor Disagree	Agree	Strongly Agree
(1)	(2)	(3)	(4)	(5)

9. Nurses are trusted by administrators. This frequently happens within the organization where I work.

Strongly Disagree	Disagree	Neither Agree Nor Disagree	Agree	Strongly Agree
(1)	(2)	(3)	(4)	(5)

10. Nurses treat each patient as an individual. This frequently happens within the organization where I work.

Strongly Disagree	Disagree	Neither Agree Nor Disagree	Agree	Strongly Agree
(1)	(2)	(3)	(4)	(5)

(continued)

11. Being there with the patient is part of nursing practice. This frequently happens within the organization where I work.

Strongly Disagree	Disagree	Neither Agree Nor Disagree	Agree	Strongly Agree
(1)	(2)	(3)	(4)	(5)

12. Nurses recognize the needs of the family. This frequently happens within the organization where I work.

Strongly Disagree	Disagree	Neither Agree Nor Disagree	Agree	Strongly Agree
(1)	(2)	(3)	(4)	(5)

13. Nurses integrate awareness of the patient's body, mind, and spirit in their practice. This frequently happens within the organization where I work.

Strongly Disagree	Disagree	Neither Agree Nor Disagree	Agree	Strongly Agree
(1)	(2)	(3)	(4)	(5)

14. Listening is a way nurses build relationships with patients. This frequently happens within the organization where I work.

Strongly Disagree	Disagree	Neither Agree Nor Disagree	Agree	Strongly Agree
(1)	(2)	(3)	(4)	(5)

15. Administrators providing support for what nurses do increases the loyalty of nurses. This frequently happens within the organization where I work.

Strongly Disagree	Disagree	Neither Agree Nor Disagree	Agree	Strongly Agree
(1)	(2)	(3)	(4)	(5)

16. Administrators empower nurses to make changes in the organization. This frequently happens within the organization where I work.

Strongly Disagree	Disagree	Neither Agree Nor Disagree	Agree	Strongly Agree
(1)	(2)	(3)	(4)	(5)

17. Nurses demonstrate compassion for what the patient is experiencing. This frequently happens within the organization where I work.

Strongly Disagree	Disagree	Neither Agree Nor Disagree	Agree	Strongly Agree
(1)	(2)	(3)	(4)	(5)

(*continued*)

18. Nurses are committed to the nursing profession. This frequently happens within the organization where I work.

Strongly Disagree	Disagree	Neither Agree Nor Disagree	Agree	Strongly Agree
(1)	(2)	(3)	(4)	(5)

19. Nurses are viewed as organizational overhead rather than organizational assets. This frequently happens within the organization where I work.

Strongly Disagree	Disagree	Neither Agree Nor Disagree	Agree	Strongly Agree
(1)	(2)	(3)	(4)	(5)

20. Support from administrators results in increased nurse retention. This frequently happens within the organization where I work.

Strongly Disagree	Disagree	Neither Agree Nor Disagree	Agree	Strongly Agree
(1)	(2)	(3)	(4)	(5)

21. Administrators recognize the value of nursing. This frequently happens within the organization where I work.

Strongly Disagree	Disagree	Neither Agree Nor Disagree	Agree	Strongly Agree
(1)	(2)	(3)	(4)	(5)

22. Awareness of the value of nursing facilitates the choices that administrators make when allocating the budget. This frequently happens within the organization where I work.

Strongly Disagree	Disagree	Neither Agree Nor Disagree	Agree	Strongly Agree
(1)	(2)	(3)	(4)	(5)

23. The integration of interpersonal resources (caring, patient education, professional nursing practice) with traditional economic resources (money, goods, services) is included in the budget. This frequently happens within the organization where I work.

Strongly Disagree	Disagree	Neither Agree Nor Disagree	Agree	Strongly Agree
(1)	(2)	(3)	(4)	(5)

24. The relational partnership between practicing nurses and administrators guides economic choice making in the organization. This frequently happens within the organization where I work.

Strongly Disagree	Disagree	Neither Agree Nor Disagree	Agree	Strongly Agree
(1)	(2)	(3)	(4)	(5)

(continued)

25. Nurses have financial knowledge to participate in organizational decision making. This frequently happens within the organization where I work.

Strongly Disagree	Disagree	Neither Agree Nor Disagree	Agree	Strongly Agree
(1)	(2)	(3)	(4)	(5)

26. A supportive relationship between the nurses and the administrators results in improved economic and patient outcomes. This frequently happens within the organization where I work.

Strongly Disagree	Disagree	Neither Agree Nor Disagree	Agree	Strongly Agree
(1)	(2)	(3)	(4)	(5)

The Relational Caring Questionnaire (Professional Form) is copyrighted. Please contact Dr. Marilyn Ray or Dr. Marian Turkel via email to formally request use of the questionnaire. Permission will be granted as long as no changes are made to the questionnaire.

Marilyn A. Ray, PhD, RN, CTN-A, FAAN
Professor Emerita
Florida Atlantic University
Christine E. Lynn College of Nursing
Boca Raton, Florida
mray@health.fau.edu

Marian C. Turkel, PhD, RN, NEA-BC, FAAN
Associate Professor
Florida Atlantic University
Christine E. Lynn College of Nursing
Boca Raton, Florida
mturkel@health.fau.edu

Relational Caring Questionnaire©
(Patient Form)

Ray and Turkel, 2005, 2007, 2017

INTRODUCTION

Nursing is important to healthcare in the United States. This questionnaire is designed to assist nursing and healthcare organizations/hospitals to understand the important components of organizational caring.

Your completion of this questionnaire implies consent to participate in this study. Assisting in this research will *not* in any way affect your status as a patient in the hospital or any healthcare facility.

This is strictly voluntary. Do not write your name on this questionnaire.

DEMOGRAPHIC INFORMATION

Directions
Mark an **X** in the box or add the information requested which applies to you

1. Gender: Female ☐   Male ☐

2. Highest Completed Education:

    Less than High School   ☐   High School/GED   ☐

    Associate Degree   ☐   Bachelor's Degree   ☐

    Master's Degree   ☐   Doctoral Degree   ☐

3. Age:

    18–25 ☐   26–35 ☐   36–45 ☐   46–55 ☐

    56–65 ☐   66–70 ☐   Over 70 ☐

4. Cultural Background: Black or African American   ☐

    (Check all that apply)   Hispanic or Latino American   ☐

                             White or Caucasian American   ☐

                             Asian American   ☐

                             North American Indian   ☐

                             Other (Specify)   (_____)

5. Number of Times Hospitalized as a Patient:

    1–5   6–10   More than 10

6. Length of Stay This Admission:

    1–3 Days   4–6 Days   7–10 Days Over 10 Days

Questionnaire Directions And Example

DIRECTIONS

Caring is important within healthcare organizations. Your responses to each statement on the following survey will help identify behaviors that are important for caring between the registered nurse (RN) and patient in a healthcare organization.

EXAMPLE

Using a pen or pencil, mark an **X** in the circle that best describes your understanding of caring in terms of your interactions with RNs in this hospital. Mark only one circle for each question. If your answer is that you "Agree" with the statement, then you would mark an **X** in the (4) for the statement as shown in the following example.

1. I am treated with respect. This frequently happens when I am a patient in this hospital.

Strongly Disagree	Disagree	Neither Agree Nor Disagree	Agree	Strongly Agree
(1)	(2)	(3)	**(X)**	(5)

Do not write your name on this questionnaire.

1. I am treated with respect. This happens when I am a patient in this hospital.

Strongly Disagree	Disagree	Neither Agree Nor Disagree	Agree	Strongly Agree
(1)	(2)	(3)	(4)	(5)

2. I am given care based on what is important to me. This happens when I am a patient in this hospital.

Strongly Disagree	Disagree	Neither Agree Nor Disagree	Agree	Strongly Agree
(1)	(2)	(3)	(4)	(5)

3. I take an active part in my own healthcare decisions. This happens when I am a patient in this hospital.

Strongly Disagree	Disagree	Neither Agree Nor Disagree	Agree	Strongly Agree
(1)	(2)	(3)	(4)	(5)

4. Knowing the nurse knows what to do for me builds my trust in the nurse. This happens when I am a patient in this hospital.

Strongly Disagree	Disagree	Neither Agree Nor Disagree	Agree	Strongly Agree
(1)	(2)	(3)	(4)	(5)

(continued)

5. The nurses treat me as a person instead of an illness. This happens when I am a patient in this hospital.

Strongly Disagree	Disagree	Neither Agree Nor Disagree	Agree	Strongly Agree
(1)	(2)	(3)	(4)	(5)

6. Interacting with the nursing staff fosters trust between the nurse and me. This happens when I am a patient in this hospital.

Strongly Disagree	Disagree	Neither Agree Nor Disagree	Agree	Strongly Agree
(1)	(2)	(3)	(4)	(5)

7. Personal interactions (e.g., eye contact or touch) help me trust my nurse. This happens when I am a patient in this hospital.

Strongly Disagree	Disagree	Neither Agree Nor Disagree	Agree	Strongly Agree
(1)	(2)	(3)	(4)	(5)

8. Nurses being there with me is a part of showing that they care. This happens when I am a patient in this hospital.

Strongly Disagree	Disagree	Neither Agree Nor Disagree	Agree	Strongly Agree
(1)	(2)	(3)	(4)	(5)

9. Nurses' teaching helps to prevent me getting sick again and having to come back to the hospital. This happens when I am a patient in this hospital.

Strongly Disagree	Disagree	Neither Agree Nor Disagree	Agree	Strongly Agree
(1)	(2)	(3)	(4)	(5)

10. When the nurse is concerned about me, I learn more from his/her teaching. This happens when I am a patient in this hospital.

Strongly Disagree	Disagree	Neither Agree Nor Disagree	Agree	Strongly Agree
(1)	(2)	(3)	(4)	(5)

11. Nurses being good at starting IVs combines compassion and skill. This happens when I am a patient in this hospital.

Strongly Disagree	Disagree	Neither Agree Nor Disagree	Agree	Strongly Agree
(1)	(2)	(3)	(4)	(5)

(continued)

12. Nurses' teaching prepares me to take care of myself at home. This happens when I am a patient in this hospital.

Strongly Disagree	Disagree	Neither Agree Nor Disagree	Agree	Strongly Agree
(1)	(2)	(3)	(4)	(5)

13. Nurses recognize the needs of my family when giving me care. This happens when I am a patient in this hospital.

Strongly Disagree	Disagree	Neither Agree Nor Disagree	Agree	Strongly Agree
(1)	(2)	(3)	(4)	(5)

14. Nurses listening to me is a part of showing that they care. This happens when I am a patient in this hospital.

Strongly Disagree	Disagree	Neither Agree Nor Disagree	Agree	Strongly Agree
(1)	(2)	(3)	(4)	(5)

15. The nurse shows compassion for what I am experiencing as a patient. This happens when I am a patient in this hospital.

Strongly Disagree	Disagree	Neither Agree Nor Disagree	Agree	Strongly Agree
(1)	(2)	(3)	(4)	(5)

The Relational Caring Questionnaire (Patient Form) is copyrighted. Please contact Dr. Marilyn Ray or Dr. Marian Turkel to formally request use of the questionnaire. Permission will be granted as long as no changes are made to the questionnaire.

Marilyn A. Ray, PhD, RN, CTN-A, FAAN
Professor Emerita
Florida Atlantic University
Christine E. Lynn College of Nursing
Boca Raton, Florida
mray@health.fau.edu

Marian C. Turkel, PhD, RN, NEA-BC, FAAN
Associate Professor
Florida Atlantic University
Christine E. Lynn College of Nursing
Boca Raton, Florida
mturkel@health.fau.edu

REFERENCES

Lane-Mathern, D. A., Casterline, G. L., & Templin, M. S. (2014). *Nurse-perception of organizational culture of caring.* Unpublished manuscript.

Ray, M. (1989). The theory of bureaucratic caring for nursing practice in the organizational culture. *Nursing Administration Quarterly, 13*(2), 31–42. doi:10.1097/00006216-198901320-00007

Ray, M. (2013). The theory of bureaucratic caring for nursing practice in the organizational culture. In M. Smith, M. Turkel, & Z. Wolf (Eds.), *Caring in nursing classics: An essential resource* (pp. 309–320). New York, NY: Springer Publishing (Reprinted from the original 1989 article).

Ray, M., & Turkel, M. (1995, September). *Nurse-patient relationship patterns: An economic resource.* Grant funded by Department of Defense, Tri-Service Nursing Research Council.

Ray, M., & Turkel, M. (1996, August). *Econometric analysis of the nurse-patient relationship I & II.* Grant funded by Department of Defense, Washington DC, Tri-Service Nursing Research Council.

Ray, M., & Turkel, M. (2000, August). *Economic and patient outcomes of the nurse-patient relationship.* Grant funded by the Department of Defense, Washington DC, Tri-Service Nursing Research Council.

Ray, M., & Turkel, M. (2005). *Final report: Economic and patient outcomes of the nurse-patient relationship.* Tri-service nursing research program abstract. Published in CINAHL, 2007.

Ray, M., Turkel, M., & Marino, F. (2002). The transformative process in workforce redevelopment. *Nursing Administration Quarterly, 26*(2), 1–14. doi:10.1097/00006216-200201000-00003

Turkel, M., & Ray, M. (2000). Relational caring complexity: A theory of the nurse–patient relationship within an economic context. *Nursing Science Quarterly, 13*(4), 307–313. doi:10.1177/08943180022107843

Turkel, M., & Ray, M. (2001). Relational complexity: From grounded theory to instrument development & theoretical testing. *Nursing Science Quarterly, 14*(4), 281–287.

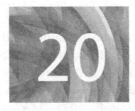

Family Caring Inventory

Anne-Marie Goff

The Family Caring Inventory is the only known instrument specifically designed to isolate and measure the concept of caring in the family. The ability to display and receive caring is the strategic core, or key factor, of healthy family functioning, especially when coping with stressful life events. The Family Caring Inventory was introduced in the second edition of this book because it has promise and potential and offers an approach to assess family caring, making it a unique and original contribution to this compilation of instruments. In the early stages of validity and reliability testing, the scale demonstrates high internal consistency reliability, with a Cronbach's alpha of .825. The Family Caring Inventory (Tool 20.1) was developed by Goff in 2002 during doctoral studies to measure adult family members' perceptions of caring as a family strength. Major changes during the past several years in healthcare, the configuration and dynamics of the family, and the nature and demands of everyday existence have influenced the availability of inherent strengths, and the ability to develop and foster additional strengths necessary for healthy family functioning (Institute of Medicine and National Research Council, 2011). Family violence, teen pregnancy, addictions, and acute and chronic illness have played a major role in the nature of family life. Dimensions of caring within the family (behaviors, thoughts, emotions, and processes) are crucial strengths in coping with both internal and external stressors. The family is viewed as a system that must have the willingness to utilize internal resources and the potential to access external resources, or social support. In order to enhance caring in the family, nurses and other healthcare professionals need to understand the structure, function, and processes that foster a healthy family environment. Assessment of the level and potential of caring behaviors may explain why some families are more vulnerable, while others are more resilient when dealing with real or perceived stressors (Henry, Sheffield Morris & Harrist, 2015; Walsh, 2016; Welch & Harrist, 2017). The development of interventions, such as education and counseling, would enhance strengths and coping mechanisms and become a key factor in the healthcare outcomes of families (Chesla, 2010).

After it was determined that an instrument to measure caring in the family did not exist, a 36-item 5-point Likert scale was developed from extensive concept analysis and both caring and family theories (Andershed & Olsson, 2009; Beavers, 1989; Beavers & Hampson, 1990; Beavers, Hampson, & Hulgus, 1985; Ford-Gilboe, 2000; Mayeroff, 1971; McCubbin, 1989; Nkongho, 1990; Olson, 1993; Powell-Cope, 1994; Swanson, 1991, 2000; Watson, 1985). Family theories and instruments involve constructs such as resilience, cohesion, social support, hardiness, adaptability, and competence, and, although a few minor attributes of caring have emerged, the concept of caring has not been isolated in the family. Caring frameworks and theories in nursing focus on the individual level, specifically the nurse–client interaction or the caregiver–client relationship (Turkel, Watson & Giovannoni, 2017; Watson, 2008, 2012). The Family Caring Inventory expands the concept of caring from the individual to the family level. Similar to negotiating partnerships in Powell-Cope's (1994) middle-range theory of the caregiving role, the Family Caring Inventory is based on a reciprocal interaction of caring. Watson's (1985) carative factors of the nurse–client relationship are adapted to the dynamics of the family unit. In addition, the instrument includes the concept of knowing, which is an isolated component of the caring process in both Powell-Cope's (1994) and Swanson's (1991) middle-range theories.

Initially, Goff developed a conceptual map of caring consisting of antecedents, attributes, and consequences. Antecedents are knowledge, experience, commitment, motivation, needs, and context (setting, population, roles, social norms, values, and culture). Several attributes, such as patience, touching, consistency, concern, and reassurance, were extracted, developed, and continuously refined, with input from both faculty and student colleagues. Consequences of family caring are viewed as resilience, cohesion, holism, growth and development, inner harmony, power, self-worth, met needs, increased knowledge, enrichment, health and healing, and development of humanity. From this conceptual map, dimensions of family caring evolved into four major categories: caring behavior or expressiveness, caring thoughts, caring feelings or emotions, and caring process. For example, consistency, interaction, projection, mutuality, transcendence, and coping/adaptation are viewed as major components of the family caring process. A series of definitions and a family caring model, Cohesive Harmony for the Family Environment, were also developed to further conceptualize the Family Caring Inventory. The model, which conceptualizes a middle-range theory of family caring, blends systems theory with a developmental framework and emphasizes both the internal and external contexts of family interaction.

Psychometric properties of The Family Caring Inventory were tested with 197 nursing students from three institutions of higher education: a community college in North Carolina and two universities in South Carolina. Participants (88.3% female) ranged in age from 18 to 66 (M = 30.2), with the largest age group between 18 and 28 (53.9%). The sample included 61.4% identifying as Caucasian, 23.9% African American or Black, 1.5% Hispanic, and 13.2% Other. Most worked full-time (28.9%), part-time (37.1%), or a few hours per week (6.1%) in healthcare areas, while 27.2% were unemployed. The majority (45.7%) reported being single, while 41.6% were married, and 9.6% divorced. The Family APGAR questionnaire (Smilkstein, 1978; Smilkstein, Ashworth, & Montano, 1982) and the Caring Ability Inventory (CAI; Nkongho, 1990) were used to determine the scale's validity. The Family APGAR measures five parameters of family functioning: Adaptability, Partnership, Growth, Affection, and Resolve. The CAI includes three subscales: Knowing, Courage, and Patience. Principal components factor analysis with varimax rotation extracted eight factors from the data, accounting for 67.17% of the variance (Polit & Yang, 2016). Four subscales emerged from these factors, with factor loadings ranging from .70 to .92. The factors are: Ability to Express Familial Emotion (M = 4.4), Comfort in Familial Relationships (M = 4.3), Level of Familial Security and Trust (M = 4.4), and Independence from Other Family Members (M = 3.7). Validity of the instrument was demonstrated by significant correlation at the .01 level with the Family APGAR (.61) and the CAI (.57). Cronbach's alpha was .825. Further testing of the Family Caring Inventory on larger and more divergent populations is necessary to establish dimensions of reliability and validity (Table 20.1). The scale demonstrates promise for future testing, refinement, and use with families in a variety of settings and circumstances in order to enhance family strengths and coping mechanisms, and to promote positive healthcare outcomes.

TABLE 20.1 Matrix of Family Caring Inventory

INSTRUMENT	AUTHOR CONTACT INFORMATION	PUBLICATION SOURCE	DEVELOPED TO MEASURE	INSTRUMENT DESCRIPTION	PARTICIPANTS	REPORTED VALIDITY/ RELIABILITY	CONCEPTUAL– THEORETICAL BASIS OF MEASUREMENT	LATEST CITATION IN NURSING LITERATURE
Family Caring Inventory (2002)	Anne-Marie Goff, PhD, RN School of Nursing University of North Carolina, Wilmington 601 S. College Road Wilmington, NC 28403 Email: goffa@ uncw.edu	Unpublished to date	Family caring as a strength as perceived by adults: caring behavior, expressiveness, caring thoughts, caring feelings or emotions, and caring process	36-item Likert-type scale measuring family caring	$N = 197$ nursing students in three schools of nursing	Cronbach's alpha = .82. Eight factors extracted (67.17% variance). Four subscales emerged with factor loading from .70 to .92. Significant correlation at .01 level. Family APGAR (.61) and Caring Ability Inventory (.57)	Developed from extensive concept analysis and both caring and family theories (Beavers, Ford-Gilboe, Mayeroff, McCubbin, Nkongo, Olson, Powell-Cope, Swanson, and Watson)	None to date

TOOL 20.1

Family Caring Inventory

Please read each of the following statements and decide how well each reflects your behaviors, thoughts, and feelings in relation to your whole family. Do not focus on individual family members. Using the response scale, please circle the degree to which you agree or disagree with each statement. There is no right or wrong answer. Please answer all of the questions. Thank you.

	1	2	3	4	5
	STRONGLY DISAGREE			STRONGLY AGREE	
1. I tell my family members that I care about them.	1	2	3	4	5
2. I like to think of myself as a person who shows other family members that I care about them.	1	2	3	4	5
3. I can turn to my family members for help when I need it.	1	2	3	4	5
4. When other family members show me that they care, I know that they mean it.	1	2	3	4	5
5. I like to think that other family members can show me that they care.	1	2	3	4	5
6. I feel secure when my family is nearby.	1	2	3	4	5
7. I consistently show my feelings.	1	2	3	4	5
8. I'm aware when I show my family members how much I care about them.	1	2	3	4	5
9. I feel more comfortable asking people outside of my family for help.	1	2	3	4	5
10. I listen when other family members need help.	1	2	3	4	5
11. I like to show other family members how much I care about them.	1	2	3	4	5
12. I feel comfortable sharing my feelings with other members of my family.	1	2	3	4	5
13. I am kind to other family members even when I don't feel like it.	1	2	3	4	5
14. It is difficult for me to understand how other family members feel about me.	1	2	3	4	5
15. I have difficulty showing my feelings to other family members.	1	2	3	4	5

(continued)

TOOL 20.1

Family Caring Inventory (*continued*)

	STRONGLY DISAGREE				STRONGLY AGREE
16. I touch other family members to show warmth and affection.	1	2	3	4	5
17. It is difficult for me to understand how I feel about other family members.	1	2	3	4	5
18. I feel hopeful even when my family and I are dealing with a difficult situation.	1	2	3	4	5
19. I help other family members with their problems.	1	2	3	4	5
20. I appreciate family members who are patient with me.	1	2	3	4	5
21. My feelings are easily hurt by other family members.	1	2	3	4	5
22. I like to encourage my family members.	1	2	3	4	5
23. I believe that family members care about me as much as I care about them.	1	2	3	4	5
24. I can tell when other family members are sad, hurt, or need help.	1	2	3	4	5
25. I am nice to other family members even when they are not nice to me.	1	2	3	4	5
26. I accept other family members the way they are.	1	2	3	4	5
27. Other family members are interested in how I feel, think, and behave.	1	2	3	4	5
28. I accept myself for who I am.	1	2	3	4	5
29. I like to protect other family members when they are sad or hurt.	1	2	3	4	5
30. It bothers me when my family members are sad, hurt, or need help.	1	2	3	4	5
31. I accept expressions of warmth and caring from other family members.	1	2	3	4	5
32. I am interested in what other family members are thinking, doing, and feeling.	1	2	3	4	5
33. When I tell family members that I care about them, I mean it.	1	2	3	4	5

(*continued*)

TOOL 20.1

Family Caring Inventory (*continued*)

	STRONGLY DISAGREE				STRONGLY AGREE
34. It is more important to show other family members that I care about them than have them tell me.	1	2	3	4	5
35. I express warmth and affection to my family members in many ways.	1	2	3	4	5
36. I feel a sense of responsibility to show other family members that I care about them.	1	2	3	4	5

REFERENCES

Andershed, B., & Olsson, K. (2009). Review of research related to Kristen Swanson's middle range theory of caring. *Scandinavian Journal of Caring Sciences, 23*(3), 598–610. doi:10.1111/j.1471-6712.2008.00647.x

Beavers, W. R. (1989). Beavers' systems model. In C. N. Ramsey (Ed.), *Family systems in medicine* (pp. 62–74). New York, NY: Guilford Press.

Beavers, W. R., & Hampson, R. B. (1990). *Successful families: Assessment and intervention*. New York, NY: Norton.

Beavers, W. R., Hampson, R. B., & Hulgus, Y. F. (1985). The Beavers' systems approach to family assessment. *Family Process, 24*, 298–405. doi:10.1111/j.1545-5300.1985.00398.x

Chesla, C. (2010). Do family interventions improve health? *Journal of Family Nursing, 16*(4), 355–377. doi:10.1177/1074840710383145

Ford-Gilboe, M. (2000). Dispelling myths and creating opportunity: A comparison of strengths of single-parent and two-parent families. *Advances in Nursing Science, 23*, 41–55. doi:10.1097/00012272-200009000-00008

Henry, C., Sheffield Morris, A., & Harrist, A. (2015, January). Family resilience: Moving into the third wave. *Family Relations: An Interdisciplinary Journal of Applied Family Studies, 64*(1), 22–43. doi:10.1111/fare.12106

Institute of Medicine and National Research Council. (2011). *Toward an integrated science of research on families: Workshop report*. Committee on the Science of Research on Families. Washington, DC: National Academies Press.

Mayeroff, M. (1971). *On caring*. New York, NY: Harper & Row.

McCubbin, M. A. (1989). Family stress and family strengths: A comparison of single- and two-parent families with handicapped children. *Research in Nursing and Health, 12*, 101–110. doi:10.1002/nur.4770120207

Nkongho, N. (1990). The caring ability inventory. In O. L. Strickland & C. F. Waltz (Eds.), *Measurement of nursing outcomes: Measuring client self-care and coping skills* (pp. 3–16). New York, NY: Springer Publishing.

Olson, D. H. (1993). Circumplex model of marital and family systems: Assessing family functioning. In F. Walsh (Ed.), *Normal family processes* (2nd ed., pp. 104–137). New York, NY: Guilford Press.

Polit, D. F., & Yang, F. M. (2016). *Measurement and the measurement of change.* Philadelphia, PA: Wolters Kluwer.

Powell-Cope, G. M. (1994). Family caregivers of people with AIDS: Negotiating partnerships with professional health care providers. *Nursing Research, 43,* 324–330. doi:10.1097/00006199-199411000-00002

Smilkstein, G. (1978). The Family APGAR: A proposal for family function test and its use by physicians. *Journal of Family Practice, 6*(6), 1231–1239.

Smilkstein, G., Ashworth, C., & Montano, D. (1982). Validity and reliability of the Family APGAR as a test of family function. *Journal of Family Practice, 15,* 303–311.

Swanson, K. (1991). Empirical development of a middle-range theory of caring. *Nursing Research, 40,* 161–166. doi:10.1097/00006199-199105000-00008

Swanson, K. (2000). A program of research on caring. In M. E. Parker (Ed.), *Nursing theories and nursing practice* (pp. 411–420). Philadelphia, PA: F. A. Davis.

Turkel, M. C., Watson, J., & Giovannoni, J. (2017). Caring science or science of caring. *Nursing Science Quarterly, 31*(1), 66–71. doi:10.1177/0894318417741116

Walsh, F. (2016). Applying a family resilience framework in training, practice and research: Mastering the art of the possible. *Family Process, 55*(4), 616–632. doi:10.1111/famp.12260

Watson, J. (1985). *Nursing: Human science and human care.* Norwalk, CT: Appleton-Century-Crofts.

Watson, J. (2008). *Nursing: The philosophy and science of caring* (2nd ed.). Boulder: University Press of Colorado.

Watson, J. (2012). *Human caring science.* Boston, MA: Jones & Bartlett.

Welch, G., & Harrist, A. (Eds.). (2017). *Family resilience and chronic illness: Interdisciplinary and translational perspectives.* Online Resource. Cham, Switzerland: Springer International Publishing.

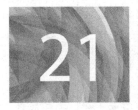

Nurse–Patient Relationship Questionnaire

Janet F. Quinn

The Nurse–Patient Relationship Questionnaire was developed to measure the caring quality of the nurse–patient relationship. To date, there have been no reliability, validity, or development efforts for refining this scale; however, it is included because of its originality and innovative promise. It has the potential to allow patients to identify and rate specific nurses on a continuum from uncaring to caring (even transpersonal caring) through a computerized instrument process.

The instrument was published as part of a paper as an example of a tool that might be useful in assessing the healing relationship (Quinn, Smith, Ritenbaugh, Swanson, & Watson, 2003). The rationale for its development was that in order to study the impact of the caring–healing relationship in clinical nursing practice, researchers need to be able to first determine the existence of such relationships. This tool can be used to rate individual nurse–patient relationships from uncaring to caring, and the scores can be correlated with a wide variety of outcome measures related to healing (Table 21.1).

The tool uses the schema proposed by Halldorsdottir (1991), based on her qualitative research on caring and the general caring theories of Watson and others (Tool 21.1). Halldorsdottir's schema of ways of being with another proposes a 5-point continuum from uncaring to caring. At the uncaring extreme of the continuum are relationships that are biocidic, or life destroying. Next are relationships that are biostatic, or life restraining. Biopassive or life-neutral relationships fall at the third point of the continuum. Next are bioactive or life-sustaining relationships. The fifth point on the continuum (the most caring) is biogenic or life-giving relationships. Terms reflective of these five points on the continuum form the 5-point scale used to rate each item. The items are drawn from the extant literature on caring and reflect commonly identified characteristics of caring. The

TABLE 21.1 Matrix of Nurse–Patient Relationship Questionnaire

INSTRUMENT	AUTHOR CONTACT INFORMATION	PUBLICATION SOURCE	DEVELOPED TO MEASURE	INSTRUMENT DESCRIPTION	PARTICIPANTS	REPORTED VALIDITY/ RELIABILITY	CONCEPTUAL– THEORETICAL BASIS OF MEASUREMENT	LATEST CITATION IN NURSING LITERATURE
Nurse–Patient Relationship Questionnaire (2003)	Janet F. Quinn, PhD, RN, FAAN 360 Lonestar Road Lyons, CO 80540 Email: janetquinnphd@ gmail.com	Quinn et al. (2003)	Quality of caring in the nurse–patient relationship	12 items 5-point Likert-type scale based on Halldorsdottir's continuum of caring	N/A	N/A	Halldorsdottir's continuum of caring and Watson's caring theory	Quinn et al. (2003)

tool is designed for patients to complete for each nurse with whom they have a relationship during a healthcare encounter.

The Nurse–Patient Relationship Questionnaire awaits refinement and testing through the use of tool development strategies (Table 21.1). The authors encourage individual researchers and systems to consider adopting and adapting this questionnaire to fit their clinical settings and computerized assessment processes.

TOOL 21.1

Nurse–Patient Relationship Questionnaire

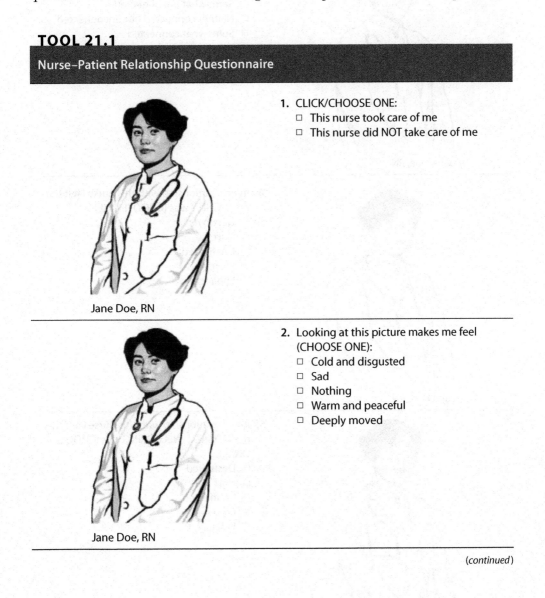

Jane Doe, RN

1. CLICK/CHOOSE ONE:
   □ This nurse took care of me
   □ This nurse did NOT take care of me

Jane Doe, RN

2. Looking at this picture makes me feel (CHOOSE ONE):
   □ Cold and disgusted
   □ Sad
   □ Nothing
   □ Warm and peaceful
   □ Deeply moved

(continued)

TOOL 21.1

Nurse–Patient Relationship Questionnaire (*continued*)

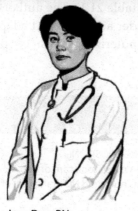

Jane Doe, RN

3. How connected to this nurse did you feel? (CHOOSE ONE):
   - ☐ Very unconnected
   - ☐ Somewhat unconnected
   - ☐ Neither connected nor unconnected
   - ☐ Somewhat connected
   - ☐ Very connected

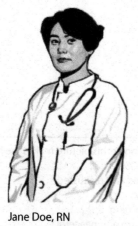

Jane Doe, RN

4. In my relationship with this nurse I felt that my DIGNITY was (CHOOSE ONE):
   - ☐ Destroyed
   - ☐ Hurt
   - ☐ Unaffected
   - ☐ Preserved
   - ☐ Enhanced

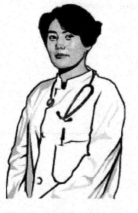

Jane Doe, RN

5. In my relationship with this nurse I felt that my PHYSICAL WELL-BEING was (CHOOSE ONE):
   - ☐ Destroyed
   - ☐ Hurt
   - ☐ Unaffected
   - ☐ Preserved
   - ☐ Enhanced

(continued)

TOOL 21.1

Nurse–Patient Relationship Questionnaire (*continued*)

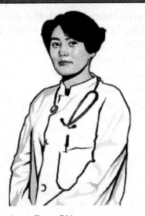

Jane Doe, RN

6. In my relationship with this nurse I felt that my EMOTIONAL WELL-BEING was (CHOOSE ONE):
   □ Destroyed
   □ Hurt
   □ Unaffected
   □ Preserved
   □ Enhanced

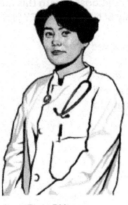

Jane Doe, RN

7. In my relationship with this nurse I felt that my SPIRITUAL WELL-BEING was (CHOOSE ONE):
   □ Destroyed
   □ Hurt
   □ Unaffected
   □ Preserved
   □ Enhanced

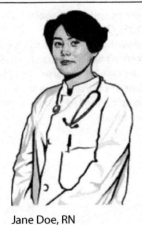

Jane Doe, RN

8. In my relationship with this nurse I felt that my HEALING was (CHOOSE ONE):
   □ Destroyed
   □ Hurt
   □ Unaffected
   □ Preserved
   □ Enhanced

(continued)

TOOL 21.1

Nurse–Patient Relationship Questionnaire (*continued*)

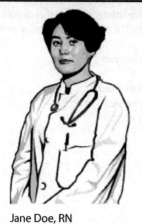

Jane Doe, RN

9. **In my relationship with this nurse I felt that my SENSE OF WHOLENESS was (CHOOSE ONE):**
   - ☐ Destroyed
   - ☐ Hurt
   - ☐ Unaffected
   - ☐ Preserved
   - ☐ Enhanced

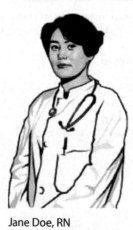

Jane Doe, RN

10. **In my relationship with this nurse I felt that my SENSE OF SAFETY was (CHOOSE ONE):**
    - ☐ Destroyed
    - ☐ Hurt
    - ☐ Unaffected
    - ☐ Preserved
    - ☐ Enhanced

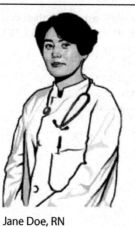

Jane Doe, RN

11. **If I were hospitalized again, I would (CHOOSE ONE):**
    - ☐ Never allow this nurse to care for me
    - ☐ Wouldn't like this nurse to care for me
    - ☐ Don't care if this nurse cares for me
    - ☐ Want this nurse to care for me
    - ☐ Would be thrilled to have this nurse care for me

(*continued*)

TOOL 21.1

Nurse–Patient Relationship Questionnaire (*continued*)

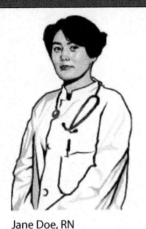

Jane Doe, RN

12. Words I would use to describe this nurse are (write in as few/many as you like):

REFERENCES

Halldorsdottir, S. (1991). Five basic modes of being with another. In D. A. Gaut & M. M. Leininger (Eds.), *Caring: The compassionate healer* (pp. 37–49). New York: National League for Nursing.

Quinn, J. F., Smith, M., Ritenbaugh, C., Swanson, K., & Watson, M. J. (2003). Research guidelines for assessing the impact of the healing relationship in clinical nursing. *Alternative Therapies in Health and Medicine, 9*(3 Suppl.), A65–A79.

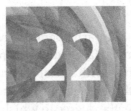

Caring Nurse–Patient Interactions Scale

Sylvie Cossette, Jacinthe Pepin, and Guillaume Fontaine

The Caring Nurse–Patient Interactions (CNPI-70) scale was developed by Cossette, Cara, Ricard, and Pepin (2005) from the theory of human caring proposed by Watson (1979, 1988). The scale was intended to facilitate research on the links between caring, as described by the 10 nursing carative factors, and patient outcomes. The items of the CNPI-70 reflect each of the 10 carative factors and are organized in 10 subscales. The scale was also designed to address practical issues that the authors felt were less well handled in previous work. Hence, the wording of items permits the scale to capture caring across different groups of informants (patients, family members, nurses, students) and for different research and educational purposes. For instance, answers can be rated in terms of satisfaction with caring attitudes, frequency of their occurrence, their importance, the extent to which respondents felt the caring attitudes were realistic in clinical settings, and nurses' and students' feelings of competence in adopting them.

An initial list of 121 items developed from the empirical and theoretical literature was reduced to 70 items following a content validity examination by 13 expert nurses. The scale was first developed in French and then back translation was used to translate the scale into English. The summary labels for the 10 subscales are humanism (6 items), hope (7 items), sensitivity (6 items), helping relationship (7 items), expression of emotions (6 items), problem solving (6 items), teaching (11 items), environment (7 items), needs (10 items), and spirituality (6 items; Tool 21.1).

Psychometric studies have been conducted with the CNPI-70, and the authors designed the CNPI-23, a shorter version of the scale in order to increase its use in clinical research settings with severely ill patients (Table 22.1). The three convenience samples for the studies described subsequently consisted of nursing students enrolled in a Canadian baccalaureate nursing program. Data were collected in 2002, 2003, and 2004.

© Springer Publishing Company DOI:10.1891/9780826195425.0022

The first study, involving 332 participants, served to assess the preliminary psychometric properties, namely face and content validity, contrasted group assessment, reliability, and links with social desirability (Cossette et al., 2005). The respondents were asked three questions for each of the 70 items concerning the importance of each attitude, the degree to which they felt competent in adopting each attitude, and the degree to which they felt it was realistic to adopt each attitude in clinical practice (ranging from "not at all" = 1 to "extremely" = 5). Cronbach's alphas for each of the 10 subscales and for each of the questions ranged from .73 to .91. Pearson's correlation coefficients between the 10 subscales ranged from .53 to .89. In many instances, the lowest coefficients (< .70) involved the relationship between the humanism factor and the spirituality carative factor, whereas the highest coefficient (.89) was found between teaching and needs. Overall, the Pearson's coefficients between social desirability and the 10 subscales assessing the importance ranged from .02 to .12, all not statistically significant ($p > .05$). The coefficients for the 10 subscales assessing how competent they felt ranged from .15 to .32 (all significant at $p < .05$). The coefficients between the realistic 10 subscales ranged from .19 to .32 (all significant at $p < .05$). Thus, although importance appears unrelated to social desirability, the nurses' competence in caring attitudes and the feasibility of their implementation are mildly related to the tendency to respond in a socially desirable manner. A contrasted group analysis was based on the hypothesis that students in the third year of the educational program based on a caring school of thought would rate adopting the caring attributes as more important and would feel more competent in adopting the caring attributes than first-year students would. Third-year students found the carative factors of humanism, hope, sensitivity, expression of emotions, teaching, and environment to be significantly ($p < .05$) more important than first-year students did. There were few differences between the two groups on competency; surprisingly, third-year students felt less competent for the spirituality factor than did first-year students. Other differences between groups (men vs. women, registered nurse students vs. nonregistered nurse students, Canadian native students vs. non–Canadian native students) are reported. No factorial analysis was performed to build the subscales of the 10 carative factors.

A second study involving 377 participants aimed to develop a shorter parallel version of the CNPI by reducing the number of items while maintaining the scale's reflection of Watson's theory (Cossette, Côté, Pepin, Ricard, & D'Aoust, 2006). Indeed, the interrelationships among the 10 subscales of the CNPI-70 were moderate to high, and the 70-item scale was judged to be difficult to use in clinical studies, particularly in those where the length of the questionnaire was an important consideration. Because it was impossible to reduce the number of items without reducing the number of subscales, the 10 carative factors were theoretically grouped into broader theoretical domains. The first three carative factors (humanism, hope, and sensitivity), which reflect the interdependent philosophical aspect of caring and the individual's value system, were grouped theoretically into a humanistic care domain. The helping relationship, expression of emotions, problem solving, and spirituality factors were grouped into a relational care domain because all emphasize major elements of a therapeutic relationship that take into account the patient's perceptions of a particular situation. The carative factors reflecting the nurse's response and the clinical skills needed to respond to patient health problems (teaching, environment, and needs) were grouped into a third caring domain: clinical care. Items were theoretically attached to their corresponding caring domains for the factorial analysis to ensure that an item initially part of a particular domain could not be retained in another domain in the shorter scale. An exploratory factor analysis with varimax rotation was performed to investigate patterns of interrelationships among items. Items were retained if they were only grouping (factor loading > .40) along with their theoretical counterpart domain. Four statistical factors emerged; these were labeled clinical care (nine items), relational care (seven items), humanistic care (four items), and comforting care (three items). The last domain, comforting care, was not anticipated but was retained since it was composed of items originally from the teaching, environment, and needs factors and in line with Watson's view of the caring relationship that protects, enhances, and preserves the patient's dignity, humanity, and wholeness. Items forming this domain were "Respecting the patient's privacy," "Taking their basic needs into account," and "Observing the treatment or medication schedule." The final CNPI-23 consists of 23 items explaining 64.45% of the variance of the score (22.56%, 22.07%, 10.41%, and 9.41%, respectively, for the first four factors; Tool 22.2). All items loaded at more than .40 on the theoretical factor to which they were primarily attached, and no items were bidimensional (i.e., they did not load at more than .40 on another domain). Pearson's correlation coefficients between the four domains were moderate (between .38 and .71).

A third sample composed of 531 participants was used to conduct a confirmatory factor analysis to evaluate the construct validity of the four-dimensional CNPI-23 (Cossette, Pepin, Côté, & de Courval, 2008). For the confirmatory factor analysis, each item was hypothesized to be related solely to its conceptual domain. Linear Structural Relations version 8.72 was used to conduct the confirmatory factor analysis. As expected with this large sample and model, the χ^2-associated p value was below the .05 significance level ($\chi^2 = 811.43$, $df = 224$, $p < .01$). However, the other indices reached acceptable levels, with .054 for the standardized root mean-squared residuals, .070 for the root mean-square error of approximation, .88 for the goodness-of-fit index, .98 for the comparative fit index, and .97 for the normal fit index. These results were considered satisfactory, given the state of the scale development. The factor loadings for all items were equal to or greater than .48 and significant at the .01 level. The factor loadings for clinical care ranged from .65 for item 5, "Know what to do in situations where one must act quickly," to .75 for item 6, "Help them with the care they cannot administer themselves." The factor loadings for relational care ranged from .71 for item 16, "Try to identify with them the consequences of their behaviors," to .82 for item 12, "Help them to clarify which things they would like significant persons to bring them," and item 13, "Help them to explore the meaning that they give to their health condition." The factor loadings for humanistic care ranged from .48 for item 20, "Not having an attitude of disapproval," to .76 for item 18, "Encouraging them to be hopeful when it is appropriate." Finally, the factor loadings for comforting care ranged from .61 for item 23, "Giving them treatments or medications at the scheduled time," to .73 for item 22, "Taking patients' basic needs into account." The alpha coefficients for the CNPI-23 ranged from .91 to .95 for the total score. The Cronbach's alphas for the four domains ranged from .82 to .93 for clinical care, .89 to .91 for relational care, .64 to .73 for humanistic care, and .61 to .74 for comforting care.

As of April 19, 2018, the articles reporting the development and validation of both versions of CNPI have been cited 130 times according to Google Scholar. An analysis of these citations reveals 60 relevant and available citing articles after duplicate removal that we can divide into seven categories: (1) cited in the background or as an example of a scale allowing the measurement of caring nurse–patient interactions; (2) cited in a systematic review; (3) used in the development of new tools, scales, or instruments; (4) translated; (5) cited in a concept analysis or qualitative study; (6) guided the development of a nursing intervention; (7) used in a study to measure caring nurse–patient interactions.

First, the CNPI articles have been cited in 29 published studies in the background or as an example of scale allowing the measurement of caring nurse–patient interactions, underlining the contribution of the CNPI in the field. Second, the CNPI articles have been cited in five systematic reviews relating to the concept of nurse–patient interaction (Fleischer, Berg, Zimmermann, Wüste, & Behrens, 2009; Müggenburg & Riveros-Rosas, 2012), ethics-of-care measurement (Kuis, Hesselink, & Goossensen, 2014), and scale development process (Morgado, Meireles, Neves, Amaral, & Ferreira, 2017). As we examined socially desirable bias in responding to our caring tool, the paper was also referred in a systematic review by van de Mortel (2008) reporting the positive relationship between social desirability and self-reported questionnaires, in about half of the papers examined in their review. Third, the CNPI has also been used in the development of nine new measures of caring or similar constructs (e.g., nurses' motivational interventions) conducted by researchers in different contexts (Blaney, 2012; Chung, Hsieh, Chen, Chang, & Hsu, 2017; Cossette & Forbes, 2012; Deschenes, Charlin, Gagnon, & Goudreau, 2011; Duffy, Hoskins, & Seifert, 2007; Fontaine et al., 2016; Hwang, Tu, Chen, & Wang, 2012; Hwang, Tu, & Wang, 2017; Piredda et al., 2017). Fourth, both the 70-item and 23-item versions of the CNPI have been translated multiple times after their initial availability in English and in French. Indeed, there are three published translations of the CNPI: in Turkish (CNPI-70; Atar & Asti, 2012),

Chinese (CNPI-23; Jiang, Ruan, Xiang, & Jia, 2015), and Slovenian (CNPI-70; Pajnkihar, Stiglic, & Vrbnjak, 2017). In addition, nonpublished translated versions of the CNPI exist in Russian (CNPI-70), Spanish (CNPI-70), and Croatian (CNPI-23). Fifth, the CNPI has been used twice in a concept analysis or qualitative study in order, for instance, to define the concept of nurse–patient interaction (Boroujeni, Mohammadi, Oskouie, & Sandberg, 2009; Fakhr-Movahedi, Salsali, Negharandeh, & Rahnavard, 2011). Sixth, the CNPI has been used twice to guide the development of a nursing intervention integrating caring components (Charchalis, 2012; Kumar & McKewan, 2011).

Importantly, the CNPI scales have been used in 11 published studies to measure caring nurse–patient interactions (Table 22.2). More specifically, the CNPI-70 has been used in three published studies among nurses (Desmond et al., 2014; Kalender, Tosun, Çınar, Bağçivan, & Yaşar, 2016; Yilmaz & Çinar, 2017) and one in a sample of nurses and patients (Delmas, O'Reilly, Iglesias, Cara, & Burnier, 2016). Similarly, the CNPI-23 has been used in five published studies among nurses (Cha, Chang, & Kim, 2014; Jiang, Yan, Xiangjing, & Jia, 2012; Jiang et al., 2015; Martin et al., 2014; Rheingans, 2012) and one in a sample of patients (Zoni et al., 2018). The use of the CNPI in these studies has allowed researchers to report correlations between caring nurse–patient interactions and personal, clinical, and organizational variables. In the personal and clinical spheres, Jiang et al. (2012) showed that more experienced nurses (age and/or work seniority) felt more competent to behave in a caring manner in three of the four subscales: clinical, relational, and humanistic as well as on the total score of competency. Moreover, more experienced nurses felt that it was more feasible to act in a caring manner in the clinical care subscale, which includes clinical activity like monitoring the health condition or giving treatment and care. The importance given to caring behaviors was not related to age or experience (Jiang et al., 2012). In another study, the clinical subscale score in the CNPI, assessing the degree to which caring attitudes and behaviors were feasible to integrate in clinical practice, was correlated with overall job satisfaction scores. This underlines that nurses' capacity and ability of integrating caring in their clinical practice is linked with their satisfaction toward their profession (Rheingans, 2012).

In the organizational domain, a Korean survey by Cha et al. (2014) reported that a fit between organizational and personal identities or values significantly related to relational subscale caring behavior with patients in hospitals. As in the study of Jiang et al. (2012), relational caring behavior was significantly correlated with older age and work experience (Cha et al., 2014). Similarly, Roch, Dubois, and Clarke (2014), reported in their study that the hospitals' organizational climate explained 11% of the variation in nurses' reported frequency of caring behaviors. Moreover, it was reported that the specialty (e.g., surgery, psychiatry) and the fact that nurses had unconscious patients in caseload explained 14% of nurses' caring behavior. Interestingly, psychiatric nurses reported performing caring practices more frequently than nurses in other specialties (Roch et al., 2014).

The CNPI-70 and the CNPI-23 were developed to reflect the 10 nursing carative factors described by Watson (1979, 1988) to facilitate research on the links between caring and patient outcomes as well as teaching caring attitudes to students. Indeed, the CNPI scales can guide nurses to adopt caring attitudes through all their actions and interventions, beyond simply being nice to the patient. This scale is also being used to orient students and faculty in teaching and learning caring attitudes (Bernard, 2006). Hence, the CNPI is, to this day, pertinent to the nursing research community. Notably, during the last 5 years, the scale was useful to the organizational domain, as it has been for the practice and the educational domains since its first publication. Another interesting observation is the translation into six languages, which increases its potential use to different cultures. While global access is to be praised, some results obtained through these translated scales might unfortunately elude us in the future.

A user guide describing the different scales, the wording of the items depending on the clientele, and the purpose of the study are available on request.

ASPECTS THAT CAN BE EVALUATED

The CNPI's items describe attitudes and behaviors that can be seen in clinical practice and that can be measured by importance, frequency, satisfaction, competency, and feasibility. It is possible to evaluate these aspects according to the perception of the patient, a member of his or her family (or any other significant person), a nurse, and a student in nursing. However, the formulation of the items varies according to the target clientele, which explains the need for three different versions.

For the patient (patient version) or a member of his or her family (family version), one can measure three aspects by adding three questions to the CNPI questionnaire.

1. To measure the importance accorded to each of these attitudes or behaviors, the following question should be inserted at the beginning: How important do you consider the attitudes and behaviors in each of the following statements to be?

2. To measure the frequency with which these attitudes and behaviors have occurred, the following question should be inserted at the beginning: How frequently do you think that the attitudes and behaviors in each of the following statements have occurred?

3. To measure the degree of satisfaction with each of these attitudes or behaviors, the following question should be inserted at the beginning: How satisfied are you with the attitudes and behaviors in each of the following statements?

For nurses and nursing students (nurse version), one can measure two aspects by adding two questions and their corresponding scales.

1. To measure the degree to which they feel competent or at ease adopting these attitudes or behaviors, the following question should be inserted at the beginning: How competent or at ease do you feel adopting the attitudes and behaviors in each of the following statements?

2. To measure the degree to which they estimate the implementation of each of these attitudes or behaviors in clinical practice to be feasible, the following question should be inserted at the beginning: In your practice, how feasible or realistic do you find the attitudes and behaviors in each of the following statements?

RATING SCALES OF THE DIFFERENT ASPECTS

The person answering the CNPI questionnaire (i.e., patient, family, nurse, or nursing student) has to circle the number from 1 to 5 that best corresponds to what he or she thinks about each of these attitudes or behaviors (Tool 22.1). The rating scales and the formulation of the statements vary according to the aspects being measured and the target clientele. It is therefore important to select the rating scale that corresponds to each aspect as well as the questionnaire corresponding to the target clientele (patient, family, or nurse version).

Rating scale for the aspects of **importance, competency,** and **feasibility**:

Not at all	A little	Moderately	A lot	Extremely
1	2	3	4	5

Rating scale for the aspect of **frequency**:

Almost never	Sometimes	Often	Very often	Almost always
1	2	3	4	5

Rating scale for the aspect of **satisfaction**:

Very unsatisfied	Unsatisfied	No opinion	Satisfied	Very satisfied
1	2	3	4	5

TABLE 22.1 Description of the Caring Nurse–Patient Interactions Scale (CNPI-70 and CNPI-23)

INSTRUMENT	AUTHOR CONTACT INFORMATION	PUBLICATION CITATION SOURCE	DEVELOPED TO MEASURE	INSTRUMENT DESCRIPTION	PARTICIPANTS	REPORTED VALIDITY/ RELIABILITY	CONCEPTUAL/ THEORETICAL BASIS OF MEASUREMENT
CNPI-70 (2005)	Sylvie Cossette, PhD, RN; Faculty of Nursing University of Montreal, Quebec, Canada	Cossette, Cara, Ricard, and Pepin (2005)	Patient's, family's, or nurse's perceptions of the importance of, feeling of competency in, and feasibility of adopting caring behaviors	Long version of the CNPI	N = 332 nursing students	Face and content validity and reliability Contrasted groups/link with social desirability	Watson's theory and the 10 carative factors
CNPI-23 (2006, 2008)	Sylvie Cossette, PhD, RN; Faculty of Nursing University of Montreal, Quebec, Canada	Cossette, Côté, Pepin, Ricard, and D'Aoust (2006) Cossette, Pepin, Côté, de Courval (2008)	Patient's, family's, or nurse's perceptions of the importance of, feeling of competency in, and feasibility of adopting caring behaviors	Short version of the CNPI	N = 377 nursing students	Face and content validity and reliability Construct validity	Four caring domains linked to Watson's theory

TABLE 22.2 Literature Synthesis: Caring Nurse–Patient Interactions (CNPI) Scale

STUDY/ COUNTRY	PURPOSE	STUDY DESIGN	PARTICIPANTS	VERSION	VALIDITY/ FIDELITY	KEY RESULTS/OBSERVATIONS RELATED TO CNPI
Cha et al. (2014) Korea	To examine the relationship between person and organizational fit on prosocial identity and various employee outcomes	Descriptive, cross-sectional study	N = 589 medical doctors, nurses, and hospital staff	CNPI-23 (Seven items only to assess relational caring behavior)	Cronbach's alpha: .95	■ Organizational prosocial identity positively related to organizational identification and caring behavior ■ Organizational identification and caring behavior increased as both personal and organizational prosocial identity increased
Delmas et al. (2016) Switzerland	To examine the feasibility, acceptability, and preliminary effects of an educational intervention based on the theory of human caring delivered to hemodialysis nurses	A mixed-design pilot study	N = 9 hemodialysis nurses; N = 22 patients	CNPI-70 (used by nurses frequency and patients)	Not reported	■ Participating nurses very often adopted caring attitudes and behaviors with the patients undergoing hemodialysis
Desmond et al. (2014) United States	To assess the effect of a one-day Watson's caring theory educational seminar with the staff to enhance patients' perceptions of care	A quasi-experimental design	N = 10	CNPI-70 (nurses' competence)	Not reported	■ Statistically significant increase in nurse's confidence in caring attitudes and behaviors was found

(continued)

259

TABLE 22.2 Literature Synthesis: Caring Nurse–Patient Interactions (CNPI) Scale *(continued)*

STUDY/ COUNTRY	PURPOSE	STUDY DESIGN	PARTICIPANTS	VERSION	VALIDITY/ FIDELITY	KEY RESULTS/OBSERVATIONS RELATED TO CNPI
Jiang et al. (2015) China	To translate the CNPI-23 to Chinese, then to investigate and analyze the caring attitude and behavior of clinical nurses in terms of importance, competency, and feasibility	Descriptive, cross-sectional study	N = 260 nurses	CNPI-23 (nurses importance competence feasibility)	Cronbach's alpha was .97 for the total scale and .92–.95 for subscales	▪ Competency scores related to caring behavior were positively correlated with age and work experience ▪ Feasibility scores for clinical care dimension of the CNPI were positively correlated with age and work experience
Kalender et al. (2016) Turkey	To assess the attitudes and behaviors of nursing students in their clinical experiences in terms of nurse–patient interactions	Descriptive, cross-sectional study	N = 200 nursing students	CNPI-70 (nurses importance competency realism)	Not reported	▪ Direct positive correlation between the CNPI scores and the attitudes and behaviors of nursing students ▪ Among the different dimensions of the CNPI, importance was the dimension the most highly rated by students.
Martin et al. (2014) United States	To examine if there is a difference in nurse attitudes and experience for those who assign Emergency Severity Index (ESI) scores accurately and those who do not assign ESI scores accurately	Descriptive, exploratory study design	N = 64 nurses	CNPI-23	Not reported	▪ Nonsignificant effect of emergency department triage experience, gender, and site of practice on attitude (CNPI-23) ▪ Years of work experience and attitude (CNPI-23) scores were negatively correlated ($r = -.78$, $p = .01$)

Study	Purpose	Design	Sample	Instrument	Reliability	Findings
Rheingans (2012) United States	To examine the influence of shared governance on nurse–patient interactions in nurses	Descriptive, cross-sectional study	N = 140 nurses	CNPI-23	Not reported	■ The CNPI-S (predominately the clinical subscale) was effective in predicting overall and some subscales of job satisfaction
Roch et al. (2014) Canada	To explain associations between organizational climate and nurses' and other workers' performance of caring practices	Mixed-methods study	N = 292 nurses	CNPI-23	Cronbach's alpha overall of .92	■ Organizational climate explained 11% of the variation in nurses' frequency of caring behavior ■ Caring behavior was affected by the interplay of organizational climate dimensions with patients' and nurses' characteristics
Yilmaz & Çinar (2017) Turkey	To examine the attitudes of senior students in the nursing department toward caring nursing–patient interactions	Descriptive, cross-sectional study	N = 57 nursing students	CNPI-70 (nurses importance competency realism)	Not reported	■ The highest average scores of the subscales were in "needs" and the lowest scores were in the "sensitivity" subscale ■ No statistically significant difference between sociodemographic characteristics of nursing students and the significance, sufficiency, and applicability dimensions of the scale

(continued)

TABLE 22.2 Literature Synthesis: Caring Nurse–Patient Interactions (CNPI) Scale (*continued*)

STUDY/ COUNTRY	PURPOSE	STUDY DESIGN	PARTICIPANTS	VERSION	VALIDITY/ FIDELITY	KEY RESULTS/OBSERVATIONS RELATED TO CNPI
Zoni et al. (2018) Switzerland	To evaluate patient self-management activities, patient perceptions of the therapeutic relationship, and satisfaction with nurse-led consultations as part of a structured, pilot program transitioning young adults with type 1 diabetes to adult-oriented community-based practices	Descriptive, cross-sectional study	*N* = 20 patients	CNPI-23	Not reported	▪ Humanistic and comforting caring attitudes/behavior received the highest ratings for importance, while the most frequently observed attitudes/behaviors were comforting care and clinical care ▪ Importance and frequency dimensions of the CNPI were strongly correlated globally ▪ The relative importance of clinical caring was significantly related to ratings of satisfaction
Pajnkihar et al. (2017) Slovenia	To translate the CNPI-70 into Slovenian and to explore relationships between the level of nursing education, the perception of nurses and nursing assistants of Watson's carative factors, and patient satisfaction	Descriptive, cross-sectional study	*N* = 1,098 nurses *N* = 1,123 patients	CNPI-70	Cronbach's alpha between subscales: .70–.94	▪ No significant relation between nurses' perception of the 10 carative factors and their level of education, except for sensibility ▪ The institution influenced nurses' perceptions of carative factors

TOOL 22.1

Caring Nurse–Patient Interactions Scale: 70-Item Version (Nurse Version)

NO.	STATEMENT	RATING SCALE				

1—Humanism: Formation of a humanistic–altruistic system of values

NO.	STATEMENT					
1.	Consider them as complete individuals; show that you are interested in more than their health problems.	1	2	3	4	5
2.	Try to see things from their point of view.	1	2	3	4	5
3.	Accept them as they are without prejudice.	1	2	3	4	5
4.	Show respect to them as well as to those closest to them.	1	2	3	4	5
5.	Do not have an attitude of disapproval.	1	2	3	4	5
6.	Be humane and warm with them and with those closest to them.	1	2	3	4	5

2—Hope: Instillation of faith–hope

NO.	STATEMENT					
7.	Show that you will be there for them if they need you.	1	2	3	4	5
8.	Encourage them to have confidence in themselves.	1	2	3	4	5
9.	Draw their attention to positive aspects concerning them and their states of health.	1	2	3	4	5
10.	Emphasize their efforts.	1	2	3	4	5
11.	Encourage them to be hopeful, when it is appropriate.	1	2	3	4	5
12.	Help them to find motivation to improve their states of health.	1	2	3	4	5
13.	Take into account what they know about their health situations.	1	2	3	4	5

3—Sensibility: Cultivation of sensitivity to one's self and to others

NO.	STATEMENT					
14.	Ask them how they would like things to be done.	1	2	3	4	5
15.	Show awareness of their feelings and of those closest to them.	1	2	3	4	5
16.	Know how to choose the right moment to discuss with them their conditions and the steps to come.	1	2	3	4	5
17.	Know how to express in an appropriate fashion your feelings toward their situations.	1	2	3	4	5
18.	Make them aware of the way those closest to them are experiencing their situations.	1	2	3	4	5
19.	Keep those closest to them up to date about their states of health (with their agreement).	1	2	3	4	5

(continued)

TOOL 22.1

Caring Nurse–Patient Interactions Scale: 70-Item Version (Nurse Version) (*continued*)

NO.	STATEMENT	RATING SCALE				

4—Helping relationship: Development of a helping–trusting, human caring relationship

NO.	STATEMENT					
20.	Listen to them attentively when they speak, as well as those closest to them.	1	2	3	4	5
21.	Introduce yourself by stating clearly your name and function.	1	2	3	4	5
22.	Answer as soon as it is convenient when they call you.	1	2	3	4	5
23.	Respect your engagements, that is to say, do what you said you would do.	1	2	3	4	5
24.	Do not seem busy or otherwise occupied when you am taking care of them.	1	2	3	4	5
25.	Do not cut them off when they speak.	1	2	3	4	5
26.	Do not confront too harshly their ideas and behaviors.	1	2	3	4	5

5—Expression of emotions: Promotion and acceptance of the expression of positive and negative feelings

NO.	STATEMENT					
27.	Encourage them to speak their thoughts and feelings freely.	1	2	3	4	5
28.	Keep calm when they are angry.	1	2	3	4	5
29.	Help them to understand the emotions they feel in their situations.	1	2	3	4	5
30.	Do not reduce your presence when they have difficult moments.	1	2	3	4	5
31.	Help them to channel their difficult emotions.	1	2	3	4	5
32.	Let them express their pain, their sadness, their fears, etc.	1	2	3	4	5

6—Problem solving: Systematic use of a creative problem-solving caring process

NO.	STATEMENT					
33.	Help them to set realistic objectives that take their health conditions into account.	1	2	3	4	5
34.	Help them to cope with the stress generated by their conditions or general situations.	1	2	3	4	5
35.	Help them to see things from a different point of view.	1	2	3	4	5
36.	Help them to recognize the means to efficiently resolve their problems.	1	2	3	4	5
37.	Try to identify with them the consequences of their behaviors.	1	2	3	4	5
38.	Inform them and those closest to them about the resources adapted to their needs (e.g., community health centers).	1	2	3	4	5

(continued)

TOOL 22.1

Caring Nurse–Patient Interactions Scale: 70-Item Version (Nurse Version) (*continued*)

NO.	STATEMENT	RATING SCALE				
	7—Teaching: Promotion of transpersonal teaching-learning					
39.	Help them to identify, formulate, and ask questions about their illnesses and treatments.	1	2	3	4	5
40.	Check if they and those closest to them have properly understood the explanations given.	1	2	3	4	5
41.	Give them the necessary information or make it available so they can make informed decisions.	1	2	3	4	5
42.	Explain to them the care or treatments beforehand.	1	2	3	4	5
43.	Do not use terms or a language that they or those closest to them do not understand.	1	2	3	4	5
44.	Provide them with the opportunity to practice self-administered care.	1	2	3	4	5
45.	Respect their pace when giving them information or answering their questions.	1	2	3	4	5
46.	Teach them how to schedule and prepare their medications.	1	2	3	4	5
47.	Give them indications and means to treat or prevent certain side effects of their medications or treatments.	1	2	3	4	5
	8—Environment: Provision for a supportive, protective, and/or corrective mental, physical, societal, and spiritual environment					
48.	Understand when they need to be alone.	1	2	3	4	5
49.	Help them to be comfortable (e.g., offer them back rubs, help them to change positions, adjust the lighting, suggest special equipment).	1	2	3	4	5
50.	Put the room back in order after having taken care of them.	1	2	3	4	5
51.	Check if their medications soothe their symptoms (e.g., nausea, pain, constipation, anxiety).	1	2	3	4	5
52.	Respect their privacy (e.g., do not expose them needlessly).	1	2	3	4	5
53.	Before leaving, check if they have everything they need.	1	2	3	4	5
54.	Help them to clarify which things they would like significant persons to bring them.	1	2	3	4	5

(*continued*)

TOOL 22.1

Caring Nurse–Patient Interactions Scale: 70-Item Version (Nurse Version) *(continued)*

NO.	STATEMENT	RATING SCALE

9—Needs: Assistance with the gratification of human needs

NO.	STATEMENT					
55.	Help them with the care they cannot administer themselves.	1	2	3	4	5
56.	Know how to give the treatments (e.g., intravenous injections, bandages).	1	2	3	4	5
57.	Know how to operate specialized equipment (e.g., pumps, monitors).	1	2	3	4	5
58.	Do treatments or give medications at the scheduled time.	1	2	3	4	5
59.	Encourage those closest to them to support them (with their agreement).	1	2	3	4	5
60.	Closely monitor their health conditions.	1	2	3	4	5
61.	Help them to feel that they have a certain control over their situations.	1	2	3	4	5
62.	Know what to do in situations where one must act quickly.	1	2	3	4	5
63.	Show ability and skill in your way of intervening with them.	1	2	3	4	5
64.	Take their basic needs into account (e.g., sleeping, hygiene).	1	2	3	4	5

10—Spirituality: Allowance for existential–phenomenological–spiritual forces

NO.	STATEMENT					
65.	Help them to feel well in their conditions.	1	2	3	4	5
66.	Recognize that prayer, meditation, or other means can help appease them and give them hope.	1	2	3	4	5
67.	Help them to explore what is important in their lives.	1	2	3	4	5
68.	Help them to explore the meaning that they give to their health conditions.	1	2	3	4	5
69.	Help them to look for a certain equilibrium/balance in their lives.	1	2	3	4	5
70.	Take into consideration their spiritual needs (e.g., prayer, meditation, participation in certain rites).	1	2	3	4	5

TOOL 22.2

Caring Nurse–Patient Interactions Scale: 23-Item Version (Nurse Version)

NO.	STATEMENT	RATING SCALE				
	A—Clinical Care					
1.	Know how to give the treatments (e.g., intravenous injections, bandages).	1	2	3	4	5
2.	Know how to operate specialized equipment (e.g., pumps, monitors).	1	2	3	4	5
3.	Check if their medications soothe their symptoms (e.g., nausea, pain, constipation, anxiety).	1	2	3	4	5
4.	Give them indications and means to treat or prevent certain side effects of their medications or treatments.	1	2	3	4	5
5.	Know what to do in situations where one must act quickly.	1	2	3	4	5
6	Help them with the care they cannot administer themselves.	1	2	3	4	5
7.	Show ability and skill in your way of intervening with them.	1	2	3	4	5
8.	Closely monitor their health conditions.	1	2	3	4	5
9.	Provide them with the opportunity to practice self-administered care.	1	2	3	4	5
	B—Relational Care					
10.	Help them to look for a certain equilibrium/balance in their lives.	1	2	3	4	5
11.	Help them to explore what is important in their lives.	1	2	3	4	5
12.	Help them to clarify which things they would like significant persons to bring them.	1	2	3	4	5
13.	Help them to explore the meaning that they gave to their health conditions.	1	2	3	4	5
14.	Help them to recognize the means to efficiently resolve their problems.	1	2	3	4	5
15.	Help them to see things from a different point of view.	1	2	3	4	5
16.	Try to identify with them the consequences of their behaviors.	1	2	3	4	5

(continued)

TOOL 22.2

Caring Nurse–Patient Interactions Scale: 23-Item Version (Nurse Version) (*continued*)

NO.	STATEMENT	RATING SCALE				

C—Humanistic Care

NO.	STATEMENT					
17.	Consider them as complete individuals; show that you are interested in more than their health problems.	1	2	3	4	5
18.	Encourage them to be hopeful, when it is appropriate.	1	2	3	4	5
19.	Emphasize their efforts.	1	2	3	4	5
20.	Do not have an attitude of disapproval.	1	2	3	4	5

D—Comforting Care

NO.	STATEMENT					
21.	Respect their privacy (e.g., do not expose them needlessly).	1	2	3	4	5
22.	Take their basic needs into account (e.g., sleeping, hygiene).	1	2	3	4	5
23.	Do treatments or give medications at the scheduled time.	1	2	3	4	5

REFERENCES

Atar, N. Y., & Asti, T. A. (2012). Bakım Odaklı Hemşire-Hasta Etkileşimi Ölçeğinin Güvenilirlik ve Geçerliği [Validity and reliability of Turkish version of the caring nurse-patient interaction scale]. *Florence Nightingale Hemşirelik Dergisi, 20*(2), 129–139.

Bernard, L. (2006). L'apprentissage du caring dans l'approche par compétences [Learning caring in the skills approach] (Master's Thesis, Université de Montréal). Retrieved from http://hdl.handle.net/1866/2334

Blaney, C. D. (2012). *The influence of changing nurse documentation practices have on patient satisfaction.* Phoenix, AZ: University of Phoenix.

Boroujeni, A. Z., Mohammadi, R., Oskouie, S. F. H., & Sandberg, J. (2009). Iranian nurses' preparation for loss: Finding a balance in end-of-life care. *Journal of Clinical Nursing, 18*(16), 2329–2336. doi:10.1111/j.1365-2702.2008.02437.x

Cha, J., Chang, Y. K., & Kim, T. Y. (2014). Person–organization fit on prosocial identity: Implications on employee outcomes. *Journal of Business Ethics, 123*(1), 57–69. doi:10.1007/s10551-013-1799-7

Charchalis, M. (2012). *Évaluation d'une intervention infirmière basée sur une approche caring et cognitive comportementale sur l'acceptation d'un défibrillateur cardiaque implantable.* Montréal, Canada: Université de Montréal.

Chung, H. C., Hsieh, T. C., Chen, Y. C., Chang, S. C., & Hsu, W. L. (2017). Cross-cultural adaptation and validation of the Chinese Comfort, Afford, Respect, and Expect scale of caring nurse–patient interaction competence. *Journal of Clinical Nursing, 27*(17–18), 3287–3297. doi:10.1111/jocn.14196

Cossette, S., Cara, C., Ricard, N., & Pepin, J. (2005). Assessing nurse–patient interactions from a caring perspective: Report of the development and preliminary psychometric testing of the Caring Nurse–Patient Interactions Scale. *International Journal of Nursing Studies, 42,* 673–686. doi:10.1016/j.ijnurstu.2004.10.004

Cossette, S., Côté, J. K., Pepin, J., Ricard, N., & D'Aoust, L.-X. (2006). A dimensional structure of nurse–patient interaction from a caring perspective: Refinement of the Caring Nurse–Patient Interaction Scale (CNPI–Short Scale). *Journal of Advanced Nursing, 55*(2), 198–214. doi:10.1111/j.1365-2648.2006.03895.x

Cossette, S., & Forbes, C. (2012). Psychometric evaluation of the caring nurse observation tool: Scale development. *International Journal for Human Caring, 16*(1), 16–23. doi:10.20467/1091-5710.16.1.16

Cossette, S., Pepin, J., Côté, J. K., & de Courval, F. (2008). The multidimensionality of caring: A confirmatory factor analysis of the Caring Nurse–Patient Interaction Short Scale. *Journal of Advanced Nursing, 61*(6), 699–710. doi:10.1111/j.1365-2648.2007.04566.x

Delmas, P., O'Reilly, L., Iglesias, K., Cara, C., & Burnier, M. (2016). Feasibility, acceptability, and preliminary effects of educational intervention to strengthen humanistic practice among hemodialysis nurses in the Canton of Vaud, Switzerland: A pilot study. *International Journal for Human Caring, 20*(1), 31–43. doi:10.20467/1091-5710.20.1.31

Deschenes, M. F., Charlin, B., Gagnon, R., & Goudreau, J. (2011). Use of a script concordance test to assess development of clinical reasoning in nursing students. *Journal of Nursing Education, 50*(7), 381–387. doi:10.3928/01484834-20110331-03

Desmond, M. E., Horn, S., Keith, K., Kelby, S., Ryan, L., & Smith, J. (2014). Incorporating caring theory into personal and professional nursing practice to improve perception of care. *International Journal for Human Caring, 18*(1), 35–44. doi:10.20467/1091-5710-18.1.35

Duffy, J. R., Hoskins, L., & Seifert, R. F. (2007). Dimensions of caring: Psychometric evaluation of the caring assessment tool. *Advances in Nursing Science, 30*(3), 235–245. doi:10.1097/01.ANS.0000286622.84763.a9

Fakhr-Movahedi, A., Salsali, M., Negharandeh, R., & Rahnavard, Z. (2011). A qualitative content analysis of nurse–patient communication in Iranian nursing. *International Nursing Review, 58*(2), 171–180. doi:10.1111/j.1466-7657.2010.00861.x

Fleischer, S., Berg, A., Zimmermann, M., Wüste, K., & Behrens, J. (2009). Nurse–patient interaction and communication: A systematic literature review. *Journal of Public Health, 17*(5), 339–353. doi:10.1007/s10389-008-0238-1

Fontaine, G., Cossette, S., Heppell, S., Boyer, L., Mailhot, T., Simard, M. J., & Tanguay, J. F. (2016). Evaluation of a web-based E-learning platform for brief motivational interviewing by nurses in cardiovascular care: A pilot study. *Journal of Medical Internet Research, 18*(8), e224. doi:10.2196/jmir.6298

Hwang, H. L., Tu, C. T., Chen, S., & Wang, H. H. (2012). Caring behaviors perceived by elderly residents of long-term care facilities: Scale development and psychometric assessment. *International Journal of Nursing Studies, 49*(2), 183–190. doi:10.1016/j.ijnurstu.2011.08.013

Hwang, H. L., Tu, C. T., & Wang, H. H. (2017). Development and psychometric evaluation of the caring scale for institutionalized elders. *Journal of Nursing Research, 25*(2), 140–147. doi:10.1097/jnr.0000000000000147

Jiang, L., Yan, H., Xiangjing, X., & Jia, Q. (2012). Status and influencing factors of nursing care behaviors of clinical nurses. *Chinese Journal of Modern Nursing, 2012*(24), 2863–2866.

Jiang, L. L., Ruan, H., Xiang, X. J., & Jia, Q. (2015). Investigation and analysis of the caring attitude and behaviour of nurses in Shanghai, China. *International Journal of Nursing Practice, 21*(4), 426–432. doi:10.1111/ijn.12287

Kalender, N., Tosun, N., Çınar, F. İ., Bağçivan, G., & Yaşar, Z. (2016). Assessing the attitudes and behaviors of nursing students according to caring nurse–patient interaction scale. *Gulhane Medical Journal, 58*(3), 277–281. doi:10.5455/Gülhane.181127

Kuis, E. E., Hesselink, G., & Goossensen, A. (2014). Can quality from a care ethical perspective be assessed? A review. *Nursing Ethics, 21*(7), 774–793. doi:10.1177/0969733013500163

Kumar, S., & McKewan, G. W. (2011). Six sigma DMAIC quality study: Expanded nurse practitioner's role in health care during and posthospitalization within the United States. *Home Health Care Management & Practice, 23*(4), 271–282. doi:10.1177/1084822310388385

Martin, A., Davidson, C. L., Panik, A., Buckenmyer, C., Delpais, P., & Ortiz, M. (2014). An examination of ESI triage scoring accuracy in relationship to ED nursing attitudes and experience. *Journal of Emergency Nursing, 40*(5), 461–468. doi:10.1016/j.jen.2013.09.009

Morgado, F. F. R., Meireles, J. F. F., Neves, C. M., Amaral, A. C. S., & Ferreira, M. E. C. (2017). Scale development: Ten main limitations and recommendations to improve future research practices. *Psicologia-Reflexao E Critica, 30*(1), 1–20. doi:10.1186/s41155-016-0057-1

Müggenburg, C., & Riveros-Rosas, A. (2012). Interacción enfermera-paciente y su repercusión en el cuidado hospitalario: Parte I. *Enfermería Universitaria, 9*(1), 36–44. doi:10.22201/eneo.23958421e.2012.1.244

Pajnkihar, M., Stiglic, G., & Vrbnjak, D. (2017). The concept of Watson's carative factors in nursing and their (dis) harmony with patient satisfaction. *PeerJ, 5*, e2940. doi:10.7717/peerj.2940

Pepin, J., Cossette, S., Ricard, N., & Côté, J. (2005, June 17). *Cultural characteristics of students enrolled in the nursing program at the Faculty of Nursing, University of Montreal.* Paper delivered at the 27th annual meeting of the International Association of Human Caring, Lake Tahoe, CA.

Piredda, M., Ghezzi, V., Fenizia, E., Marchetti, A., Petitti, T., De Marinis, M. G., & Sili, A. (2017). Development and psychometric testing of a new instrument to measure the caring behaviour of nurses in Italian acute care settings. *Journal of Advanced Nursing, 73*(12), 3178–3188. doi:10.1111/jan.13384

Rheingans, J. I. (2012). The alchemy of shared governance: Turning steel (and sweat) into gold. *Nurse Leader, 10*(1), 40–42. doi:10.1016/j.mnl.2011.11.007

Roch, G., Dubois, C. A., & Clarke, S. P. (2014). Organizational climate and hospital nurses' caring practices: A mixed-methods study. *Research in Nursing & Health, 37*(3), 229–240. doi:10.1002/nur.21596

van de Mortel, T. F. (2008). Faking it: Social desirability response bias in self-report research. *Australian Journal of Advanced Nursing, 25*(4), 40–48.

Watson, J. (1979). *Nursing: The philosophy and science of caring.* Boston, MA: Little, Brown.

Watson, J. (1988). *Nursing. Human science and human care. A theory of nursing.* New York, NY: National League for Nursing.

Yilmaz, D., & Çinar, H. G. (2017). Examination of attitudes of nursing department senior students towards caring nurse–patient interaction. *Journal of Human Sciences, 14*(4), 3300–3309. doi:10.14687/jhs.v14i4.4911

Zoni, S., Verga, M. E., Hauschild, M., Aquarone-Vaucher, M. P., Gyuriga, T., Ramelet, A. S., & Dwyer, A. A. (2018). Patient perspectives on nurse-led consultations within a pilot structured transition program for young adults moving from an academic tertiary setting to community-based type 1 diabetes care. *Journal of Pediatric Nursing-Nursing Care of Children & Families, 38*, 99–105. doi:10.1016/j.pedn.2017.11.015

Development of the Caring Factor Survey (CFS), an Instrument to Measure Patient's Perception of Caring

John W. Nelson, Jean Watson, and Inova Health

The Caring Factor Survey (CFS) is a tool that examines the construct of "caritas," which literally means "divine care/love." A "construct" is an attribute of people reflected in testing (Cronbach & Meehl, 1955). In this case, it is the testing of nurses' use of physical, mental, and spiritual caring behaviors as reported by the patients for whom they provide care. Caritas is a construct that is premised on Watson's current views of caring in healthcare (Watson, 2005). The CFS was created by the instrument's original authors Karen Drenkard, John Nelson, Gene Rigotti, and Jean Watson to be readily available in the public domain. The CFS was created to be used by either patients or family members of patients. This brief chapter will review the initial psychometric testing of the CFS that was a result of studies conducted in 2006 and 2007.

At the time of the development of the CFS, at least 21 instruments had been developed to assess and measure caring. Six of the known instruments to measure caring were derived from Watson's original theory of caring and the 10 carative factors (Watson, 2002). (Carative factors, according to Watson, are elements that exist within the interaction between patient and nurse.) However, none of the instruments to date had incorporated Watson's contemporary theoretical concepts of caritas that acknowledge connections between caring and love and self-caring practices within explicit references of spirituality.

The CFS was originally written with 20 statements, two statements for each of the caritas processes. The method was selected with the goal to decrease the

20 items to 10 items, with each item reflecting each of the 10 caritas processes articulated by Watson's most recent views of caring in healthcare (Watson, 2005) from the patient's perspective. This item-reduction method is utilized in new instrumentation development (Cronbach & Meehl, 1955).

The CFS uses a 1–7 Likert-type scale, with higher scores indicating a greater sense of caring from the patient's perspective. All statements were phrased positively. Patients or patients' family members were asked to respond to each statement. Numbers 1 to 3 on the scale indicated levels of disagreement; number 1 indicated the strongest level of disagreement, number 2 moderate disagreement, and number 3 slight disagreement. Numbers 5 to 7 indicated levels of agreement with the statement of caring; number 7 indicated the strongest level of agreement, number 6 moderate agreement, and number 5 slight agreement. Number 4 was used only if the respondent felt neutral about the statement.

VALIDITY

Several aspects of validity were established, including face, content, criterion, and predictive. Validity will establish that the CFS indeed measures caring as reported by the patient.

Face Validity

The first 20 statements, two for each aspect of caritas, were formulated by John Nelson and sent to Jean Watson to establish face validity. "Face validity" refers to whether an instrument appears to measure the construct of interest (Polit & Hungler, 1999). After face validity was established, the additional two authors of the CFS were asked to assist with content validity.

Content Validity

"Content validity" refers to the adequacy of an instrument to represent all possible questions to acquire information about the topic of interest (Polit & Hungler, 1999). Content validity of the CFS was established by asking four experts in the caritas processes: Karen Drenkard and Gene Rigotti of Inova Health, John Nelson of Heathcare Environment, Inc., and theorist Jean Watson. After a total of nine revisions to the 20 questions, all of these experts, who are also the authors of the CFS, were in 100% agreement that the content of each statement reflected the caritas processes:

- "Practice of loving kindness" by staff was assessed via items 1 and 3.
- "Instilling faith and hope" was addressed via statements 5 and 7.
- "Spiritual beliefs and practices" were assessed using statements 9 and 11.

- "Developing a helping–trusting relationship between patient and nurse" was assessed using items 13 and 15.

- "Promotion and acceptance of positive and negative feeling" was assessed with items 17 and 19.

- "Using a caring process for decision making" was assessed using items 2 and 4.

- "Performing teaching and learning that addresses the individual needs and learning styles" was assessed using items 6 and 8.

- "Creation of a healing environment for the physical and spiritual self" as perceived by the patient was assessed by questions 10 and 12.

- "Assistance with physical, emotional, and spiritual human needs" as perceived by the patient was assessed using statements 14 and 16.

- "Allowing room for miracles to take place" as perceived by the patient was assessed using statements 18 and 20.

More detailed explanations of the caritas processes are described on Watson's website: www.watsoncaringscience.org.

Criterion Validity

To assess for "criterion validity," the CFS was measured against a selected well-validated caring tool that was perceived to be the most similar to the CFS, the Caring Assessment Tool (CAT II)© (Duffy, 2002). The CAT II was developed to measure the caring processes proposed within the work of Watson and was viewed as the ideal candidate to establish criterion validity.

The CAT II was developed in 1990 to measure patients' perceptions of nurse–caring behaviors (Duffy, 1990). (This should not be confused with patient satisfaction as that is a different construct.) The items in the CAT II were developed from the caring theory as defined by Watson, with each of the 10 carative factors represented. Originally, the CAT II had 130 items. Through content analysis, 30 were deleted. The remaining 100 items composed the present instrument used for this study (Duffy, 2002). Dr. Watson was herself one of the validators of the CAT II. Internal consistency has been measured at ~.9776 in several studies (Andrews, Daniels, & Hall, 1996; Duffy 2002).

Pearson's correlation was used to evaluate the relationship between the CFS and the CAT II when being measured at the same time, on the same patients, on the same units of care. A correlation of .80 or greater, which is considered a strong correlation (Glasnapp & Poggio, 1985), was chosen to evaluate whether the two instruments were indeed measuring the same construct. A significance of $p < .10$ was chosen because levels of significance less than .05 were judged to be too stringent, causing more type II errors. (Type II errors occur when a false null hypothesis is accepted [Howell, 1997].) It was recognized that .10 was a liberal

p-level to use. Considering that this was an exploratory study, relationships that may exist within the study's theoretical framework may have been missed if a stricter p-level of .05 had been used. The relationship between the CFS and CAT II was assessed (using Pearson's correlation) on eight patient care units. Analysis was done at the unit level. The correlation between the two instruments was found to be .69, significant at the .10 level ($p = .06$).

Predictive Validity

"Predictive validity" is indicated by the consistency of the measurement and observed predicted operations. Predictive validity of the CFS was determined by evaluating CFS survey outcomes between four patient care units that experienced a caring intervention and four control units. There were 96 patients in the treatment units and 64 in the control units. All were medical–surgical units. The treatment units had higher scores on the CFS on 9 of the 10 factors measured, including the total CFS score. A comparison of mean scores from the treatment and control groups indicated that the treatment group was more satisfied than the control group with the overall perception of care (mean scores 5.64 and 5.52, respectively). This difference of .12 on a scale of 1–7 was not statistically significant.

RELIABILITY TESTING

"Reliability" refers to the degree of consistency with which an instrument measures the attribute of interest (Polit & Hungler, 1999). Reliability was established by evaluating internal consistency, which is a method to evaluate how each of the items relates to each other and to the total score. In addition, Cronbach's alpha was assessed, which determines how consistent responders understood the questions.

The correlation of each paired statement was examined to identify whether they measured the same caring behavior. It was desired to have correlations of .80 or higher, which indicates a high correlation (Glasnapp & Poggio, 1985). In 2007, at Wyoming Medical Center, there were 232 patients and 79 family members who responded to the CFS. Nine of the ten paired statements were found to have a correlation greater than .80 (using Pearson's r), indicating they measured the same factor. Only the paired statements that measured Promotions of Feelings fell below .80 with a correlation of .74. The paired statements for the 79 family members were also found to have correlations greater than .80. Only the paired statements for Support of Spiritual Belief and Creating a Healing Environment fell below .80, at .77 and .75, respectively. All of these correlations within the Wyoming Medical Center study were found to be statistically significant at the .001 level.

Internal Consistency was evaluated using a zero-order correlation table (Sramek & Legler, 2007). Item-to-total correlations for all 20 of the statements were found to range between .81 and .91 for the patients and .80 and .93 for family members. Interitem correlations for all 20 statements were between .58 and .92 for the patients and .49 and .93 for family members. All of these correlations were found to be significant at the .001 level of significance.

A Cronbach's alpha of .70 was accepted as minimum for this new 20-item scale. Polit and Hungler (1996) assert that an alpha less than .70 should be considered risky (Polit, 1996). Items were evaluated to determine whether deleting them would result in an increase in the alpha value. The Cronbach's alpha was tested in three studies in the United States. The first was conducted in 2006 in an East Coast healthcare system on eight medical-surgical patient care units. The study tested results of an intervention of implementing caring behaviors in nursing staff. There were 96 patients in the treatment group and 64 in the control group. The Cronbach's alpha was assessed and found to be .97. No item, if deleted, would have resulted in an increase of the Cronbach's alpha. In a second study in 2007 at New York Presbyterian Hospital in New York City, 84 patients were given the CFS in a baseline assessment of caring behaviors. The Cronbach's alpha of the CFS was found to be .97. The third study was conducted at Wyoming Medical Center where 232 patients and 79 family members responded to the CFS. The Cronbach's alpha for patients was found to be .98 and for family members was also found to be .98.

DISCUSSION AND IMPLICATIONS

Development of psychometrically sound instruments is essential to articulate the place care has within the increasingly mechanistic environment of healthcare. Direct care providers must find ways to examine the impact of caring using scientifically sound methods. Use of the CFS will assist those who want to use brief, psychometrically tested instruments to measure patients' subjective perceptions of care. It may also be used in conjunction with other caring instruments to strengthen the scientific argument that the construct of caring is indeed being measured. The limitations of the CFS include being a new instrument with more validity and reliability testing needed.

The CFS has recently been translated into Filipino and Italian languages and is currently being tested psychometrically. Use of caring instruments across cultures will facilitate examination of what is important in caring and healing across the globe. In addition, examination of which aspects of the caring behaviors that are rated high and low can be evaluated in order to refine specific caring behaviors, whether it be problem solving between nurse and patient, effective teaching, or spiritual care.

Furthermore, enhancement of care may impact human resource and operational outcomes within the hospital or healthcare system. Creation of such data may be used to articulate the return on investment that result from caring behaviors. It is the hope of the authors of the CFS that measurement of being connected to the direct care provider can become a central outcome measure as it has been articulated by the patient as the most important aspect of being within a hospital (Picker/Commonwealth, 1993). The authors assert that it is through the caring processes that humans can heal as whole persons in the way they believe is appropriate. The development of measures of care is an essential aspect of the evaluation and progression of research in processes of caring.

UPDATE OF CFS

Construct validation of the instrument was conducted by DiNapoli, Turkel, Nelson, and Watson (2010). The construct validation by DiNapoli et al. (2010) was used to reduce the 20-item survey to a 10-item survey. Results of the 10-item composite measure revealed good model fit (DiNapoli et al., 2010).

The CFS has been used to study the patients' perception of caring when implementing the processes of care according to Watson (Turner & Toomer, 2012) or models and frameworks of care that are consistent or combined with Watson's processes of caritas, including Primary Nursing (Persky, Felgen, & Nelson, 2012), Relationship-Based Care (Foerster, 2011; Hozak & Brennan, 2012; Testa, 2017), Patient-Centered Care (Moran, 2012), and Partners in Care (Julian & Bott, 2012). Some researchers have used the CFS to test implementation of interventions to impact specific processes of caring, like creation of a caring/healing environment (Spies Ingersoll & Schaper, 2012). The CFS has also been used to study the profile of nurses effective in caring (Persky, Nelson, & Bent, 2008), how caring for the patient relates to job satisfaction (Berry et al., 2013), and how emotional intelligence of nurses relates to caring (Araque, 2015). The impact of architecture has also been studied as it relates to being able to care for the patient, as measured by the CFS (Hozak, Nelson, & Gregory, 2016). Meehan (2015) compared the CFS to four other measures of caring.

Internationally, the CFS has been translated into several languages or into dialects outside the United States. Published international studies include those in Italy (Masera, 2012), the Philippines (Reyes et al., 2012), Thailand (Piyasiripan, Isaraporn, Onnon, & Jinda, 2012), United Kingdom (Tinker, Sweetham, & Nelson, 2012), and China (Zhu, Lok, Cheong, Lao, & Cheong, 2012). There have also been studies to compare patients' report of caritas across countries: China, Italy, Philippines, and the United States (Nelson et al., 2012).

The CFS has also been used in specific contexts to test the processes of caring. Contexts include hospice (Sollami & Cutrera, 2012), long-term care (Phillips & Rieg, 2012), care of patients receiving electroconvulsive therapy (McDavitt & Glynn, 2012), patients with coronary heart disease (Piyasiripan et al., 2012), and labor and delivery (Rogers & Fahimi, 2010).

The CFS has been used to create six derivation works, including caring for self (Lawrence & Kear, 2012), caring for coworkers (Lawrence & Kear, 2012), caring of the manager (Olender & Phifer, 2012), and caring of the preceptor (Testerman, 2012). There is also a version to examine the care providers' perspectives of caring for patients (Johnson, 2012). The final derivation work is used to examine the caring behavior of the last care provider who cared for the patient (Legler, Sramek, Conklin, & Nelson, 2012). There are multiple studies that use these derivation works but are not included in this chapter. A search for the CFS or any derivation work in Google Scholar will provide many more resources for building an argument on the impact of the caritas processes being enacted on self and others.

REFERENCES

Andrews, L. W., Daniels, P., & Hall, A. G. (1996). Nurse caring behaviors: Comparing five tools to define perceptions. *Ostomy/Wound Management, 42*(5), 28–30.

Araque, J. B. (2015). *Nurse emotional intelligence and patients' perceptions of caring: A quantitative study.* Tempe, AZ: University of Phoenix.

Berry, D. M., Kaylor, M. B., Church, J., Campbell, K., McMillin, T., & Wamsley, R. (2013). Caritas and job environment: A replication of Persky et al. *Contemporary Nurse: A Journal for the Australian Nursing Profession, 43*(2), 237–243. doi:10.5172/conu.2013.43.2.237

Cronbach, L. J., & Meehl, P. E. (1955). Construct validity in psychological tests. *Psychological Bulletin, 52,* 281–302. doi:10.1037/h0040957

DiNapoli, P., Turkel, M., Nelson, J. W., & Watson, J. (2010). Measuring the caritas processes: Caring Factor Survey. *International Journal for Human Caring, 14*(3), 15–20. doi:10.20467/1091-5710.14.3.15

Duffy, J. R. (1990). An analysis of the relationships among nurse caring behaviors and selected outcomes of care in hospitalized medical and/or surgical patients. Unpublished doctoral dissertation, Catholic University of America, Washington, DC, p. 216.

Duffy, J. R. (2002). *Caring assessment tools. Assessing and measuring caring in nursing and health science.* New York, NY: Springer Publishing.

Foerster, B. J. (2011). Relationship-based care: Effects on patient satisfaction. *Electronic Theses and Dissertations.* Retrieved from https://openprairie.sdstate.edu/etd/934

Glasnapp, D. R., & Poggio, J. P. (1985). *Essentials of statistical analysis for the behavioral sciences.* Columbus, OH: Merrill Publishing.

Howell, D. C. (1997). *Statistical methods for psychology* (4th ed.). Belmont, MA: Duxbury.

Hozak, M. A., & Brennan, M. (2012). Caring at the core: Maximizing the likelihood that a caring moment will occur. In J. W. Nelson & J. Watson (Eds.), *Measuring caring: International research on Caritas as Healing* (pp. 195–223). New York, NY: Springer Publishing.

Hozak, M. A., Nelson, J., & Gregory, D. (2016). Relationship of hospital architecture to staff caring for self, caring for patients and job satisfaction. *Interdisciplinary Journal of Partnership Studies, 3*(1). doi:10.24926/ijps.v3i1.121

Johnson, J. (2012). Creation of the caring factor survey—Care provider version. In J. W. Nelson & J. Watson (Eds.), *Measuring caring: International research on Caritas as Healing* (pp. 40–42). New York, NY: Springer Publishing.

Julian, D., & Bott, M. J. (2012). "Partners in care": Patient and staff responses to a new model of care delivery. In J. W. Nelson & J. Watson (Eds.), *Measuring caring: A compilation of international research on Caritas as Healing* (pp. 225–247). New York, NY: Springer Publishing.

Lawrence, I., & Kear, M. (2012). The practice of loving kindness to self and others as perceived by nurses and patients in the Cardiac Interventional Unit. In J. W. Nelson & J. Watson (Eds.),

Measuring caring: International research on Caritas as Healing (pp. 36–39). New York, NY: Springer Publishing.

Legler, P., Sramek, D., Conklin, S., & Nelson, J. W. (2012). Patient and nurse perception of the individual caring relationship. In J. W. Nelson & J. Watson (Eds.), *Measuring caring: International research on Caritas as Healing* (pp. 43–46). New York, NY: Springer Publishing.

Masera, G. (2012). First measurement of Caritas in Italy. In J. W. Nelson & J. Watson (Eds.), *Measuring caring: International research on Caritas as Healing* (pp. 291–296). New York, NY: Springer Publishing.

McDavitt, C., & Glynn, P. (2012). Caring in the context of curing: What are patient's perceptions of nurse caring when receiving ECT in the PACU? In J. W. Nelson & J. Watson (Eds.), *Measuring Caring: International research on Caritas as Healing* (pp. 421–425). New York, NY: Springer.

Meehan, M. (2015). *Called to Caring: A Tool to Assess Awareness and Attitudes in Baccalaureate Nursing Students at Point Loma Nazerene University*. Lenexa, KS: Point Loma Nazarene University.

Moran, K. (2012). A patient-centered medical home (PCMH) care delivery innovation that improves outcomes. Retrieved from www.doctorsofnursingpractice.org website: http://www.doctorsofnursingpractice.org/wp-content/uploads/2014/01/A_PCMH_Care_Delivery_Innovation_That_Improves_Outcomes_8-8-12.pdf

Nelson, J. W., Persky, G., Sramek, D., Masera, G., Ga, M. M., Zhu, M. M. X., . . . Sollami, A. (2012). Comparison of Caritas in health care facilities in China, Italy, the Philippines, and the United States as perceived by patients. In J. W. Nelson & J. Watson (Eds.), *Measuring Caring: International research on Caritas as Healing* (pp. 337–356). New York, NY: Springer Publishing.

Olender, L., & Phifer, S. (2012). Development of the caring factor survey, caring of the manager. In J. W. Nelson & J. Watson (Eds.), *Measuring caring: International research on Caritas as Healing* (pp. 57–62). New York, NY: Springer Publishing.

Persky, G., Felgen, J., & Nelson, J. W. (2012). Measuring caring in primary nursing. In J. W. Nelson & J. Watson (Eds.), *Measuring caring: International research on Caritas as Healing* (pp. 65–86). New York, NY: Springer Publishing.

Persky, G., Nelson, J. W., Watson, J., & Bent, K. (2008). Creating a profile of a nurse effective in caring. *Nursing Administration Quarterly, 32*(1), 15–20. doi:10.1097/01.naq.0000305943.46440.77

Phillips, M. M., & Rieg, L. A. (2012). The presence of caring among long-term care nurses in the United States. In J. W. Nelson & J. Watson (Eds.), *Measuring caring: International research on Caritas as Healing* (pp. 389–396). New York, NY: Springer Publishing.

Picker/Commonwealth. (1993). *Through the patient's eyes*. San Francisco, CA: Jossey-Bass.

Piyasiripan, N., Isaraporn, O., Onnon, N., & Jinda, S. (2012). Caring behaviors of staff nurses as perceived by coronary heart disease patients in tertiary care hospital in the lower northern part of Thailand. *Cebu Normal Univeristy (CNU) Journal of Higher Education, 6*, 113–133.

Polit, D. F. (1996). *Data analysis and statistics for nursing research*. Stamford, CT: Appleton & Lange.

Polit, D. F., & Hungler, B. P. (1996). *Essentials of nursing research* (6th ed.). Philadelphia, PA: Lippincott.

Polit, D. F., & Hungler, B. P. (1999). *Nursing research*. Philadelphia, PA: Lippincott.

Reyes, P. C. V., Avecilla, D. M. S., Cruz, M. S. S., Ramos, F. R. S., Rubis, E. O., Villamero, J. C. G., & Ga, M. M. (2012). Utilization of the clinical Caritas process in a selected tertiary hospital in the Philippines. In J. W. Nelson & J. Watson (Eds.), *Measuring Caring: International research on Caritas as Healing* (pp. 297–302). New York, NY: Springer Publishing.

Rogers, S. M., & Fahimi, B. (2010). Impact of intentional caring behaviors on a labor and delivery unit. *Journal of Obstetric, Gynecologic, and Neonatal Nursing, 39*(s1), S115. doi:10.1111/j. 1552-6909.2010.01129.x

Sollami, A., & Cutrera, C. (2012). The holistic perspective of nursing, The Caring Factor Survey in a hospital in Italy. In J. W. Nelson & J. Watson (Eds.), *Measuring caring: International research on Caritas as Healing* (pp. 373–378). New York, NY: Springer Publishing.

Spies Ingersoll, S., & Schaper, A. M. (2012). Therapeutic music pilot in the context of Human Caring theory. In J. W. Nelson & J. Watson (Eds.), *Measuring Caring: International research on Caritas as Healing* (pp. 257–268). New York, NY: Springer Publishing.

Sramek, D., & Legler, P. (2007). *Measuring the impact of an intervention to refine caring.* Casper: Wyoming Medical Center.

Testa, D. (2017). Development and psychometric evaluation of the nurse's perception of the relationship-based care environment scale. *International Journal for Human Caring, 21*(4), 193–199.

Testerman, R. (2012). Preceptor caring attributes as perceived by graduate nurses. In J. W. Nelson & J. Watson (Eds.), *Measuring caring: International research on Caritas as Healing* (pp. 47–52). New York, NY: Springer Publishing.

Tinker, A., Sweetham, J., & Nelson, J. (2012). Reflection as a process to understand caring behaviors during implementation of Relationship-Based Care in a community health service in England. In J. W. Nelson & J. Watson (Eds.), *Measuring caring: International research on Caritas as Healing* (pp. 303–318). New York, NY: Springer Publishing.

Turner, J., & Toomer, L. (2012). The caring moment and Participative Action Reearch (PAR) in outcomes management. In J. W. Nelson & J. Watson (Eds.), *Measuring caring: International research on Caritas as Healing.* New York, NY: Springer Publishing.

Watson, J. (2002). *Assessing and measuring caring in nursing and health science.* New York, NY: Springer Publishing.

Watson, J. (2005). *Caring science as sacred science.* Philadelphia, PA: F. A. Davis.

Zhu, M. M. X., Lok, G. K. I., Cheong, S. W., Lao, S. S. W., & Cheong, J. P. L. (2012). A Chinese cultural perspective of nursing care in Macau, China. In J. W. Nelson & J. Watson (Eds.), *Measuring Caring: International research on Caritas as Healing* (pp. 319–334). New York, NY: Springer

Student Perspectives
of Caring Online

Kathleen L. Sitzman

The Student Perspectives of Caring Online tool was developed by Dr. Kathleen Sitzman, based upon her early interest in how nursing faculty may convey and model caring in online education. This focus deepened during her doctoral studies at the University of Northern Colorado.

This Caring Online tool was first published and is based on two pilot studies that explored student perceptions related to caring behaviors demonstrated by nursing instructors in online classroom settings (Leners & Sitzman, 2006; Sitzman & Leners, 2006). A 25-item Likert-type survey for a larger study was created based on the findings of the two pilot studies. In the larger study, emailed messages requesting participation were sent to 750 undergraduate registered nurse (RN) students in five different institutions of higher education, and 122 students completed the survey (Sitzman, 2010). After the larger study was completed, internal consistency (the degree to which items within one tool all measure the same attribute—which in this case was caring online) was assessed using Cronbach's alpha. This analysis was performed in the Statistical Package for the Social Sciences (SPSS) Base 10, with the result being alpha = .8313. An alpha equal to or greater than .70 indicates adequate internal consistency. Construct and content validity were achieved during the pilot study process and subsequent development of the main survey items.

One open-ended question at the end of the survey asked the following: "In addition to the behaviors listed above, are there any other things an instructor might do in an online teaching situation that would convey caring to you?" (Sitzman, 2010, p. 174). Of the 122 respondents, 85 answered the open-ended question at the end of the survey (Sitzman, 2010). Responses to the open-ended question demonstrated consensus that the survey items adequately assessed caring in online classroom settings and also provided additional empirical validation and depth to the tool.

Since the tool was first published, the author has received many requests to use the scale from nurses completing dissertation work, to nursing instructors interested in learning more about what they can do to convey and sustain caring in their own nursing classrooms. For example, Mann (2014) published a research study that utilized this tool with 48 RN–bachelor of science in nursing (BSN) students at a historically Black university. Results validated findings in the Sitzman (2010) study.

Online education technology and practices are continually evolving. This tool can and should be adapted to reflect ongoing changes related to online education. The author requests that she be contacted for permission, support, and advice regarding use of the tool (Tool 24.1).

TOOL 24.1

Student Perspectives of Caring Online

Please place a check mark in the box on the right that best describes the level of importance of each instructor behavior listed on the left.

NI = Not important, SI = Somewhat important, MI = Moderately important, EI = Extremely important.

INSTRUCTOR BEHAVIOR	NI	SI	MI	EI
Responds to postings and emails within 24–48 hours.	☐	☐	☐	☐
Responds to postings and emails on weekends.	☐	☐	☐	☐
Mindfully addresses student challenges as soon as they become evident, for example, if a student has not been online for a week, calls to find out why and offers support to help the student get back on track.	☐	☐	☐	☐
Recounts challenges experienced in the online classroom setting and shares remedies that have worked for self and other students.	☐	☐	☐	☐
Expresses the belief that students will be successful in the online setting.	☐	☐	☐	☐
Writes out and posts clear instructions regarding schedules and due dates.	☐	☐	☐	☐
Provides students with a detailed class calendar that includes all due dates for postings, papers, and projects.	☐	☐	☐	☐
Writes out and posts clear instructions regarding acceptable social behavior in the online classroom.	☐	☐	☐	☐
Writes out and posts clear instructions regarding acceptable length/quality of required online communications (postings, papers, projects, emails, etc.)	☐	☐	☐	☐
Provides students with the opportunity for face-to-face meetings at the beginning of the semester if possible.	☐	☐	☐	☐
If face-to-face meetings are not possible, arranges for a web camera exchange between individual students and instructor so that each student has a chance to "see" and interact with the instructor in real time.	☐	☐	☐	☐
Provides scheduled telephone availability so that students know when the instructor will be available to speak to them.	☐	☐	☐	☐
Provides an email address outside the course homepage.	☐	☐	☐	☐
Provides students with a discussion board thread dedicated to student questions and concerns only.	☐	☐	☐	☐

(continued)

TOOL 24.1

Student Perspectives of Caring Online (*continued*)

INSTRUCTOR BEHAVIOR	NI	SI	MI	EI
Provides virtual office hours with scheduled chats.	☐	☐	☐	☐
Posts a casual (conversational) personal introduction via the online posting forum in the first week or two of class.	☐	☐	☐	☐
Shares informal glimpses of self by posting fun/personal photographs.	☐	☐	☐	☐
Discusses hobbies or extracurricular interests.	☐	☐	☐	☐
Discusses past scholarly work and professional experiences.	☐	☐	☐	☐
Provides (at a minimum) weekly praise and encouragement to individuals and/or groups for work that is well done.	☐	☐	☐	☐
Provides supportive/corrective guidance to individual students via personal email or telephone rather than in any public venue, that is, chat or postings.	☐	☐	☐	☐
When responding to student work, refers to specifics so that students know their work has been thoroughly read.	☐	☐	☐	☐
Verbalizes enthusiasm for learning.	☐	☐	☐	☐
Demonstrates respect for the learning process by exhibiting excellence in creating/presenting online content.	☐	☐	☐	☐

In the space provided, please respond to the following question:

In addition to the behaviors listed above, are there any other things an instructor might do in an online teaching situation that would convey caring to you?

A subset of respondents will be asked to participate in an email interview. If you are willing to participate in the email interview portion of this study, will you please provide your contact information in the following space, including your name and email address?

TABLE 24.1 Matrix of Student Perspectives of Caring Online

INSTRUMENT	AUTHOR CONTACT INFORMATION	PUBLICATION SOURCE	DEVELOPED TO MEASURE	INSTRUMENT DESCRIPTION	PARTICIPANTS	REPORTED VALIDITY/ RELIABILITY	CONCEPTUAL– THEORETICAL BASIS OF MEASUREMENT	LATEST CITATION IN NURSING LITERATURE
Student Perspectives of Caring Online	Kathleen Sitzman, PhD, RN, PhD, CNE, ANEF, FAAN Phone: (801) 791-1177 Email: sitzmank@ ecu.edu; Kathy. sitzman@ gmail.com	Sitzman (2007)	Nursing students' perspectives of caring online behaviors demonstrated by nursing instructors	24 items on a 4-point Likert-type scale and one open-ended question	122 undergraduate nursing students from five different institutions of higher education from an emailed request sent to 750 prospective respondents	Cronbach's alpha reported at .8313. Two pilot studies completed to inform the construction and content of the final tool	Watson's Human Caring Theory	Mann (2014) Sitzman (2010)

REFERENCES

Leners, D., & Sitzman, K. (2006). Graduate student perceptions: Feeling the passion of caring online. *Nursing Education Perspectives, 27*(6), 315–319.

Mann, J. C. (2014). A pilot study of RN-BSN completion students' preferred instructor online classroom caring behaviors. *Association of Black Nursing Faculty (ABNF) Journal, 25*(2), 33–39.

Sitzman, K. (2007). *Bachelor of science in nursing student perceptions of caring online* (Doctor of Philosophy Dissertation). University of Northern Colorado, College of Natural and Health Sciences, School of Nursing, Nursing Education, Greeley, CO.

Sitzman, K. (2010). Student-preferred caring behaviors for online nursing education. *Nursing Education Perspectives, 31*(3), 171–178.

Sitzman, K., & Leners, D. (2006). Student perceptions of caring in online baccalaureate education. *Nursing Education Perspectives, 27*(5), 254–259.

The Nurse's Perception of the Relationship-Based Care Environment Scale

Denise Testa

The theoretical basis of the Nurse's Perception of the Relationship-Based Care Environment (NPRBCE) scale incorporates nursing theories of caring and literature on relationship-based (centered) care. A literature review about caring and relationships in healthcare was undertaken and clearly demonstrated that nurse–patient, nurse–nurse, and nurse–colleague relationships are considered critically important for the well-being of both patients and providers (Dossey & Keegan, 2013; Jones, 2013; Koloroutis, 2004; Swanson, 1991; Tresolini & Pew-Fetzer Task Force, 1994; Watson, 1989, 2008). Additionally, extant literature supports the idea that the environment in which care occurs must support caring relationships if high-quality patient-centered care is to be delivered (Koloroutis, 2004; Testa & Emery, 2014; Tresolini & Pew-Fetzer Task Force, 1994, Watson, 2008). A theoretical representation (Figure 25.1), based on literature review and a prior qualitative study (Testa & Emery, 2014), was created to delineate the critical relationships between nurses and others in the healthcare setting (Testa, 2017). The four dimensions of this representation, nurse to patient; nurse to other disciplines; nurse to organization; and nurse to nurse including the self, were the basis of item development for the NPRBCE scale.

CONCEPTUAL BASIS OF THE NPRBCE SCALE

The dimensions of the theoretical representation (Figure 25.1) differ from and expand on previous descriptions of relationship-based care (RBC) in two ways. Firstly, the provider is specifically defined as the nurse, and secondly the element "nurse to organization" has been included as part of the RBC environment.

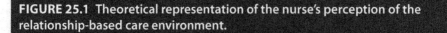

FIGURE 25.1 Theoretical representation of the nurse's perception of the relationship-based care environment.

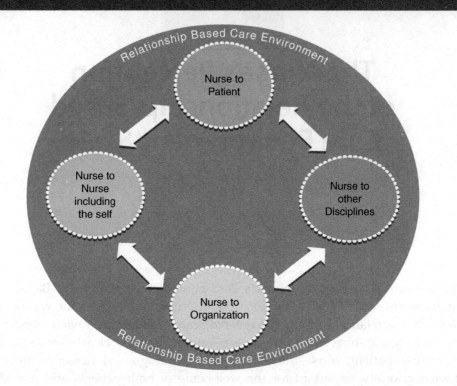

Operational definitions of the four dimensions are as follows: Nurse to patient is the relationship wherein nurses come to know the patient as a whole person through active listening, caring, and intentional presence.

"Nurse to nurse" is the ability of nurses to care for, understand, and respect other nurses and the self. "Nurse to other disciplines" is collaborative decision making with mutual respect for the knowledge, expertise, and values of other disciplines. "Nurse to organization" is the nurse's ability to participate in an environment that allows nurses to lead policy and practice initiatives, attain adequate resources for patient care, and be respected by the organization as leaders in care.

ITEM DEVELOPMENT AND CONTENT VALIDITY

Items were developed for each of the four dimensions (nurse to patient; nurse to other disciplines; nurse to organization; and nurse to nurse including the self), and content validity was determined by an expert panel of registered nurses (RNs). Seven nurse experts were asked to determine how well the specific items represented the universe of possible items in each of the four dimensions. Each panel member individually scored every item for relevance, readability, and understandability. At the end of the scoring, panel members were asked if there were any other important aspects of the dimension that should be included. In this way, the panel determined the content validity of the items. After minor rewording there was 100% consensus by the expert nurse panel that all items were relevant and fully measured the dimension; therefore the Content Validity Index was 1.0.

TESTING AND RELIABILITY

The NPRBCE scale was tested on a sample of all direct care nurses at two hospitals in the Northeast between January 1 and March 29 of 2016. Surveys were administered via email and 476 nurses responded to the survey. Four hundred and seventy-three surveys had no missing data and these complete surveys were included in data analysis. In order to determine the extent to which the dimensions of the NPRBCE scale could be demonstrated, Principal Component Analysis with varimax rotation was undertaken. The scree test graphing the eigenvalues indicated a five-, six-, or seven-component solution. Each of these was examined and the five-component solution made the best conceptual sense; therefore, a second Principal Component Analysis specifying five components was performed. Fourteen items were eliminated because they had factor loading cut-offs below .5, low total-item correlations, and did not affect the conceptual integrity of the scale. As a result of the data analysis, the scale was refined to 56 items. The five components were given labels to best reflect that component. Those five labels are as follows: nurse to other disciplines; nurse to organization; nurse to nurse; nurse to patient: respect for the patient; nurse to patient: knowing the patient. Cronbach's alpha was computed at .96 for the scale as a whole with a range of .86 to .93 for the five scale components. Table 25.1 summarizes these findings. Component one (nurse to other disciplines) contained 15 items and explained 12% of variance; component two (nurse to organization) comprised 13 items and explained an additional 11.4% of variance; component three (nurse to nurse including the self) was defined by 10 items and explained an additional 8.9% of variance; component four (nurse to patient, knowing the patient) comprised 10 items and explained an additional 8.3% of variance; component five (nurse to patient, respect for the patient) comprised eight items and explained an additional 8.2% of variance.

DISCUSSION AND IMPLICATIONS

The psychometric evaluation of the NPRBCE scale supports the theoretical representation (Figure 25.1). Interestingly, the component "nurse to patient" was split into two parts, "nurse to patient: knowing the patient" and "nurse to patient: respect for the patient." Although initially surprising that the component was split, upon further consideration it has been recognized that both knowing and

TABLE 25.1 Matrix of Nurse's Perception of Relationship-Based Care Environment Scale

INSTRUMENT	AUTHOR CONTACT INFORMATION	PUBLICATION SOURCE	DEVELOPED TO MEASURE	INSTRUMENT DESCRIPTION	PARTICIPANTS	REPORTED VALIDITY/ RELIABILITY	CONCEPTUAL– THEORETICAL BASES OF MEASUREMENT	LATEST CITATION IN NURSING LITERATURE
Nurse's perception of the relationship-based care environment	Denise Testa, PhD, CRNA William F. Connell School of Nursing Boston College 140 Commonwealth Ave. Chestnut Hill, MA 02477 Email: denise .testa@bc.edu	Testa (2017)	Relationships between nurses and others in healthcare setting	56-item, 6-point Likert scale (1 = strongly disagree to 6 = strongly agree) Five subscales: nurse to other disciplines; nurse to organization; nurse to nurse including the self; nurse to patient, knowing the patient; nurse to patient: respect for the patient	473 complete surveys from direct care registered nurses	Expert panel Reviewed items and content validity index = 1. Principal component analysis determined that five factors explained 48.8% of the variance Cronbach's alpha for total scale = .96 Cronbach's alpha for five individual subscales ranged from .88 to .93	Nurse caring theories and relationship-based care literature	Testa (2017)

respecting the patient are essential parts of the nurse–patient relationship. Nurses gain insight into their patients' wellness/illness experiences through relationships wherein the patient is both known and respected (Jones, 2013; Watson, 1979, 1989, 2008). The NPRBCE scale provides a method to evaluate a broadened conceptualization of nurses' relationships with others in the complex healthcare environment. The NPRBCE instrument (Tool 25.1) is a newly developed tool and further testing is needed to establish reliability and validity in varied healthcare settings. Future research efforts may utilize data resultant from this scale to evaluate interventions and application of nursing models that seek to improve caring relationships in healthcare settings.

TOOL 25.1

Nurse's Perception of the Relationship Based Environment scale

Section 1

Please read each statement and indicate the degree to which you agree or disagree with that statement.

SD=Strongly Disagree, D=Disagree, sD=Somewhat Disagree, sA= Somewhat Agree, A=Agree, SA=Strongly Agree

		SD	D	sD	sA	A	SA
On my unit:		SD	D	sD	sA	A	SA
1.	I respect my patients' goals.	SD	D	sD	sA	A	SA
2.	I show authentic interest in the lives of my patients.	SD	D	sD	sA	A	SA
3.	I show interest in my patients' perceptions of their illnesses.	SD	D	sD	sA	A	SA
4.	I accept my patients' beliefs and values without judgment.	SD	D	sD	sA	A	SA
5.	My intentional presence with my patients brings them comfort.	SD	D	sD	sA	A	SA
6.	I validate the unique experiences of my patients.	SD	D	sD	sA	A	SA
7.	I actively listen to the words of my patients.	SD	D	sD	sA	A	SA
8.	My interactions with my patients are genuine.	SD	D	sD	sA	A	SA
9.	I partner with my patients to identify problems that compromise their health.	SD	D	sD	sA	A	SA
10.	My plan of care is guided by the patients' preferences.	SD	D	sD	sA	A	SA
11.	I focus on knowing what is important to my patients.	SD	D	sD	sA	A	SA
12.	I take the time to listen attentively to my patients.	SD	D	sD	sA	A	SA
13.	I have enough time to come to know my patients.	SD	D	sD	sA	A	SA
14.	I come to know my patients as unique individuals.	SD	D	sD	sA	A	SA
15.	I am aware of my patients' spiritual beliefs.	SD	D	sD	sA	A	SA

(continued)

TOOL 25.1

Nurse's Perception of the Relationship Based Environment scale (*continued*)

		SD	D	sD	sA	A	SA
16.	I engage in uncovering the meaning of illness for my patients.	SD	D	sD	sA	A	SA
17.	I adapt the environment of care to best fit with the pattern of my patients' lives.	SD	D	sD	sA	A	SA
18.	I am fully attentive to the meaning of health for my patients.	SD	D	sD	sA	A	SA
19.	I have a trusting relationship with members of other disciplines.	SD	D	sD	sA	A	SA
20.	Nurses collaborate with other disciplines to make decisions about patient care.	SD	D	sD	sA	A	SA
21.	Nurses share important information about patients with other disciplines.	SD	D	sD	sA	A	SA
22.	Other disciplines share important information about patients with nurses.	SD	D	sD	sA	A	SA
23.	Nurses and other disciplines have shared goals.	SD	D	sD	sA	A	SA
24.	If conflict arises between nurses and other disciplines, it is managed well.	SD	D	sD	sA	A	SA
25.	Nurses work with other disciplines to discuss patient care concerns.	SD	D	sD	sA	A	SA
26.	Nurses and members of other disciplines exchange ideas to determine the future direction of patient care.	SD	D	sD	sA	A	SA
27.	Nurses respect the perspective of other disciplines.	SD	D	sD	sA	A	SA
28.	Members of other disciplines respect the perspective of nurses.	SD	D	sD	sA	A	SA
29.	During interdisciplinary rounds nurses participate in discussion about the patients' plan of care.	SD	D	sD	sA	A	SA
30.	Nurses and members of other disciplines support each other.	SD	D	sD	sA	A	SA
31.	Nurses and members of other disciplines help each other whenever possible.	SD	D	sD	sA	A	SA
32.	Nurses respect the knowledge of other disciplines.	SD	D	sD	sA	A	SA
33.	Other disciplines respect the knowledge of nurses.	SD	D	sD	sA	A	SA
34.	I have a trusting relationship with other nurses.	SD	D	sD	sA	A	SA
35.	Nurses trust one another.	SD	D	sD	sA	A	SA
36.	Nurses share the goal of providing holistic care for their patients.	SD	D	sD	sA	A	SA
37.	Nurses respect one another regardless of differences in age.	SD	D	sD	sA	A	SA
38.	Nurses respect one another regardless of differences in educational level.	SD	D	sD	sA	A	SA

(*continued*)

TOOL 25.1

Nurse's Perception of the Relationship Based Environment scale (*continued*)

	SD	D	sD	sA	A	SA
39. Nurses manage conflict effectively.	SD	D	sD	sA	A	SA
40. Nurses think that their relationships with other nurses are important.	SD	D	sD	sA	A	SA
41. Nurses work together to provide holistic care for patients.	SD	D	sD	sA	A	SA
42. Nurses communicate effectively with one another.	SD	D	sD	sA	A	SA
43. Nurses openly share ideas regarding patient care with other nurses.	SD	D	sD	sA	A	SA

Section 2

In this section the response format is the same but the items are preceded by the phrase "In this organization."

SD=Strongly Disagree, D=Disagree, sD=Somewhat Disagree, sA= Somewhat Agree, A=Agree, SA=Strongly Agree

	SD	D	sD	sA	A	SA
In this organization:	SD	D	sD	sA	A	SA
44. Nursing knowledge is valued by leadership.	SD	D	sD	sA	A	SA
45. Nurses have time to know their patients as persons.	SD	D	sD	sA	A	SA
46. Relationships between nurses and patients are fostered.	SD	D	sD	sA	A	SA
47. Relationships between nurses and other disciplines are promoted.	SD	D	sD	sA	A	SA
48. Relationships between and among disciplines are a priority.	SD	D	sD	sA	A	SA
49. Nurses participate in decisions about allocation of resources.	SD	D	sD	sA	A	SA
50. The time I spend with my patients is valued by the leadership.	SD	D	sD	sA	A	SA
51. An environment has been created that supports the professional judgment of nurses.	SD	D	sD	sA	A	SA
52. There is enough time to discuss patient care issues with my colleagues.	SD	D	sD	sA	A	SA
53. The environment supports continuity in patient care.	SD	D	sD	sA	A	SA
54. The perspective of bedside nurses is respected.	SD	D	sD	sA	A	SA
55. I am able to advocate for my patients.	SD	D	sD	sA	A	SA
56. I am able to access the resources that my patients need.	SD	D	sD	sA	A	SA

REFERENCES

Dossey, B. M., & Keegan, L. (2013). *Holistic nursing*. Burlington, MA: Jones & Bartlett.

Jones, D. A. (2013). Nurse-patient relationship: Knowledge transforming practice at the bedside. In J. I. Erickson, D. A. Jones, & M. Ditomassi (Eds.), *Fostering nurse led care* (pp. 85–117). Indianapolis, IN: Sigma Theta Tau International.

Koloroutis, M. E. (2004). *Relationship-based care: A model for transforming practice*. Minneapolis, MN: Creative Health Care Management.

Swanson, K. M. (1991). Empirical development of a middle range theory of caring. *Nursing Research, 40*(3), 161–166. doi:10.1097/00006199-199105000-00008

Testa, D. (2017). Development and psychometric evaluation of the nurse's perception of the relationship-based care environment scale. *International Journal for Human Caring, 21*(4), 193–199. doi:10.20467/1091-5710.21.4.193

Testa, D., & Emery, S. (2014). Understanding the perceptions and experiences of Certified Registered Nurse Anaesthetists regarding handovers: A focus group study. *Nursing Open, 1*(1), 32–41. doi:10.1002/nop2.9

Tresolini, C., & Pew-Fetzer Task Force. (1994). *Health professions education and relationship centered care*. San Francisco, CA: Pew Health Professions Commission.

Watson, J. (1979). *Nursing: The philosophy and science of caring*. Boston, MA: Little Brown.

Watson, J. (1989). Watson's philosophy and theory of human caring in nursing. In J. Riehl-Sisca (Ed.), *Conceptual models for nursing practice* (3rd ed., pp. 207–219). Norwalk, CT: Appleton & Lange.

Watson, J. (Ed.). (2008). *Assessing and measuring caring in nursing and health science* (2nd ed.). New York, NY: Springer Publishing.

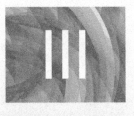

Challenges, Opportunities, and Future Directions

The Evolution of Measuring Caring: Moving Toward Construct Validity

Carolie Coates

For the first edition of *Assessing and Measuring Caring in Nursing and Health Sciences*, I prepared a summary chapter on the state of construct validity in the progress toward quantitative assessment of caring in nursing. At that point there were 21 different caring measures, some of which had multiple forms. The metaphor I used at the time of the first edition was that of a patchwork quilt; each author prepared his or her unique block of the quilt in relative isolation. Today, the second edition includes updated information on the original 21 measures and 6 additional ones for a grand total of 27. The metaphor that springs to mind now is that of an extensive colorful tile mosaic. The quality of the work is definitely more solid and substantial than that reported in 2002. Some portions of the mosaic are very complex and differentiated, representing sophisticated measurement development. Other parts of the mosaic display rudimentary and uneven patterns, and there are gaps in the representations—this represents less developed caring measurement endeavors. Some of the patterns were created by experienced teams of researchers, and others by individuals. Some patterns incorporate new pieces of tile (i.e., new research studies). Some parts of the mosaic remain untouched after several years. However, there are linkages among the various mosaic patterns.

The purpose of the validity summary in the first edition was to provide a vehicle for organization, description, and analysis of the measures. The purpose of this chapter is to provide a point of view about construct validity and caring measurement research.

Today the authors of the measurements are linked by a common book and by the Internet, but they still experience severe problems of limited funding and limited opportunities to perform large-scale psychometric studies with the rigor expected from the scientific community. As we embrace a fairly accepted view today that validity and reliability issues should be viewed as a continuum, we must ask, Where are we on this continuum? Goodwin's (1997) comments that validity is a unitary concept, although various types of evidence referred to in the literature as content, criterion-related, and construct validity need to be sought by measurement developers, are still pertinent. Reliability of an instrument is viewed as a part of an instrument's construct validity. The challenge remains for each instrument developer to build a case or complex web of evidence (based on his or her own research or the research of others) from a variety of approaches, using different samples of respondents, contexts, and research questions. This process will provide evidence for the construct validity of each instrument. The use of multiple studies with appropriate measures of instrument validity and a wealth of evidence as to content, criterion, and construct validity is evidence of a greater degree of construct validity. While each measure may be at a different point on a conceptualized construct validity continuum, at least the goal is more clearly in sight than it was in 2002.

In the first edition, I attempted to impose order and organization by using a 5-point rating scale to rate the degree to which a given instrument demonstrated, in its development or refinement, a series of characteristics that have been associated in psychometric literature with higher degrees of construct validity. The following guidelines are psychometric methods and processes associated with instrument construct validity:

1. Theoretical linkage to a well-articulated theory—the degree to which the instrument is anchored in a theoretical framework. In the majority of instruments, that theory has been Watson's theory of caring.

2. Content validity—the degree to which the instrument underwent content validity verification during the development phase. Content experts or other informed sources are often used to operationalize this process. Note that content validity assessment can verify the proposed conceptual domain of the instrument. In some cases, the process of content validity verification can refine the definition and scope of the instrument.

3. Pilot testing—the degree to which the instrument was developed from an extensive pool of well-crafted items related to the concept being measured.

4. Sample size and quality—the degree to which large appropriate samples were utilized to develop or refine the instrument.

5. Reliability assessment—the degree of instrument stability or internal consistency. Most often scale reliability is operationalized as assessment of a scale's internal consistency (Cronbach's alpha). Measurement experts often hold .80 as the minimal level for acceptable internal consistency. It should also be noted that the alpha should be calculated for each study and sample, as it can vary with each usage. Researchers often talk as if a pattern of good alpha results (.80 or higher) in a series of studies indicates

that an instrument possesses a high degree of reliability. With refinement, a process of removing items that do not contribute to internal consistency, reported alphas may increase over time from less acceptable levels (e.g., .60) to more acceptable ranges in the .80s or .90s. Split-half and test–retest methods to assess scale reliability are employed less frequently in instrument development.

6. Factor analysis—the degree to which an instrument is measuring what it purports to measure (i.e., that it has construct validity). Analysis of the resultant factors, the percentage of variance accounted for by the factors, the pattern of items loading on each factor, and the relationships among the factors can inform instrument development and refinement decisions. Theory and conceptual frameworks provide the structure against which the resultant factor structure can be compared. The more the factors make conceptual sense and are related to theory, the more confident one can be that the instrument has construct validity.

7. Known group validity—the ability of a scale to demonstrate sufficient statistical significance between at least two groups of subjects known to be either high or low on the assessed concept. This method has been used fairly rarely so far in the caring measurement literature, as many of the studies are single-sample studies. In theory it could be used in caring research by a priori identification of caring nurses or care units.

8. Convergent or concurrent validity—the testing of the relationships (typically correlational in nature) between the target instrument and other reliable and valid instruments. Predictions as to the nature of the relationship between the target measure and the validating measure come from theory or previous research. A related concept is criterion-related validity, which measures whether the validity of the target measure is assessed in relationship to accepted criterion measures. As the complexity of descriptive quantitative research studies increases in the field of caring measurement, instances of concurrent validity increase. ("Gold standard" construct validity demonstration would employ convergent/divergent validity analysis and would assess the discriminant validity power of the target instrument in large and complex studies. This level of sophistication remains fairly rare in psychometric literature.)

9. Predictive validity—the degree to which an instrument demonstrates that it is an effective predictor of performance on another measure at some future date. The prediction is rooted in theory or previous research. This type of measurement sophistication is fairly rare in the caring measurement literature.

This list should not be viewed as a checklist, but as a guide for assessing indicants of the degree of construct validity of an instrument. Given the complexity of the studies presented in this volume, I believe a simplistic rating system would not do justice in analyzing either the summative or the dynamic nature of the degree of construct validity possessed by any given measure. However, it is clear that since almost all the scales utilize a Likert scale format, they must be held to rigorous quantitative criteria for construct validity.

As we consider the elusive, desired goal of construct validity for each instrument, it is a given that it is a relative, nonstatic concept. Most of the instruments have reported acceptable levels of reliability. For potential users of instruments, the most important issues regarding the degree of construct validity are the definition of the conceptual domain of the instrument, the degree to which it is grounded in theory, and whether or not there exists a portfolio of research evidence that would suggest to a fair-minded judge that the instrument measures what it purports to measure.

Another lens for assessing the quality or sophistication of measurement research studies is complexity of research design. It is very clear that the majority of studies involving the development or refinement of caring measures are descriptive and correlational in nature. The fact that a number of the measures correlate in predictable ways with other measures in the nursing arena is very encouraging. However, the lack of replication remains troubling.

Very few researchers have been able to move toward more sophisticated research designs to assess pre–post change or to predict a pattern of change. Almost no studies utilizing an experimental or quasi-experimental design are in evidence. Thus, there is little evidence as to how sensitive most of the instruments may be to change. Most of the time the caring measures are treated as descriptive variables at a single point in time, not as mediating or outcome variables.

Recall that the goal of moving toward construct validity for a given measure is to assemble a case based on a wealth of quality research studies. One of our research design goals is to triangulate sources by replicating the studies with a diversity of appropriate samples. Research designs that are eventually able to triangulate sources and methods are still on the horizon. When our measures are methodologically defensible, then hopefully some large-scale multivariable and multi-institutional studies will be initiated. So far, funding support for methodological work in caring assessment appears to be very limited. Despite the limitations, the task of a test author is to continue to build the case for construct validity through complex and reliable patterns of measurement evidence (either from one's own initiative or from the work of other researchers).

As a measurement developer, I have given the issue of construct validity much consideration. My advice is that since we are competing in a methodology that is very dependent on quality psychometrics, we have no choice but to increase the quality of our studies and our analyses. This point is made with the conviction that no measurement research is worthy of the exhaustive work it takes to work toward construct validity unless the foundational theoretical and conceptual work is first rate.

RECOMMENDATION 1

My quest brought me to a recent article by a group of researchers facing a somewhat similar dilemma. Frost, Reeve, Liepa, Stauffer, and Hays (2007) recently offered some conclusions with regard to the work on reliability and validity of patient-reported outcome measures. They have suggested that some guidelines be set for sufficient evidence of reliability and validity before any clinical trial studies in the area of patient-reported outcome measures are conducted. My major recommendation is that caring instrument developers begin to adopt these guidelines as well. Some examples would be the adoption of a minimum reliability threshold of .70 and a minimum sample size for testing of 200 cases. Results should be replicated in at least one additional sample. At least one full report on the development and one on the use of the instrument would be necessary to evaluate the psychometric properties. A number of the caring instruments have met these criteria, and they could be goals for refinement of other instruments. My recommendation is that caring researchers make a concerted effort to improve the quality of published research studies on caring measures. Some of the instruments in this volume have already achieved an impressive track record and are moving toward a fairly sophisticated level of construct validity, while others are taking the first step on a path to instrument development and refinement.

RECOMMENDATION 2

My second major recommendation is to continue to pursue the merits of blending quantitative measurement of caring with qualitative methodologies such as the use of focus groups, semi-structured interviews, observations, and stories from relevant sources such as nursing students, nursing staff, and patients. (A few small studies with this blended design format are in evidence in the study of caring efficacy in Chapter 14.) In my view, the understanding and measurement of caring can only be enhanced by the use of blended quantitative and qualitative research methodologies.

SUGGESTIONS FOR USERS OF THIS EDITION

My suggestions for using this volume, based on my experiences with nursing students in using the first edition, would be to first be very clear about what aspect of caring you wish to assess. For example, caring behaviors are not the same as caring efficacy. Carefully review the definitions and theoretical grounding of the potential choices. Read the items to make your own assessment as to the degree of content validity and the usability/suitability of the instrument for your particular research questions and samples. Then go to the articulated case for construct validity made by the instrument developer. Utilize your research sophistication to make your choices. While we have high goals for the future in our progress toward construct validity, current developers will attest to how difficult it has been to accomplish what we have. For most of us, the work gets conducted with limited resources and reliance on convenience samples. Given all of that, it is absolutely amazing that so many experienced and novice researchers have accomplished so much in the past 10 to 15 years. Perhaps this second edition will stimulate even more research collaboration. And yes, there is always the possibility of yet another caring measure—just keep your conceptual work paramount!

REFERENCES

Frost, M. H., Reeve, B. B., Liepa, A. M., Stauffer, J. W., & Hays, R. D. (2007). What is sufficient evidence for the reliability and validity of patient-reported outcome measures? *Value in Health, 10* (Suppl. 2), S94–S105. doi:10.1111/j.1524-4733.2007.00272.x

Goodwin, L. D. (1997). Changing concepts of measure validity. *Journal of Nursing Education, 36*(3), 102–107.

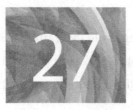

Postscript: Thoughts on Caring Theories and Instruments for Measuring Caring

Jean Watson

As we review the development and evolution of the caring instruments, it helps to summarize the relationships between extant caring theories and specific instruments as they have evolved to date and continue to evolve. As noted in the discussions and the matrix cells, some instruments are guided formally by an identified theory, some by multiple theories. Others are more empirically derived, while still others are reported to be atheoretical in origin. This chapter offers a general overview of the theoretical connections and origins of the diverse instruments and seeks a more coherent view of the relationship between extant theories of caring and specific instruments. This focus contributes to both the disciplinary and professional foundation of nursing as a developing and growing science with caring as a core concept that transcends and unifies all aspects of healthcare. Please note that the categorizations for how to locate and identify the specific instruments and related theories are nonexclusive and overlapping.

A number of the instruments refer to the general caring theory literature and the conceptual aspects of caring without use of any specific theory as a basis for formal instrumentation. I refer to these instruments using multiple concepts from extant caring theories as broad guiding frameworks, as well as empirical strategies for item development. These are:

- CARE-Q, CARE/SAT, and Modified CARE-Q (Larson, 1984; Larson & Ferketich, 1993; Lee et al., 2006)
- Professional Caring Behaviors (developed by Horner and published by Harrison [1995])

- Client Perception of Caring Scale (McDaniel, 1990)
- Caring Dimensions Inventory (Watson & Lea, 1997)
- Caring Attributes, Professional Self-Concept, and Technological Influences Scale (Arthur et al., 1999)
- Methodist Health Care System Nurse Caring Instrument (Shepherd, Rude, & Sherwood, 2000)

Some instruments were developed through the formal identification and derivation of items from a specific caring theory or other relevant theories. These theories and the instruments are:

- Bandura's social learning theory from social psychology: Caring Efficacy Scale (Coates, 1996)
- Howard's humanistic theory from psychology: Holistic Caring Inventory (Latham, 1988)
- Mayeroff's philosophy: Caring Ability Inventory (Nkongho, 1990); Nyberg Caring Assessment Scale (Nyberg, 1990)
- Paterson and Zderad's humanistic nursing theory: Caring Behaviors of Nurses Scale (Hinds, 1988)
- Swanson's caring theory: Caring Professional Scale (Swanson, 2000a)
- Halldorsdottir's caring research: Nurse–Patient Relationship Questionnaire (Quinn et al., 2003)
- Turkel and Ray's relational caring complexity theory: Relational Caring Questionnaires (Turkel & Ray, 2001)
- Combination of family and caring theories: Family Caring Inventory (Goff, Chapter 21)

It is interesting to discover that the most frequently reported theory in the caring instrument literature that informed the development of caring tools was Watson's theory of caring and the 10 carative factors. When used in nursing research, this instrument development and testing could be considered one form of empirical validation of Watson's theory. For example, the following instruments were based on Watson's theory of human caring and/or the 10 carative factors:

- Caring Behaviors Inventory (Wolf, 1986)
- Caring Behaviors Assessment Tool (Cronin & Harrison, 1988)
- Nyberg Caring Assessment Scale (Nyberg, 1990)
- CAT, CAT-admin, and CAT-edu (Duffy, 1992, 2002; Duffy, Hoskins, & Seifert, 2007)
- Caring Efficacy Scale (Coates, 1996, 1997)

■ Caring Nurse–Patient Interactions Scale (Cossette, Côté, Pepin, Ricard, & D'Aoust, 2006)

■ Caring Behaviors Inventory—Short Form (Wu, Larrabee, & Putnam, 2006)

■ Caring Factor Survey (DiNapoli, Nelson, Turkel, & Watson, 2010)

The following instruments can be characterized as primarily empirically based and largely atheoretical:

■ Caring Dimensions Inventory (Watson & Lea, 1997)

■ Caring Attributes, Professional Self-Concept, and Technological Influences Scale (Arthur et al., 1999)

■ CARE-Q and modified forms (Larson, 1984; Lee, Larson, & Holzmer, 2006)

Yet even these most empirically derived caring instruments were informed, although indirectly, by early writings in the field of caring and by concepts embedded in those theoretical and general writings in the literature.

There are no hard conclusions that can be drawn about the relationship between caring theory and caring instruments, except that, from the state of the science to date, the following instruments seem to stand out as the most theoretically grounded:

■ *Mayeroff Caring Concepts & Philosophy*, Nkongho Caring Ability Inventory

■ *Paterson and Zderad Humanistic Nursing*

■ Hinds's Caring Behavior of Nurses Scale

■ *Swanson Caring Theory*, Swanson Caring Professional Scale

■ *Watson's Caring Theory*

■ Wolf Caring Behavior Inventory

■ Cronin & Harrison Caring Behavior Nurses Scale

■ Nyberg Caring Attributes Scale

■ Duffy Caring Assessment Tool (CAT-IV, CAT-admin, and CAT-edu)

■ Coates's Caring Efficacy Scale

■ Wu, Larrabee, and Putnam Caring Behavior Inventory

■ Nelson, Watson, InovaHealth Caring Factor Survey

The instruments that are most empirically grounded based on studies with large samples are:

■ Caring Dimensions Inventory (Watson & Lea, 1997)

■ Caring Attributes, Professional Self-Concept, and Technological Influences Scale (Arthur et al., 1999)

■ Caring Professional Scale (Swanson, 2000)

The only instruments that focus on organization and climate for caring are:

- Peer Group Caring Interaction Scale (Hughes, 1993)
- Organizational Climate for Caring Questionnaire (Hughes, 1998)
- Relational Caring Questionnaires (Ray & Turkel, 2001)

The most educationally relevant instruments are:

- Student Perceptions to Caring Online
- Peer Group Caring Interaction Scale (Hughes, 1998)
- CAT-edu (Duffy, 2007)
- Caring Efficacy Scale (Coates, 1996)

Those instruments most tested and based in clinical nursing practices are:

- CARE-Q and Modified CARE-Q (Larson, 1984)
- Caring Behaviors Assessment Tool (Cronin & Harrison, 1988)
- Caring Assessment Tools (Duffy, 2002)
- Caring Attributes, Professional Self-Concept, and Technological Influences Scale (Arthur et al., 1999)
- Caring Professional Scale (Swanson, 2000)
- Methodist Health Care System Nurse Caring Instrument (Shepherd, Rude, & Sherwood, 2000)
- Caring Factor Survey (Nelson et al., 2008)

The instruments most congruent with assessing caring at the administrative level are:

- Nyberg Caring Assessment Scale (Nyberg, 1990)
- CAT-admin (Duffy, 2007)
- Organizational Climate for Caring Questionnaire (Hughes, 1993)
- Relational Caring Questionnaires (Ray & Turkel, 2001)

As one can readily see, several of the instruments fall into more than one category based on their origin and use. Some have mixed use for students, clients, and nurses themselves, as they can be used interchangeably for different audiences. While various extant caring theories are acknowledged and used as a basis for the instruments in this book, there are other contemporary theories of caring upon which research is based that do not rely on empirical measures.

By way of closing remarks, I offer the following reflections for the future of caring theory, instrumentation, and research. Rather than perpetuating a dualistic worldview that separates theory from practice and research and isolates instrumentation and measurement from theoretical and conceptual relevance, different theories and measurement traditions need to begin to more systematically inform each other. The artificial dichotomy between qualitative and quantitative research and methods no longer can be sustained in such a complex world of clinical care. We have reached the paradoxical point that brings us both confusion and clarity in the phenomena we are studying and our methods. This paradoxical turn now invites an inclusion of all sources of data, both conventional and original. This new horizon is required if we are to move forward with meaningful forms of inquiry about the still largely unstudied human phenomena of caring, healing processes, and outcomes. Therefore, multiple theories, methods, and measurements can begin to inform, enrich, and sharpen each other's focus. Models of integration benefit from new developments; the different extant theories and research traditions, as well as new models emerging on the horizon, can generate new and diverse research and data sources.

The relationship and interplay between caring theories and diverse approaches to measurement can lead to refinements, expansion, further explication, and validation of both current and emergent theories, as well as sophistication of instrumentation. The next generation of theory, research, methods, and measurements needs conceptual and operational space to develop and validate new grand theories, mini-theories, middle-range theories, and situation-specific theories; this can be achieved through the exploration and uncovering of old and new relationships and new understandings about the phenomenon of caring between and among different populations and different human experiences.

The next generation of caring research and instrument development needs freedom for researchers and instrument developers to pursue directions and multiple methods that explore the caring phenomenon in diverse practice domains, in educational caring curricula/pedagogies, and in administrative, environmental, structural, and system–organizational–computerized designs, thus revealing and improving our knowledge of those caring practices operating at the ontological level, where caring is lived.

The current cultural demands for evidence and outcomes invite and require innovative and substantive approaches for exploring clinical research questions and multiple conceptual and operational approaches to assessment, evaluation, and measurement. Thus, the demand for theory-guided, theory-based, and theory-located contexts for evidence becomes even greater. Without a theoretical context for study, evidence becomes a hollow pursuit and does not build the discipline or the profession.

There is intellectual room and freedom in nursing science, and all sciences in this new millennium turn to explore greater depths of construct and concept and empirical validity of caring. This is an era in which to consider conceptual triangulation, theoretical–empirical triangulation, and instrument triangulation. This is a moment to dare to move between and beyond methods and dated research traditions. This is a time to entertain parallel and multisite studies, a period in history when we are called to reflect upon data and evidence from numbers, facts, texts, experience, self-reports, observations, narratives, stories, interviews, dialogues, photos, videos, and perhaps even cyberspace, where physiological, technological, epistemological, and ontological dimensions converge.

All these challenges await nursing and all health professions. This work is embedded, grounded, and located in nursing science, but it is not just nursing—this work is by its very nature interdisciplinary, interprofessional, and even transdisciplinary; it resides in that indeterminate zone of science and practice where all health practitioners and all patients ultimately live.

Finally, this work has just begun. This second edition attests to the growing need for an interest and activities in this area of caring research. The phenomenon of caring in nursing and healthcare awaits these new research innovations and new methodologies for assessing caring. In the meantime, the extant contemporary caring instruments that have been developed await a new generation of replication; theoretical, conceptual, and empirical triangulation; and continued validation and refinement. This is especially relevant with respect to new views of construct validity as well as the multiple meanings and approaches to assessing caring. Again, we must remind ourselves that, in the end, all caring measurements are only one indicator of a human experience and ontological phenomenon that offers at best some snapshots of a dynamic human dimension of *being* and *becoming*. Nevertheless, if we fail to incorporate caring into contemporary nursing and health sciences research, a core and vital aspect of nursing and healthcare will remain unarticulated, unexplored, excluded, and unknown.

REFERENCES

Arthur, D., Pang, S., Wong, T., Alexander, M. F., Drury, J., Eastwood, H., . . . & O'Brien, A. (1999). Caring attributes, professional self concept and technological influences in a sample of Registered Nurses in eleven countries. *International Journal of Nursing Studies, 36*(5), 387–396.

Coates, C. J. (1996). *Development of the Caring Efficacy Scale: Self-report and supervisor versions.* Unpublished manuscript. Denver, CO: University of Colorado Health Sciences Center.

Coates, C. J. (1997). The Caring Efficacy Scale: Nurses' self-reports of caring in practice settings. *Advanced Practice Nursing Quarterly, 3*(1), 53–59.

Cossette, S., Côté, J. K., Pepin, J., Ricard, N., & D'Aoust, L.-X. (2006). A dimensional structure of nurse–patient interaction from a caring perspective: Refinement of the Caring Nurse–Patient Interaction Scale (CNPI–Short Scale). *Journal of Advanced Nursing, 55*(2), 198–214. doi:10.1111/j.1365-2648.2006.03895.x

Cronin, S. N., & Harrison, B. (1988). Importance of nurse caring behaviors as perceived by patients after myocardial infarction. *Heart and Lung, 17,* 374–380.

DiNapoli, P., Nelson, J. W., Turkel, M., & Watson, J. (2010). Measuring the caritas processes: Caring Factor Survey. *International Journal of Human Caring, 14*(3), 16–21.

Duffy, J. (1992). The impact of nurse caring on patient outcomes. In D. A. Gaut (Ed.), *The presence of caring in nursing* (pp. 113–136). New York, NY: National League for Nursing.

Duffy, J. (2002). Caring assessment tools. In J. Watson (Ed.), *Instruments for assessing and measuring caring in nursing and health sciences* (pp. 120–150). New York, NY: Springer Publishing.

Duffy, J., Hoskins, L. M., & Seifert, R. F. (2007). Dimensions of caring: Psychometric properties of the Caring Assessment Tool. *Advances in Nursing Science, 30*(3), 1–12. doi:10.1097/01.ans.0000286622.84763.a9

Harrison, E. (1995). Nurse caring and the new health care paradigm. *Journal of Nursing Care Quality, 9*(4), 14–23. doi:10.1097/00001786-199507000-00004

Hinds, P. S. (1988). The relationship of nurses' caring behaviors with hopefulness and health care outcomes in adolescents. *Archives of Psychiatric Nursing, 2*(1), 21–29.

Hughes, L. (1993). Peer group interactions and the students-perceived climate for caring. *Journal of Nursing Education, 32*(2), 78–83.

Hughes, L. C. (1998). Development of an instrument to measure caring peer group interactions. *Journal of Nursing Education, 37*(5), 202–207.

Larson, P. (1984). Important nurse caring behaviors perceived by patients with cancer. *Oncology Nursing Forum, 11*, 46–50.

Latham, C. L. (1988, March). *Measurement of caring in recipient-provider interactions.* Paper presented at the Second Measurement of Clinical and Educational Nursing Outcomes Conference, San Diego, CA.

Lee, M. H., Larson, P. J., & Holzemer, W. L. (2006). Psychometric evaluation of the modified CARE-Q among Chinese nurses in Taiwan. *International Journal for Human Caring, 10*(4), 8–13. doi:10.20467/1091-5710.10.4.8

McDaniel, A. (1990). The caring process in nursing: Two instruments for measuring caring behaviors. In O. Strickland & C. Waltz (Eds.), *Measurements of nursing outcomes* (pp. 17–27). New York, NY: Springer Publishing.

Nkongho, N. O. (1990). The caring ability inventory. In O. L. Strickland & C. F. Waltz (Eds.), *Measurement of nursing outcomes: Measuring client self-care and coping skills* (pp. 3–16). New York, NY: Springer Publishing.

Nyberg, J. (1990). The effects of care and economics on nursing practice. *Journal of Nursing Administration, 20*(5), 13–18. doi:10.1097/00005110-199005000-00006

Quinn, J. F., Smith, M., Ritenbaugh, C., Swanson, K., & Watson, M. J. (2003). Research guidelines for assessing the impact of the healing relationship in clinical nursing. *Alternative Therapies in Health and Medicine, 9*(3), A65–A79.

Shepherd, M., Rude, M., & Sherwood , G. (2000, July 2). *Patient satisfaction with nurses' caring: Instrument development for a nursing quality indicator.* Rhythms of Caring: A Cadence for a New Century, 22nd International Association for Human Caring Research Conference, Boca Raton, FL.

Swanson, K. (2000a). Predicting depressive symptoms after miscarriage: A path analysis based on the Lazarus paradigm. *Journal of Women's Health & Gender-Based Medicine, 9*(2), 191–206. doi:10.1089/152460900318696

Turkel, M. C., & Ray, M. A. (2001). Relational complexity: From grounded theory to instrument development and theoretical testing. *Nursing Science Quarterly, 14*(4), 281–287. doi:10.1177/08943180122108571

Watson, R., & Lea, A. (1997). The Caring Dimensions Inventory. (CDI): Content validity, reliability, and scaling. *Journal of Advanced Nursing, 25*, 87–94. doi:10.1046/j.1365-2648.1997.1997025087.x

Wolf, Z. R. (1986). The caring concept and nurse identified caring behaviors. *Topics in Clinical Nursing, 8*, 84–93.

Wu, Y., Larrabee J., & Putman, H. (2006). Caring Behaviors Inventory: A reduction of the 42-item instrument. *Nursing Research, 55*(1), 18–25. doi:10.1097/00006199-200601000-00003

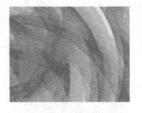

Appendix

Master Matrix of All
Measurement Instruments

Master Matrix Blueprint of All Instruments for Measuring Caring

INSTRUMENT	AUTHOR CONTACT INFORMATION	PUBLICATION SOURCE	DEVELOPED TO MEASURE	INSTRUMENT DESCRIPTION	PARTICIPANTS	REPORTED VALIDITY/ RELIABILITY	CONCEPTUAL-THEORETICAL BASIS OF MEASUREMENT	LATEST CITATION IN NURSING LITERATURE
Caring Assessment Instrument (1984)	Patricia Larson, DNSc, RN, FAAN University of California, San Francisco School of Nursing Department of Physiology Nursing. Box 0610-N611Y San Francisco, CA 94143-0610 Email: pattwkw@msn.com	Larson, P. (1984). Important nurse-caring behaviors perceived by patients with cancer. *Oncology Nursing Forum, 11(6),* 46–50.	Perceptions of nurse-caring behaviors	Q-Sort 50 cards into 7 piles/7-point scale to prioritize perception of nurse-caring behaviors The most commonly used instrument, both nationally and internationally, although it is noted to be confusing, ambiguous, and time consuming	N = 57 oncology patients	Expert panel test–retest Content and face validity	General references to nursing theories of caring A priori development Guided by care needs of cancer patients	Chinese version of CARE-Q Holroyd, E., Yue-kuen, C., Sau-wai, C., Fung-shan, L., & Wai-wan, W. (1998). A Chinese cultural perspective of nursing care behaviors in an acute setting. *Journal of Advanced Nursing, 28(6),* 1289–1294.

| CARE-Q (1986) | Patricia Larson, DNSc, RN, FAAN

University of California, San Francisco School of Nursing

Department of Physiology Nursing.

Box 0610-N611Y

San Francisco, CA 94143-0610

Email: pattwkw@msn.com | Larson, P. (1986). Cancer nurses' perception of caring. *Cancer Nursing, 9(2)*, 86–91. | Perceptions of nurse-caring behaviors | Q-Sort | N = 57 oncology nurses | Extension of Larson (1984)

See Larson (1984) | See Larson (1984) | See Larson (1984) | See Larson (1984) |
|---|---|---|---|---|---|---|---|---|---|

(continued)

Master Matrix Blueprint of All Instruments for Measuring Caring (*continued*)

INSTRUMENT	AUTHOR CONTACT INFORMATION	PUBLICATION SOURCE	DEVELOPED TO MEASURE	INSTRUMENT DESCRIPTION	PARTICIPANTS	REPORTED VALIDITY/ RELIABILITY	CONCEPTUAL- THEORETICAL BASIS OF MEASUREMENT	LATEST CITATION IN NURSING LITERATURE
CARE-Q	Patricia Larson, DNSc, RN, FAAN

University of California, San Francisco School of Nursing

Department of Physiology Nursing.

Box 0610 N 611Y San Francisco, CA 94143-0610

Email: pattwkw@ msn.com | Larson, P. (1987). Comparison of cancer patients, and professional nurses' perceptions of important nurse-caring behaviors. *Heart and Lung, 16(2),* 187–193. | Identifies nurse-caring behaviors | Q-Sort | *N* = 57 oncology nurses

N = 57 oncology patients | See Larson (1984) | See Larson (1984) | See Larson (1984) |

CARE-Q Replication Study and Use	D. Mayer, PhD, RN, Clinical Specialist Massachusetts General Hospital	Mayer, D. (1987). Oncology nurses, vs. cancer patients' perception of nurse caring behaviors: A replication study. *Oncology Nursing Forum, 14*(3), 48–52.	Evaluate nurse-caring behaviors	Q-Sort	$N = 28$ oncology nurses $N = 54$ oncology patients	Content and face validity Test–retest reliability (refers to Larson, 1984, original testing)	Replication of instrument plus extension of conceptual foundation of original Larson version of CARE-Q	See Larson (1984)
CARE-Q	Nori Komorita, PhD, RN; Kathleen Doehring, MS, RN; and Phyllis Hirchert, MS, RN Urbana Regional Program College of Nursing University of Illinois, Urbana	Komorita, N., Doehring, K., & Hirchert, P. (1991). Perceptions of caring by nurse educators. *Journal of Nursing Education, 30*(1), 23–29.	Nurse educators' perceptions of caring behaviors	Q-Sort	$N = 110$ nurse educators	Refers to Larson's (1984) original work	Caring in relation to nursing education No new reliability or validity reported for nursing educational use	See Larson (1984)

(continued)

Master Matrix Blueprint of All Instruments for Measuring Caring (continued)

INSTRUMENT	AUTHOR CONTACT INFORMATION	PUBLICATION SOURCE	DEVELOPED TO MEASURE	INSTRUMENT DESCRIPTION	PARTICIPANTS	REPORTED VALIDITY/ RELIABILITY	CONCEPTUAL- THEORETICAL BASIS OF MEASUREMENT	LATEST CITATION IN NURSING LITERATURE
CARE-Q	Antonia Mangold, MSN, RN Oncology Clinical Staff Nurse Thomas Jefferson University Hospital, Philadelphia, PA	Mangold, A. (1991). Senior nursing students' and professional nurses' perception of effective caring behaviors: A comparative study. *Journal of Nursing Education, 30*(3). 134–139.	Identifies and compares nursing students' and RNs' perceptions of caring behaviors	Q-Sort	*N* = 30 nursing students	See Larson (1984) Original citation for test–retest reliability	Larson's original conceptual basis Informed by Watson's 10 carative factors	See Larson (1984)

CARE-Q
Original

Hulela, E. B., Seboni, N. M., & Akinsola, H. A. (2000). The perception of acutely ill patients about the caring behavior of nurses in Botswana. *West African Journal of Nursing, 11*(2), 24–30.

Gardner, A., Goodsell, J., Duggan, T., Murtha, B., Peck, C., & Williams, J. (2001). "Don't call me Sweetie!" Patients differ from nurses in their perceptions of caring. *Collegian, 8*(3), 32–38.

(continued)

Master Matrix Blueprint for All Instruments for Measuring Caring (*continued*)

INSTRUMENT	AUTHOR CONTACT INFORMATION	PUBLICATION SOURCE	DEVELOPED TO MEASURE	INSTRUMENT DESCRIPTION	PARTICIPANTS	REPORTED VALIDITY/ RELIABILITY	CONCEPTUAL- THEORETICAL BASIS OF MEASUREMENT	LATEST CITATION IN NURSING LITERATURE
CARE-Q	Louise von Essen, MS, and Per-Olow Sjödén, PhD Center for Caring Sciences Uppsala University Akademiska Hospital S-751 85 Uppsala, Sweden Email: Louise-von.essen@ccs .uu.se	von Essen, L., & Sjödén, P. (1991a). The importance of nurse-caring behaviors as perceived by Swedish hospital patients and nursing staff. *International Journal of Nursing Studies, 28*(3), 267–281.	Perceived caring behaviors by nurses and patients	Q-Sort International Swedish version	*N* = 81 oncology, general surgery, and orthopedic patients *N* = 105 nurses	No reliability or validity reported for Swedish version Refers to information reported by Larson (1981, 1984)	Affective components of care and a caring relationship	Chang, Y., Lin, Y., Chang, H., & Lin, C. (2005). Cancer patient and staff ratings of caring behavior: Relationship to level of pain intensity. *Cancer Nursing, 28*(5), 331–339.

Larsson, G., Peterson, V. W., Lampic, C., von Essen, L., & Sjödén, P. (1998). Cancer patient and staff ratings of the importance of caring behaviors and their relations to patient anxiety and depression. *Journal of Advanced Nursing, 27,* 855–864.

(continued)

Master Matrix Blueprint for All Instruments for Measuring Caring (continued)

INSTRUMENT	AUTHOR CONTACT INFORMATION	PUBLICATION SOURCE	DEVELOPED TO MEASURE	INSTRUMENT DESCRIPTION	PARTICIPANTS	REPORTED VALIDITY/ RELIABILITY	CONCEPTUAL-THEORETICAL BASIS OF MEASUREMENT	LATEST CITATION IN NURSING LITERATURE
CARE-Q	Louise von Essen, MS, and Per-Olow Sjödén, PhD Center for Caring Sciences Uppsala University Akademiska Hospital S-751 85 Uppsala, Sweden Email: Louise-von.essen@ccs.uu.se	von Essen, L., & Sjödén, P. (1991). Patient and staff perceptions of caring: Review and replication. *Journal of Advanced Nursing, 16*(11), 1363–1374.	Perceived caring behaviors by nurses and patients (Swedish population)	International version Q-Sort of same items of 7-point scale (Swedish version) Replication of 1991 study Questionnaires with items of Q-Sort	*N* = 73 nurses *N* = 86 medical patients	See von Essen and Sjödén (1991a)		Larsson, G., Peterson, V. W., Lampic, C., von Essen, L., & Sjödén, P. (1998). Cancer patient and staff ratings of the importance of caring behaviors and their relations to patient anxiety and depression. *Journal of Advanced Nursing, 27*, 855–864.

CARE-Q	Kathryn Rosenthal, MS, RN University of Colorado Rosenthal, K. (1992). Coronary care patients' and nurses' perceptions of important nurse-caring behaviors. *Heart and Lung, 21*(6), 536–539.	Examines the relationship of patient-perceived and nurse-perceived caring behaviors	Q-Sort	$N = 30$ coronary nurses $N = 30$ coronary patients	See Larson (1984, 1987)	General nursing caring literature (Larson, 1984, 1987, for tool) Watson et al. included in background of study	None to date
CARE-Q	Louise von Essen, MS, and Per-Olow Sjödén, PhD Center for Caring Sciences Uppsala University Akademiska Hospital S-751 85 Uppsala, Sweden Email: Louise-von.essen@ccs.uu.se von Essen, L., & Sjödén, P. (1993). Perceived importance of caring behaviors to Swedish psychiatric inpatients and staff, with comparisons to somatically ill samples. *Research in Nursing & Health, 16,* 293–303.	Nurse-caring behaviors as perceived by psychiatric patients compared with somatically ill patients	Q-Sort Comparative study with different patient populations International Swedish version of tool Modified for psychiatric patients (Used free response format)	$N = 63$ psychiatric nurses, RNs, and students $N = 61$ mental health patients	Discussion of difficulty with Q-Sort Found to be unreliable due to forced distribution Discusses internal consistency using a free response format	General nursing caring literature (Larson, 1984, 1987, for tool) Watson et al. included in background of study Perception of caring relationship and caring behaviors	Larsson, G., Peterson, V. W., Lampic, C., von Essen, L., & Sjödén, P. (1998). Cancer patient and staff ratings of the importance of caring behaviors and their relations to patient anxiety and depression. *Journal of Advanced Nursing, 27,* 855–864.

(continued)

| Master Matrix Blueprint for All Instruments for Measuring Caring *(continued)* | | | | | | | | |
INSTRUMENT	AUTHOR CONTACT INFORMATION	PUBLICATION SOURCE	DEVELOPED TO MEASURE	INSTRUMENT DESCRIPTION	PARTICIPANTS	REPORTED VALIDITY/ RELIABILITY	CONCEPTUAL-THEORETICAL BASIS OF MEASUREMENT	LATEST CITATION IN NURSING LITERATURE
CARE-Q	Margaret K. Smith, MSN, RN Assistant Nurse Manager. Nursing Home Care Unit VA Palo Alto Health Care System Menlo Park, CA	Smith, M., & Sullivan, J. (1997). Nurses' and patients' perceptions of most important caring behaviors in a long-term care setting. *Geriatric Nursing, 18(2),* 70–73.	Compare rankings of caring behaviors as perceived by patients and nurses	50 items with six subscales Q-Sort	$N = 12$ men and 2 women patients $N = 15$ RNs from nursing home care unit at Veterans Affairs Medical Center	Content validity addressed Reliability and validity not addressed	No theoretical/ conceptual model mentioned	
CARE/SAT Questionnaire (1993)	Patricia Larson, DNSc, RN, FAAN, and Sandra Ferketick, PhD, RN College of Nursing University of Arizona, Tucson, AZ	Larson, P., & Ferketich, S. (1993). Patients' satisfaction with nurses' caring during hospitalization. *Western Journal of Nursing Research, 15(6),* 690–707.	Patient satisfaction with nursing care	Descriptive correlational study Visual analog scale adapted from CARE-Q; 29 items	$N = 268$ patients	Cronbach's alpha Construct and concurrent validity reported Factor analysis = 3 factors to account for variance	Caring Behaviors Original	Manojlovich, M. (2005). The effect of nursing leadership on hospital nurses' professional practice behaviors. *Journal of Nursing Administration, 35(7/8),* 366–374.

Modified CARE-Q (2006)	Mei-Hua Lee, P. Larson, and W. L. Holzemer Mei-Hua Lee 8250 Hardester Drive Sacramento, CA 95828 Email: mefalee@yahoo.com	Lee, M.-H., Larson, P. J., & Holzemer, W. L. (2006). Psychometric evaluation of the modified CARE-Q among Chinese nurses in Taiwan. *International Journal for Human Caring*, 10(4), 8–13.	Modified for Chinese nurses in Taiwan	Adapted from original CARE-Q into a 7-point Likert scale	N = 770 nurses	Test–retest reliability .0803 between Chinese version and original English version Internal consistency coefficient alpha .97 for total modified CARE-Q; .82–.92 subscales	Original work of Larson, with adaptation. Also available in Chinese version upon request	Lee, M.-H., Larson, P. J., & Holzemer, W. L. (2006) Psychometric evaluation of the modified CARE-Q among Chinese nurses in Taiwan. *International Journal for Human Caring,10(4),* 8–13.

(continued)

Master Matrix Blueprint for All Instruments for Measuring Caring (*continued*)

INSTRUMENT	AUTHOR CONTACT INFORMATION	PUBLICATION SOURCE	DEVELOPED TO MEASURE	INSTRUMENT DESCRIPTION	PARTICIPANTS	REPORTED VALIDITY/ RELIABILITY	CONCEPTUAL-THEORETICAL BASIS OF MEASUREMENT	LATEST CITATION IN NURSING LITERATURE
Caring Behaviors of Nurses' Scale (1985, 1988)	Pamela S. Hinds, PhD, RN, FAAN Director of Nursing Research St. Jude Children's Research Hospital 332 North Lauderdale Memphis, TN 38105 Email: Pam .Hinds@stjude .org	Hinds, P. S. (1988). The relationship of nurses' caring behaviors with hopefulness and health care outcomes in adolescents. *Archives of Psychiatric Nursing, 2*(1), 21–29.	Caring behaviors of nurses within intersubjective human relationships	Inductively based 22-item visual analog scale, with possible range of 0 to 100 (highest score indicates the respondent feels more cared for by nurse)	*N* = 25 inpatient adolescents in substance abuse treatment unit in the Southwest	Reported to have face and content validity, form equivalence, and internal consistency (Hinds, 1985) Cronbach's alpha of .86 for two data collection points for adolescent study (1988)	Existential-humanistic nursing (Paterson & Zderad, 1976) intersubjective relationship of caring	Hinds, P. S. (1988). The relationship of nurses' caring behaviors with hopefulness and health care outcomes in adolescents. *Archives of Psychiatric Nursing, 2*(1), 21–29.

Dorsey, C., Phillips, K. D., & Williams, C. (2001). Adult sickle cell patients' perceptions of nurses' caring behaviors. *Association of Black Nursing Faculty (ABNF) Journal, 12*(5), 95–100.

Pragmatic content analysis and semantic content analysis achieved with pre-established criterion levels of .8 or higher across the data collection points

Intercoder reliability and stability

(continued)

Master Matrix Blueprint for All Instruments for Measuring Caring (*continued*)

INSTRUMENT	AUTHOR CONTACT INFORMATION	PUBLICATION SOURCE	DEVELOPED TO MEASURE	INSTRUMENT DESCRIPTION	PARTICIPANTS	REPORTED VALIDITY/ RELIABILITY	CONCEPTUAL-THEORETICAL BASIS OF MEASUREMENT	LATEST CITATION IN NURSING LITERATURE
Nyberg Caring Assessment Scale (1989, 1990)	Jan Nyberg, PhD, RN	Nyberg, J. (1990). The effects of care and econom-ics on nurs-ing practice. *Journal of Nursing Ad-ministration, 20*(5), 13–18.	Caring attributes of nurses (more subjective human element than behaviors)	20 items on 5-point Likert scale Four separate rating scales on items	*N* = 135 nurses from ran-dom sample mailing of questionnaire	Cronbach's alpha reported at .87–.98 No discussion of construct or content validity, except use of theory factors, previously tested (Cronin & Harrison, 1988)	Draws directly from caring theory literature Specific items from Watson's carative factors; others from Noddings, Gaut, and Mayeroff	Nyberg, J. (1990). The effects of care and economics on nursing prac-tice. *Journal of Nursing Admin-istration, 20*(5), 13–18. McCartan, P. J., & Hargie, O. D. (2004). Assertiveness and caring: Are they compatible? *Journal of Clinical Nursing, 13*(6), 707–713.

Instrument	Author/Contact	Concept measured	Administration	Sample	Reliability	Other	Source
Caring Ability Inventory (1990)	Ngozi O. Nkongho, PhD, RN Associate Professor Lehman College Department of Nursing The City University of New York Bronx, NY 10468 Phone: 718-960-8794	Nkongho, N. (1990). The Caring Ability Inventory. In O. L. Strickland & C. R. Waltz (Eds.) *Measurement of nursing outcomes* (Vol. 4, pp. 3–16). New York, NY: Springer Publishing.	Ability to care when involved in a relationship	Self-administered 7-point Likert with 37 items	$N = 462$ college students, varied majors	Cronbach's alpha for each factor (range: .71–84)	General review of caring theory literature	Nkongho, N. (1990). The Caring Ability Inventory. In O. L. Strickland & C. R. Waltz (Eds.), *Measurement of nursing outcomes* (Vol. 4, pp. 3–16). New York, NY: Springer Publishing.

(continued)

Master Matrix Blueprint for All Instruments for Measuring Caring (continued)

INSTRUMENT	AUTHOR CONTACT INFORMATION	PUBLICATION SOURCE	DEVELOPED TO MEASURE	INSTRUMENT DESCRIPTION	PARTICIPANTS	REPORTED VALIDITY/ RELIABILITY	CONCEPTUAL-THEORETICAL BASIS OF MEASUREMENT	LATEST CITATION IN NURSING LITERATURE
Caring Ability Inventory (1990)				Major factors: knowing, courage, patience Measured with subscales	N = 75 nurses attending a professional conference	Factor analysis for collapsing items Content validity established with experts Test-retest r = .64–.80 Construct validity between group discrimination and correlation established with Tennessee Self-Concept Scale	Development informed by Mayeroff's eight critical elements of caring Simmons, P. R., & Cavanaugh, S. (2000). Relationships among student and graduate caring ability and professional school climate. Journal of Professional Nursing, 16(2), 76–83.	Hegedus, K. S. (1999). Providers' and consumers' perspective of nurses' caring behaviours. Journal of Advanced Nursing, 30(5), 1090–1096.

Cossette, S., Côté, J. K., Pepin, J., Ricard, N., & D'Aoust, L.-X. (2006). A dimensional structure of nurse–patient interaction from a caring perspective: Refinement of the Caring Nurse–Patient Interaction Scale (CNPI-Short Scale). *Journal of Advanced Nursing, 55*(2), 198–214.

Fjortoft, N. (2000). Caring pharmacists, caring teachers. *American Journal of Pharmaceutical Education, 68*(1), 1–2.

Barrera, O., Galvis, L., Moreno, F., Pinto, A. N., Pinzón, R, Romero, G., & Sánchez, M. (2006). Caring ability of family caregivers of chronically diseased people. *Investigación y Educación en Enfermería, 24*(1), 36–46.

(continued)

Master Matrix Blueprint for All Instruments for Measuring Caring (continued)

INSTRUMENT	AUTHOR CONTACT INFORMATION	PUBLICATION SOURCE	DEVELOPED TO MEASURE	INSTRUMENT DESCRIPTION	PARTICIPANTS	REPORTED VALIDITY/ RELIABILITY	CONCEPTUAL- THEORETICAL BASIS OF MEASUREMENT	LATEST CITATION IN NURSING LITERATURE
Caring Behavior Checklist	Anna McDaniel, PhD, RN, FAAN Dean and the Linda Harman Aiken Professor University of Florida College of Nursing, Gainesville, Florida Email: annammcdaniel@ufl.edu Phone: 352-273-6324	McDaniel, A. M. (1990). The caring process in nursing: Two instruments for measuring caring behaviors. In O. Strickland & C. Waltz (Eds.), *Measurement of nursing outcomes* (pp. 17–27). New York, NY: Springer Publishing.	Caring process (external observable)	12 items of observable caring behaviors; dichotomous scoring of each item by trained observers	105 BSN students from two traditional BSN programs	Interrater reliability .92 overall on 12 items Content validity index .80	Informed by philosophical views in general caring literature Interest in *caring about* as well as *caring for* guided instrument development	Dunnington, R. M., & Farmer, S. R. (2015). Caring behaviors among student nurses interacting in scenario-based high fidelity human patient simulation. *International Journal for Human Caring, 19,* 44–49. doi:10.20467/1091-5710-19.4.44 Jasmine, T. (2007). *The elderly client's perception of caring behaviors.* Retrieved from ProQuest Dissertations & Theses database. (UMI No. 3283698).

Owens, R. A. (2006). The caring behaviors of the home health nurse and influence on medication adherence. *Home Healthcare Nurse, 24*(8), 517–526.

(continued)

Master Matrix Blueprint for All Instruments for Measuring Caring *(continued)*

INSTRUMENT	AUTHOR CONTACT INFORMATION	PUBLICATION SOURCE	DEVELOPED TO MEASURE	INSTRUMENT DESCRIPTION	PARTICIPANTS	REPORTED VALIDITY/ RELIABILITY	CONCEPTUAL-THEORETICAL BASIS OF MEASUREMENT	LATEST CITATION IN NURSING LITERATURE
Client Perception of Caring Scale	Anna McDaniel, PhD, RN, FAAN Dean and the Linda Harman Aiken Professor University of Florida College of Nursing, Gainesville, Florida Email: annammc daniel @ufl.edu Phone: 352-273-6324	McDaniel, A. M. (1990). The caring process in nursing: two instruments for measuring caring behaviors. In O. Strickland & C. Waltz (Eds.). *Measurement of nursing outcomes* (pp. 17–27). New York, NY: Springer Publishing.	Clients' perceptions of nurse caring (detect both caring and noncaring behaviors as perceived by clients)	Designed to be used with CBC in hospital setting 10 items rated on 6-point scale (scores ranging from 10 to 60)	Junior-level nursing students in BS nursing program (N not given)	Content validity index = 1.00 Alpha .81 reliability Item-to-total correlation .41 Construct validity not significant after correction with empathy scale	General caring theory literature Conceptual model of caring process developed to guide instrument	Jasmine, T. (2007). *The elderly client's perception of caring behaviors.* Retrieved from ProQuest Dissertations & Theses database. (UMI No. 3283698). Owens, R. A. (2006). The caring behaviors of the home health nurse and influence on medication adherence. *Home Healthcare Nurse, 24*(8), 517–526.

Peer Group Caring Interaction Scale and Organizational Climate for Caring Questionnaire (1993, 1998)	Linda Hughes, PhD[‡]	Organizational Climate for Caring Questionnaire used by W. Gabbert in dissertation research with online nursing students (hybrid version) Email: Wrennah .gabbert@ angelo.edu

(continued)

[‡] Deceased

Master Matrix Blueprint for All Instruments for Measuring Caring (*continued*)

INSTRUMENT	AUTHOR CONTACT INFORMATION	PUBLICATION SOURCE	DEVELOPED TO MEASURE	INSTRUMENT DESCRIPTION	PARTICIPANTS	REPORTED VALIDITY/ RELIABILITY	CONCEPTUAL- THEORETICAL BASIS OF MEASUREMENT	LATEST CITATION IN NURSING LITERATURE
Caring Efficacy Scale (CES; 1992, 1995)	Carolie Coates, PhD Research and Measurement Consultant 1441 Snowmass Ct. Boulder, CO 80303 Phone: 303-499-5756 Email: Coatescj@ home.com	Coates, C. (1997). The Caring Efficacy Scale: Nurses' self-reports of caring in practice settings. *Advanced Practice Nursing Quarterly, 3*(1), 53–59.	Assess conviction or belief in one's ability to express a caring orientation, develop caring relationship with patients	Original instrument had 46 items Current instrument has 12 items 6-point Likert-type scale Current instrument has 30 items (both self-report and supervisor format)	*N* = 110 nursing students *N* = 119 alumni *N* = 117 alumni employers *N* = 67 clinical supervisors	Cronbach's alpha Form A = .85 Form B = .88 Form B (short version) = .84 Content validity against theory and Watson's carative factors Significant positive correlation between clinical evaluative tool (alpha .85 and .95) and CES	Bandura's social psychology Self-Efficacy Scale and Watson's caring theory and 10 carative factors	Coates, C. (1997). The Caring Efficacy Scale: Nurses' self-reports of caring in practice settings. *Advanced Practice Nursing Quarterly, 3*(1), 53–59. Sadler, J. (2003). A pilot study to measure the caring efficacy of baccalaureate nursing students. *Nursing Education Perspectives, 24*(6), 295–299.

Instrument	Contact/Reference	Construct	Description	Sample	Statistics	Comments	Citation
Caring Dimensions Inventory (1997)	Roger Watson, PhD, RN, FAAN, Editor, *Journal of Clinical Nursing* Professor of Nursing School of Nursing and Midwifery The University of Sheffield Sheffield, UK S10 2TN Phone: +44-114-222-9848 Fax: +44-114-222-9712 Email: Roger .watson@ sheffield.ac.uk Watson, R., & Lea, A. (1997). The Caring Dimensions Inventory (CDI): Content validity, reliability and scaling. *Journal of Advanced Nursing, 25,* 87–94.	Perceptions of caring from large sample of nurses	5-point Likert scale with 41 questions (25 core questions regarding perceptions of caring)	$N = 1,452$ nurses and nursing students	Cronbach's alpha = .91 Mokken Scaling and Spearman's correlation of age Kruskal-Wallis one-way ANOVA for males versus females ($p < .05$) for age and sex differences in perceptions of caring	Empirical approach, versus theoretical basis, although caring theory that supported operationalizing of caring was influential	Lea, A., Watson, R., & Deary, I.J. (1998). Caring in nursing: A multivariate analysis. *Journal of Advanced Nursing, 28(3),* 662–671.

(continued)

Master Matrix Blueprint for All Instruments for Measuring Caring (continued)

INSTRUMENT	AUTHOR CONTACT INFORMATION	PUBLICATION SOURCE	DEVELOPED TO MEASURE	INSTRUMENT DESCRIPTION	PARTICIPANTS	REPORTED VALIDITY/ RELIABILITY	CONCEPTUAL- THEORETICAL BASIS OF MEASUREMENT	LATEST CITATION IN NURSING LITERATURE
	Amandah (Lea) Hoogbruin, PhD, MScN, BScN, RN Nursing Faculty Kwantlen University College 12666–72nd Avenue Surrey, B.C. V3W 2 MB Email: Amandah .hoogbruin@ kwantlen.ca							Watson, R., Deary, I. J., & Hoogbruin, A. L. (2001). A 35-item version of the Caring Dimensions Inventory (CD-35) multivariate analysis and application to a longitudinal study involving nursing students. *International Journal of Nursing Studies, 38(5),* 511–521.

Watson, R.
(2003).
Intrarater
reliability of
the Caring
Dimensions
Inventory
and Nursing
Dimensions
Inventory.
*Journal
of Clinical
Nursing, 12*(5),
786–787.

(continued)

Master Matrix Blueprint for All Instruments for Measuring Caring (*continued*)

INSTRUMENT	AUTHOR CONTACT INFORMATION	PUBLICATION SOURCE	DEVELOPED TO MEASURE	INSTRUMENT DESCRIPTION	PARTICIPANTS	REPORTED VALIDITY/ RELIABILITY	CONCEPTUAL-THEORETICAL BASIS OF MEASUREMENT	LATEST CITATION IN NURSING LITERATURE
Caring Dimensions Inventory (1997)								Watson, R., Hoogbruin, A. L., Rumeu, C., Beunza, M., Barbarin, B., MacDonald, J., & McCready, T. (2003). Differences and similarities in the perception of caring between Spanish and UK nurses. *Journal of Clinical Nursing, 12*(1), 85–92.

Caring Attributes, Professional Self-Concept, and Technological Influences Scale (2001)	David Arthur, PhD, RN Professor and Dean School of Nursing and Midwifery The Aga Khan University Karachi Pakistan Email: david.arthur@aku.edu	Arthur, D., Pang, S., Wong, T., Alexander, M. F., Drury, J., Eastwood, K., ...Xiao, S. (1999). Caring attributes, professional self-concept and technological influences in a sample of registered nurses in eleven countries. *International Journal of Nursing Studies, 36,* 387–396.	Multidimensional construct of caring internationally	Uses three subscales of caring attributes and three subscales of 13 theoretical items, 41 practical items, and 7 pedagogical items	$N = 1,957$ RNs from 11 countries (Hong Kong, Australia, Canada, China, Korea, New Zealand, Philippines, Scotland, Singapore, South Africa, Sweden)	Cronbach's alpha .75, overall PSCNI = .89, TIQ = .75, TISQ = .94, CAQ = .88	Items designed to reflect theoretical, practical, and pedagogical perspectives of caring. Items in three categories generated by caring theory literature (e.g., Leininger, Benner, Watson, Morse)	Arthur, D., Pang, S., Wong, T., Alexander, M. F., Drury, J., Eastwood, K., ...Xiao, S (1999). Caring attributes, professional self-concept and technological influences in a sample of registered nurses in eleven countries. *International Journal of Nursing Studies, 36,* 387–396.

(continued)

Master Matrix Blueprint for All Instruments for Measuring Caring (*continued*)

INSTRUMENT	AUTHOR CONTACT INFORMATION	PUBLICATION SOURCE	DEVELOPED TO MEASURE	INSTRUMENT DESCRIPTION	PARTICIPANTS	REPORTED VALIDITY/ RELIABILITY	CONCEPTUAL-THEORETICAL BASIS OF MEASUREMENT	LATEST CITATION IN NURSING LITERATURE
CAPST-2 (2001)	David Arthur, PhD, RN Professor and Dean School of Nursing and Midwifery The Aga Khan University Karachi Pakistan Email: david .arthur@aku .edu	Arthur, D., Pang, S., & Wong, T. (2001). The effect of technology on the caring attributes of an international sample of nurses. *International Journal of Nursing Studies, 38,* 37–43.	Multidimensional construct of caring across cultures and in different branches of nursing	31 items measure caring attributes in four dimensions: caring communication, caring involvement, caring advocacy, and learning to care	*N* = 1,957 RNs from 11 countries (Hong Kong, Australia, Canada, China, Korea, New Zealand, Philippines, Scotland, Singapore, South Africa, Sweden)	Caring communication: 10 items (α = .84, factor analysis % of variance = 15.96) Caring involvement: 8 items (α = .79, factor analysis % of variance = 11.67) Caring advocacy: 7 items (α = .78, factor analysis % of variance = 9.83) Learning to care: 5 items (α = .62, factor analysis % of variance = 7.02)	Items designed to reflect theoretical, practical, and pedagogical perspectives of caring Items in three categories generated by caring theory literature (e.g., Leininger, Benner, Watson, Morse) Refined by psychometric analysis and factor analysis	Arthur, D., & Randle, J. (2007). The professional self-concept of nurses: A review of the literature from 1992–2006. *Australian Journal of Advanced Nursing, 24*(3), 60–64.

Caring Professional Scale (2000)	Kristine Swanson, PhD	Swanson, K. (2000).	Consumers' ratings of healthcare providers on their practice relationship	14-item 5-point Likert scale	$N = 185$ women who had experienced miscarriage	Construct and content validity established through correlation with Barret-Lennart Relationship Inventory subscale of empathy ($r = .61\ p < .001$)	Swanson's caring theory	Swanson, K. (2000). A program of research on caring. In M. E. Parker (Ed.), *Nursing theories and nursing practice* (pp. 31–60). Philadelphia, PA: F. A. Davis.
	Professor of Nursing, Chair of Family and Child Nursing	Predicting depressive symptoms after miscarriage: A path analysis based on the Lazarus Paradigm. *Journal of Women's Health & Gender-Based Medicine, 9*(2), 191–206.		Items derived from Swanson's caring theory, and empirical research, that reflects the empirically derived subcategories of knowing, being with, doing for, enabling, and maintaining belief				
	University of Washington					Cronbach's alpha = .74–.96 for advanced practice nurses, .97 for nurses, and .96 for physicians		
	Box 357262							
	Seattle, WA 98195							
	Phone: 206-543-8228							
	Fax: 206-543 6656							
	Email: kswanson@u .washington .edu							

(continued)

Master Matrix Blueprint for All Instruments for Measuring Caring (continued)

INSTRUMENT	AUTHOR CONTACT INFORMATION	PUBLICATION SOURCE	DEVELOPED TO MEASURE	INSTRUMENT DESCRIPTION	PARTICIPANTS	REPORTED VALIDITY/ RELIABILITY	CONCEPTUAL-THEORETICAL BASIS OF MEASUREMENT	LATEST CITATION IN NURSING LITERATURE
Relational Caring Questionnaire–Professional Form (2001)	Marilyn Ray, PhD, RN, CTN, FAAN Professor Emerita Florida Atlantic University Christine E. Lynn College of Nursing 8487 Via D'Oro Boca Raton, FL 33433 Phone: 561-470-8109 Email: mray@health.fau.edu	Turkel, M., & Ray, M. (2001). Relational complexity: From grounded theory to instrument development & theoretical testing. *Nursing Science Quarterly, 14(4),* 281–287.	Organizational caring (professional form) and nurse-caring behavior (patient form)	Professional form: 26 items, 5-point Likert scale	Qualitative research from 1995 to 2001 with over 250 registered nurses, patients, and administrators from seven diverse hospitals	Professional form reliability .86 Content validity established by panel of six experts ≥75% items very relevant	Qualitative research findings from interviews with over 250 registered nurses, patients, and administrators	Turkel, M., & Ray, M. (2001). Relational complexity: From grounded theory to instrument development & theoretical testing. *Nursing Science Quarterly, 14(4),* 281–287.

| Relational Caring Questionnaire–Patient Form (2001) | Marian Turkel, PhD, RN, NEA-BC, FAAN Associate Professor Florida Atlantic University Christine E. Lynn College of Nursing 8487 Via D'Oro Boca Raton, FL 33433 Work: 561-297-3264 Cell: 312-203-3944 Email: mturkel@health.fau.edu | Ray, M., & Turkel, M. (2005). *Final report: Economic and patient outcomes of the nurse-patient relationship.* Tri-service nursing research program abstract. Published in CINAHL, 2007. | Patient form: 15 items, 5-point Likert scale | Psychometric testing from 1996 to 2003 with 447 RNs and administrators and 234 patients from seven diverse hospitals | Convergent or concurrent validity determined with Valentine Caring Questionnaire .14 Construct validity, exploratory factor analysis | Turkel, M., & Ray, M. (2000). Relational caring complexity: A theory of the nurse–patient relationship within an economic context. *Nursing Science Quarterly, 13*(4), 307–313. | Ray, M., & Turkel, M. (2005). *Final report: Economic and patient outcomes of the nurse-patient relationship.* Tri-service nursing research program abstract. Published in CINAHL, 2007. |

(continued)

343

Master Matrix Blueprint for All Instruments for Measuring Caring (continued)

INSTRUMENT	AUTHOR CONTACT INFORMATION	PUBLICATION SOURCE	DEVELOPED TO MEASURE	INSTRUMENT DESCRIPTION	PARTICIPANTS	REPORTED VALIDITY/ RELIABILITY	CONCEPTUAL-THEORETICAL BASIS OF MEASUREMENT	LATEST CITATION IN NURSING LITERATURE
Relational Caring Questionnaire–Patient Form (2001)						Four factors explained 47% of the variance. First factor loading coefficient .490; reliability .73 Second factor loading coefficient .515; reliability .83 Third factor loading coefficient .569; reliability .78 Fourth factor loading coefficient .481; reliability .72 Patient form reliability .86 Content validity established by panel of six experts	Ray, M., Turkel, M., & Marino, F. (2002). The transformative process in workforce redevelopment. *Nursing Administration Quarterly, 26*(2), 1–14.	Final report, National Technical Information Service. U.S. Government Repository, 2007.

≥75% items very relevant

Convergent or concurrent validity determined with Valentine Caring Questionnaire .54

Construct validity, exploratory factor analysis

Four factors explained 64% of the variance.

Based on analysis, three factors retained

First factor loading coefficient .483; reliability .94

Second factor loading coefficient −.565; reliability .85

Third factor loading coefficient −.596; reliability .81

(continued)

Master Matrix Blueprint for All Instruments for Measuring Caring (continued)

INSTRUMENT	AUTHOR CONTACT INFORMATION	PUBLICATION SOURCE	DEVELOPED TO MEASURE	INSTRUMENT DESCRIPTION	PARTICIPANTS	REPORTED VALIDITY/ RELIABILITY	CONCEPTUAL-THEORETICAL BASIS OF MEASUREMENT	LATEST CITATION IN NURSING LITERATURE
Relational Caring Questionnaire–Professional Form (2001, 2005, 2007)	Marilyn Ray, PhD Professor Emerita Florida Atlantic University Christine E. Lynn College of Nursing 8487 Via D'Oro Boca Raton, FL 33433 Phone: 561-470-8109 Email: mturkel@ health.fau.edu	Turkel, M., & Ray, M. (2001). Relational complexity: From grounded theory to instrument development & theoretical testing. *Nursing Science Quarterly, 14(4),* 281–287.	Organizational caring (professional form) and nurse-caring behavior (patient form)	Professional form: 26 items, 5-point Likert scale	Qualitative research from 1995 to 2001 with over 250 registered nurses, patients, and administrators from seven diverse hospitals	Professional form reliability .86	Qualitative research findings from interviews with over 250 registered nurses, patients, and administrators	Turkel, M., & Ray, M. (2001). Relational complexity: From grounded theory to instrument development & theoretical testing. *Nursing Science Quarterly, 14(4),* 281–287.

Relational Caring Questionnaire–Patient Form (2001, 2005, 2007)	Marian Turkel, PhD, RN, NEA-BC, FAAN Associate Professor Florida Atlantic University Christine E. Lynn College of Nursing 8487 Via D'Oro Boca Raton, FL 33433 Work: 561-297-3264 Cell: 312-203-3944 Email: mturkel@health.fau.edu	Ray, M., & Turkel, M. (2005). *Final report: Economic and patient outcomes of the nurse-patient relationship.* Tri-service nursing research program abstract. Published in CINAHL, 2007.	Patient form: 15 items, 5-point Likert scale	Psychometric testing from 1996 to 2003 with 447 RNs and administrators and 234 patients from seven diverse hospitals	Content validity established by panel of six experts ≥75% items very relevant Convergent or concurrent validity determined with Valentine Caring Questionnaire .14	Turkel, M., & Ray, M. (2000). Relational caring complexity: A theory of the nurse–patient relationship within an economic context. *Nursing Science Quarterly, 13*(4), 306–313. Ray, M., Turkel, M., & Marino, F. (2002). The transformative process in workforce redevelopment. *Nursing Administration Quarterly, 26*(2), 1–14.	Ray, M., & Turkel, M. (2005). *Final report: Economic and patient outcomes of the nurse–patient relationship.* Tri-service nursing research program abstract. Published in CINAHL, 2007. Final report. National Technical Information Service.

(continued)

Master Matrix Blueprint for All Instruments for Measuring Caring (continued)

INSTRUMENT	AUTHOR CONTACT INFORMATION	PUBLICATION SOURCE	DEVELOPED TO MEASURE	INSTRUMENT DESCRIPTION	PARTICIPANTS	REPORTED VALIDITY/ RELIABILITY	CONCEPTUAL- THEORETICAL BASIS OF MEASUREMENT	LATEST CITATION IN NURSING LITERATURE
						Construct validity, exploratory factor analysis		U.S. Government Repository, 2007.
						Four factors explained 47% of the variance		
						First factor loading coefficient .490; reliability .73		
						Second factor loading coefficient .515; reliability .83		
						Third factor loading coefficient .569; reliability .78		

Fourth factor
loading
coefficient
.481; reliability
.72

Patient form
reliability
.86 Content
validity
established
by panel of six
experts

≥75% items
very relevant

Convergent or
concurrent
validity
determined
with Valentine
Caring
Questionnaire
.54

(continued)

Master Matrix Blueprint for All Instruments for Measuring Caring (*continued*)

INSTRUMENT	AUTHOR CONTACT INFORMATION	PUBLICATION SOURCE	DEVELOPED TO MEASURE	INSTRUMENT DESCRIPTION	PARTICIPANTS	REPORTED VALIDITY/ RELIABILITY	CONCEPTUAL-THEORETICAL BASIS OF MEASUREMENT	LATEST CITATION IN NURSING LITERATURE
Relational Caring Question-naire– Patient Form (2001, 2005, 2007)						Construct validity, exploratory factor analysis Four factors explained 64% of the variance Based on analysis, three factors retained First factor loading coefficient .483; reliability .94 Second factor loading coefficient −.565; reliability .85 Third factor loading coefficient −.596; reliability .81		

| Family Caring Inventory (2002) | Anne-Marie Goff, PhD, RN

School of Nursing, University of North Carolina, Wilmington

601 S. College Road

Wilmington, NC 28403

Email: goffa@ uncw.edu | Unpublished to date | Family caring as a strength as perceived by adults: caring behavior, expressiveness, caring thoughts, caring feelings or emotions, and caring process | 36-item Likert-type scale measuring family caring | $N = 197$ nursing students in three schools of nursing | Cronbach's alpha = .82.

Eight factors extracted (67.17% variance)

Four subscales emerged with factor loading from .70 to .92

Significant correlation at .01 level

Family Apgar (.61) and Caring Ability Inventory (.57) | Developed from extensive concept analysis and both caring and family theories

Beavers, Ford-Gilboe, Mayeroff, McCubbin, Nkongo, Olson, Powell-Cope, Swanson, and Watson | None to date |

(continued)

Master Matrix Blueprint for All Instruments for Measuring Caring (*continued*)

INSTRUMENT	AUTHOR CONTACT INFORMATION	PUBLICATION SOURCE	DEVELOPED TO MEASURE	INSTRUMENT DESCRIPTION	PARTICIPANTS	REPORTED VALIDITY/ RELIABILITY	CONCEPTUAL-THEORETICAL BASIS OF MEASUREMENT	LATEST CITATION IN NURSING LITERATURE
Nurse-Patient Relationship Question-naire (2003)	Janet F. Quinn, PhD, RN, FAAN 360 Lonestar Road Lyons, CO 80540 Email: janetquinnphd @gmail.com	Quinn, J. F., Smith, M., Ritenbaugh, C., Swanson, K., & Watson, M. J. (2003). Research guidelines for assessing the impact of the healing relationship in clinical nursing. *Alternative Therapies in Health and Medicine,* 9(3 Suppl.), A65–A79.	Quality of caring in the nurse–patient relationship	12 items 5-point Likert-type scale based on Halldorsdottir's continuum of caring	N/A	N/A	Halldorsdottir's continuum of caring and Watson's caring theory	Quinn, J. F., Smith, M., Ritenbaugh, C., Swanson, K., & Watson, M. J. (2003). Research guidelines for assessing the impact of the healing relationship in clinical nursing. *Alternative Therapies in Health and Medicine,* 9(3 Suppl.), A65–79.

| CNPI-70 (2006) | Sylvie Cossette, PhD, RN; Chantal Cara, PhD, RN; Nicole Ricard, PhD, RN; and Jacinthe Pepin, PhD, RN / Faculty of Nursing University of Montreal, Quebec, Canada | Cossette, S., Cara, C., Ricard, N., & Pepin, J. (2005). Assessing nurse–patient interactions from a caring perspective: Report of the development and preliminary psychometric testing of the Caring Nurse–Patient Interactions Scale. *International Journal of Nursing Studies, 42,* 673–686. | Patient's, family's, or nurse's perceptions of the importance of, feeling of competency in, and feasibility of adopting caring behaviors | Long version of the CNPI | *N* = 332 nursing students | Face and content validity and reliability / Contrasted groups/link with social desirability | Watson's theory and the 10 carative factors | Pepin, J., Cossette, S., Ricard, N., & Côté, J. (2005, June 17). *Cultural characteristics of students enrolled in the nursing program at the Faculty of Nursing, University of Montreal.* Paper delivered at the 27th annual meeting of the International Association of Human Caring, Lake Tahoe, CA. |

(continued)

Master Matrix Blueprint for All Instruments for Measuring Caring (*continued*)

INSTRUMENT	AUTHOR CONTACT INFORMATION	PUBLICATION SOURCE	DEVELOPED TO MEASURE	INSTRUMENT DESCRIPTION	PARTICIPANTS	REPORTED VALIDITY/ RELIABILITY	CONCEPTUAL-THEORETICAL BASIS OF MEASUREMENT	LATEST CITATION IN NURSING LITERATURE
Student Perspectives of Caring Online	Kathleen Sitzman, PhD, RN, PhD, CNE, ANEF, FAAN Phone: (801) 791-1177 Email: sitzmank@ecu.edu; Kathy.sitzman@gmail.com	Sitzman, K (2007). Bachelor of Science in Nursing Student Perceptions of Caring Online (Doctor of Philosophy Dissertation). University of Northern Colorado, College of Natural and Health Sciences, School of Nursing, Nursing Education.	Nursing students' perspectives of caring online behaviors demonstrated by nursing instructors.	24 items on a 4-point Likert-type scale and one open-ended question.	122 undergraduate nursing students from five different institutions of higher education from an e-mailed request sent to 750 prospective respondents	Cronbach's alpha reported at .8313. Two pilot studies completed to inform the construction and content of the final tool.	Watson's Human Caring Theory	Mann, J. C. (2014). A pilot study of RN-BSN completion students' preferred instructor online classroom caring behaviors. *Association of Black Nursing Faculty (ABNF) Journal, 25*(2), 33–39. Sitzman, K. (2010). Student-preferred caring behaviors for online nursing education. *Nursing Education Perspectives, 31*(3), 171–178.

Scale	Author/Contact	Citation	Construct	Items/Response Format	Sample	Psychometrics	Theoretical Basis	Reference
Nurse's Perception of the Relationship-Based Care Environment	Denise Testa, PhD, CRNA William F. Connell School of Nursing Boston College 140 Commonwealth Ave. Chestnut Hill, MA 02477 Email: denise.testa@bc.edu	Testa, D. (2017) Development and psychometric evaluation of the nurse's perception of the Relationship-Based Care Environment Scale. *The International Journal for Human Caring, 21*(4), 193–199.	Relationships between nurses and others in healthcare setting	56-item, 6-point Likert scale (1 = strongly disagree to 6 = strongly agree) Five subscales: nurse to other disciplines; nurse to organization; nurse to nurse including the self; nurse to patient, knowing the patient; nurse to patient, respect for the patient	473 surveys with no missing data from direct care nurses	Expert panel reviewed items and content validity index = 1 Principal component analysis determined that five factors explained 48.8% of variance Cronbach's alpha for total scale = .96 Cronbach's alpha for five individual subscales ranged from .88 to .93	Nurse caring theories and relationship-based care literature	Testa, D. (2017) Development and psychometric evaluation of the nurse's perception of the Relationship-Based Care Environment Scale. *The International Journal for Human Caring, 21*(4), 193–199.

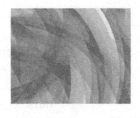

Index